Paramedic Care

Principles & Practice

Special Considerations/Operations

Instructor's Resource Manual

Third Edition

Tony Crystal, ScD, EMT-P, RPhT

Bryan E. Bledsoe, DO, FACEP, EMT-P

Emergency Physician
Midlothian, Texas
and
Professor, Health Sciences
University of Nevada, Las Vegas
Las Vegas, Nevada

Robert S. Porter, MA, NREMT-P

Senior Advanced Life Support Educator
Madison County Emergency Medical Services
Canastota, New York
and
Flight Paramedic
AirOne, Onondaga County Sheriff's Department
Syracuse, New York

Richard A. Cherry, MS, NREMT-P

Clinical Assistant Professor of Emergency Medicine
Technical Director for Medical Simulation
Upstate Medical University
Syracuse, New York

D1451045

PEARSON
Prentice
Hall

Upper Saddle River, New Jersey 07458

Publisher: *Julie Levin Alexander*
Publisher's Assistant: *Regina Bruno*
Executive Editor: *Marlene McHugh Pratt*
Senior Managing Editor for Development: *Lois Berlowitz*
Project Manager: *Triple SSS Press Media Development, Inc.*
Editorial Assistant: *Sean Karpowicz*
Director of Marketing: *Karen Allman*
Executive Marketing Manager: *Katrin Beacom*
Marketing Specialist: *Michael Sirinides*
Managing Editor for Production: *Patrick Walsh*
Production Liaison: *Faye Gemmellaro*
Production Editor: *Roxanne Klaas/S4Carlisle Publishing Services*
Manufacturing Manager: *Ilene Sanford*
Manufacturing Buyer: *Pat Brown*
Senior Design Coordinator: *Christopher Weigand*
Cover Design: *Jill Little*
Cover Image: *Ray Kemp/911 Imaging*
Composition: *S4Carlisle Publishing Services*
Printer/Binder: *Bind-Rite Graphics*
Cover Printer: *Phoenix Color*

NOTICE ON CPR AND ECC

The national standards for Cardiopulmonary Resuscitation (CPR) and Emergency Cardiovascular Care (ECC) are reviewed and revised on a regular basis and may change slightly after this manual is printed. It is important that you know the most current procedures for CPR and ECC, both for the classroom and your patients. The most current information may always be downloaded from *www.bradybooks.com* or obtained from the appropriate credentialing agency.

NOTICE ON CARE PROCEDURES

This instructor's resource manual reflects current EMS practice based on the 1998 U.S. Department of Transportation's EMT-Paramedic National Standard Curriculum. It is the intent of the authors and publisher that this manual be used as part of a formal EMT-Paramedic program taught by qualified instructors and supervised by a licensed physician. The procedures described in this manual are based upon consultation with EMT and medical authorities. The authors and publisher have taken care to make certain that these procedures reflect currently accepted clinical practice; however, they cannot be considered absolute recommendations.

The material in this manual contains the most current information available at the time of publication. However, federal, state, and local guidelines concerning clinical practices, including, without limitation, those governing infection control and universal precautions, change rapidly. The reader should note, therefore, that the new regulations may require changes in some procedures.

It is the responsibility of the reader to familiarize himself or herself with the policies and procedures set by federal, state, and local agencies as well as the institution or agency where the reader is employed. The authors and the publisher of this manual disclaim any liability, loss, or risk resulting directly or indirectly from the suggested procedures and theory, from any undetected errors, or from the reader's misunderstanding of the text. It is the reader's responsibility to stay informed of any new changes or recommendations made by any federal, state, and local agency as well as by his or her employing institution or agency.

Pearson Prentice Hall™ is a trademark of Pearson Education, Inc.
Pearson® is a registered trademark of Pearson plc.
Prentice Hall® is a registered trademark of Pearson Education, Inc.

Pearson Education Ltd., London
Pearson Education Singapore, Pte. Ltd.
Pearson Education Canada, Inc.
Pearson Education—Japan
Pearson Education Australia Pty, Limited
Pearson Education North Asia Ltd., Hong Kong
Pearson Educación de Mexico, S.A. de C.V
Pearson Education Malaysia, Pte. Ltd.
Pearson Education, Upper Saddle River, New Jersey

10 9 8 7 6 5 4 3 2 1
ISBN: 0-13-514129-X
ISBN: 978-0-13-514129-8

Dedication

This Instructor's Resource Manual is dedicated to all the hard-working EMS educators who strive to enhance the quality of EMS education and provision in their communities. And to my wife, children, and granddaughter, who both tolerate and inspire my labors toward a better future for EMS.

CONTENTS

©2009 Pearson Education, Inc.
Paramedic Care: Principles & Practice, Vol. 5, 3rd. Ed.

ACKNOWLEDGMENTS

With this 3rd edition of *Paramedic Care: Principles & Practice Instructor's Resource Manual,* exciting new ideas and approaches have been introduced to better equip instructors to educate and train EMT-Paramedics. Since the 1st edition, many individuals have strengthened the educational foundation on which this IRM is built. It is important to acknowledge those who have given so much of their talents and insight to this current edition and those who have contributed to the previous editions as well.

LESSON DEVELOPMENT SPECIALIST

David M. Habben, NREMT-P
EMS Instructor/Consultant
Boise, Idaho

TEACHING STRATEGIES SPECIALIST

Heather Davis, MS, NREMT-P
Education Program Director
Los Angeles County Fire Department
Los Angeles, California

TEST ITEM SPECIALIST

We also wish to thank the following for coordination of test questions in the *Prentice Hall TestGen* that accompanies Volume 5, *Special Considerations/Operations.* The quality of work was excellent, and her assistance is appreciated.

Melissa Alexander-Shook, EdD, NREMT-P
Director, EMS Academy
University of New Mexico
Albuquerque, New Mexico

LETTER TO INSTRUCTOR

As we enter the 21st century, dynamic changes will be taking place in Emergency Medical Services and health care in general. With shorter hospital stays, an increase in home care activities, and the general changes in society, the number and types of patients receiving prehospital care are increasing. We have come a long way from "The White Paper" of 1966 (*Accidental Death and Disability: The Neglected Disease of Modern Society*) to the present, and we still have a long way to go. The skills needed and types of treatment rendered by EMS personnel have changed in recent years and will continue to change. Skills and treatment modalities once reserved for physicians and other specialists are now being performed by EMT-Paramedics, EMT-Intermediates, and EMT-Basics.

The National Highway Traffic Safety Administration has developed a series of documents to help guide our path. The *EMS Agenda for the Future* serves as a guideline for EMS providers, health care organizations and institutions, governmental agencies, and policy makers committed to improving health care in their communities and to ensure that EMS efficiently contributes to that goal. The *EMS Education Agenda for the Future* serves as a guideline that provides EMS educational outcomes designed to meet the needs of the public. This system also emphasizes the integration of EMS within the overall health care system. The *National EMS Research Agenda* serves as a guideline for EMS research and for elevating the science of EMS and prehospital care to the next level. The *Trauma System Agenda for the Future* documents the importance of full implementation of quality trauma systems across the United States to provide optimal care for injured patients and to enhance the country's readiness to respond to future acts of terrorism. The *National EMS Scope of Practice Model* provides the framework for the future development of the National EMS Education Standards.

Instructor's Resource Manual, Volume 5, has been developed to provide you with resources needed to effectively present the materials related to *Special Considerations/Operations*. The *Special Considerations/Operations* IRM not only covers the materials in the National Standard Curriculum, but incorporates numerous references to a variety of Brady/Prentice Hall Health products to enhance student education, evaluate student progress, and provide for remediation of materials, as needed. These materials have been developed by a team of EMS educators and production professionals to bring you state-of-the-art resources for today's EMS educational programs.

Tony Crystal, ScD, EMT-P, RPhT
St. Mary's Hospital
Decatur, Illinois

PREFACE

How to Integrate This Manual with Paramedic Care: Principles & Practice, 3rd Edition Brady Learning Materials

USING YOUR STUDENT TEXT FEATURES

The key to keeping your students engaged is often knowing when and how to integrate their assigned chapter materials into your lectures and discussions. Here are tips on the key text features and how to use them.

- **DOT Objectives.** This feature references the appropriate curriculum objectives contained in each chapter. The list of objectives includes the DOT objective in addition to the page reference on which the objective is covered. Student understanding of the link between these objectives and ultimately their exams is a giant step toward understanding how to study for the exams.

- **Key Terms.** Tell your students that these key terms will be found in each chapter and to use the page references on which the terms first appear. It's often easier than sending them to the index.

- **Case Study.** Real-life anecdotes, experiences, and advice shared by experienced providers in the field are intended to set the stage for the chapter they introduce. The case study feature provides students with realistic and honest perceptions of prehospital care from many points of view. It is a way of mentoring students so they can have a better understanding of EMS.

- **Patho Pearls.** This special feature offers a snapshot of pathological considerations students will encounter in the field.

- **Cultural Considerations.** This new feature conveys different experiences and issues to consider when providing care for patients from other cultures.

- **Legal Notes.** This special feature presents instances in which legal or ethical considerations should be evaluated.

- **Running Glossary.** This feature highlights terms and definitions directly next to the paragraph in which the terms are first presented. This is another quick reference for saving time and reinforcing difficult-to-remember medical terminology and EMS references.

- **Figures.** Updated illustrations and photos help to explain, enhance, and demonstrate key concepts.

- **Tables.** The tables summarize and condense difficult or complex subjects. Some contain photos to enhance and better explain content. Many EMT-Paramedic students are visual learners and may require a boost to their reading skills. As the saying goes, a picture is worth a thousand words, and students find that when they see information in a graphic manner, the material is better understood.

- **Content Review.** Lists, mnemonics, and summaries of key information for quick reference and review make the Content Review a concise feature.

- **Procedures.** Key information and step-by-step approaches are summarized and presented for easy reference in illustrated procedures. In presenting the materials to teach EMT-Paramedics, it is understood that it sometimes can take many words to thoroughly cover a topic. This may sometimes overwhelm students and hinder their ability to sort out the more important information they need. Students need to be able to integrate the didactic material so they can apply it to the psychomotor skills they are expected to perform. Procedures are resources that help to facilitate this educational process, and instructors should consider using them as part of their toolbox.

- **Summary.** Students need a concise review of important chapter information. The Summary is intended to briefly recap the topic of the chapter and flag important points. It is a quick review but certainly does not cover any specific point in depth. Students should find it helpful in bringing together the many pieces of information that a chapter covers. It is an excellent reinforcement tool. Encourage students to read the summaries and reflect back on the chapters to identify those areas that require more study in order for them to better understand the material.

- **Review Questions.** These ask students to recall certain information and to apply the principles they've just learned.
- **You Make the Call.** This feature asks students to think critically and thoughtfully, applying their new knowledge to more complex subjects.

USING THE PACKAGE

This section offers examples and ideas on how to combine or mix and match the *Paramedic Care: Principles & Practice,* 3rd edition suite of products or "toolbox" into your classroom. The following offers ideas on how to enhance your classroom with each product.

- **Student CD.** This all-new in-text CD contains multiple-choice quizzes, case studies with questions and rationales, interactive animations and exercises, virtual tours, a drug guide, EMS scenes, and an audio glossary. Assign its use during or after each chapter. The Student CD has been designed specifically for this text. It is a tool for those students who benefit from using a computer as part of their learning style. Those who take advantage of this CD will find it not only will help with retention of the course material but it also will be fun to use. Encourage students to take advantage of this resource. Use this CD for those difficult-to-learn concepts; they are brought to life with video and animation.
- **Workbook.** The workbook contains matching exercises, multiple-choice questions, short-answer questions, street scenes questions, labeling exercises, case studies and questions, references to other resources, and skill performance checklists. Students should be strongly encouraged to use the workbook side-by-side with the text. Those students who need more direct mentoring may require specific assignments to complete in order for this resource to be most effective for them.
- **EMT Achieve: Paramedic Test Preparation.** This program enables students to practice test-taking online. Four 180-question tests contain questions across the major content areas found in national and state examinations. In addition, each content area has two 25-question tests. Once students take a test, they can see their results, targeting areas of improvement. Before going on to another test, they can take quizzes in each of the content areas. All test questions have rationales and are reinforced with text, photos, illustrations, and video clips. Visit *www.prenhall.com/emtachieve.*
- **TestGen.** The TestGen has been thoroughly updated and reviewed. It contains more than 2,000 exam-style questions, including references to DOT objectives and the student text. The questions in the TestGen are well-designed multiple-choice questions that represent a complete cross-section of the course objectives. Consider composing tests of various lengths throughout the course at regular intervals so students can be evaluated on as much of the course material as possible. TestGen will allow students to become comfortable with the multiple-choice format and style of testing; it is the one most commonly used for state certification examinations and the National Registry.
- **Companion Website.** This site contains quizzes, labeling exercises, links, and state EMS office listings. This tool is another important resource for students who have access to the Internet. Visit *www.bradybooks .com/paramedic.* If students have not already discovered this site on their own, show them where it is located. Also, if students don't have access to the Internet, consider helping them "make the connection."
- **PowerPoint® Presentation.** Every chapter of this PowerPoint® Presentation has been updated. All include additional illustrations and photos as well as a new Image Bank containing all artwork from the textbooks. PowerPoint® slides are a wonderful tool to help teach topics in an EMT-Paramedic course, and there are several advantages to using them.

  First, many are developed specifically for this particular textbook and work extremely well with the ancillary materials provided to assist students and support instructors. The slides flow with the topics of the textbook in order to provide continuity. Second, the slides have been designed from an educational perspective for an instructor by an instructor. Third, this presentation is also customizable. You can delete or add slides and even delete or add photographs or other resources. Personalize them for your classroom without starting from scratch. These slides are meant to give you a base to work from;

©2009 Pearson Education, Inc.
Paramedic Care: Principles & Practice, Vol. 5, 3rd. Ed.

changes to text and photographs and insertion or deletion of text can be done easily. Here are some tips for using slides:

- Use them sparingly.
- Review well in advance.
- Test equipment before class.
- Have a backup plan in case of equipment failure.
- Don't use as a screen a whiteboard or wall that will cause a glare.
- Pay attention to the lighting level in the room.

- **OneKey.** This new distance learning program for didactic portions of the course is offered on one of three platforms: Course Compass, Blackboard, or WebCT. OneKey includes the IRM, PowerPoints®, TestGen, and Companion Website for instruction. You can use this learning program for all your needs in one place. Features include:
  - Course outline
  - Online grade book, which automatically keeps track of students' performance on quizzes, class participation, and attendance
  - Ability to upload questions authored off line and to randomize question order for each student
  - Ability to add your own URLs and course links, set up discussion boards, modify navigation features
  - A virtual classroom for real-time sessions and communication with students
  - Web links
  - Ability to include your teaching assistants into course creation/management

- **Advanced Life Support Skills.** This highly visual manual guides readers through 26 practical skills in detail. Step-by-step procedures are shown in full color and are accompanied by rationales. In addition, each skill includes Key Terms, Objectives, Introduction, Equipment, Assessment, Overview, Rationales, Problem Solving, Ongoing Assessment, Geriatric/Pediatric Notes, Case Studies, and Review Questions. This accessible, easy-to-follow format helps readers understand what, how, and why each skill is performed and is perfect for initial or refresher training.

- **Advanced Life Skills Review.** Over 150 minutes of video show 26 skills close-up, step-by-step for thorough review, so that students can see exactly how skills should be performed. A companion to the Advanced Life Support Skills text, this powerful package is all students need to study for their practical exams.

- **Brady Skills Series: Advanced Life Support.** Over 3 hours of video on 4 tapes/CDs, contains 26 skills in the following format:
  - *Introduction*—what you'll see; indications, contraindications, assessment, as appropriate; also to include video clips for actual scenes
  - *Equipment*—to include variations; photos/illustrations and text
  - *Overview*—quick run through the entire skill
  - *Skill Close-up*—step-by-step for each skill with commentary by authors, and problem solving—by the authors

ADDITIONAL RESOURCES

- **SUCCESS! for the Paramedic, 4th edition (ISBN 0132385503).** This is the text for helping students pass national and state examinations. All items are written and tested by educators and offer proven authoritative information. This text blends a collection of practice exam questions with helpful test-taking tips and student hints. Rationales are also provided for all answers.

- **Paramedic National Standards Self-Test, 5th edition (ISBN 0131999877).** This self-test format enables students to target areas for further study. Includes multiple-choice and scenario-based questions to sharpen test-taking skills, and provides a section on preparing for practical exams.

TIPS FOR PROGRAM/CLASSROOM SUCCESS

ABOUT THE 1998 EMT-PARAMEDIC CURRICULUM

The *Instructor's Resource Manuals* that accompany *Paramedic Care: Principles & Practice*, 3rd edition build on the knowledge and skills gained by experienced instructors who have taught the EMT-Paramedic National Standard Curriculum (NSC). Their knowledge of the curriculum, coupled with extensive field and/or instructional experience, has shaped the many materials included in this manual.

This educational program is based upon the 1998 U.S. Department of Transportation EMT-Paramedic: National Standard Curriculum and is divided into five volumes. The first volume is entitled *Introduction to Advanced Prehospital Care* and addresses the fundamentals of paramedic practice, including pathophysiology, pharmacology, medication administration, and advanced airway management. The second volume, *Patient Assessment*, builds on the assessment skills of the EMT-Basic with special emphasis on advanced patient assessment at the scene. The third volume, *Medical Emergencies*, is the most extensive and addresses paramedic-level care of medical emergencies. Particular emphasis is placed on the most common medical problems and serious emergencies, such as respiratory and cardiovascular emergencies. The fourth volume, *Trauma Emergencies*, discusses advanced prehospital care from the mechanism of injury analysis to shock/trauma resuscitation. The final volume in the series, *Special Considerations/Operations*, includes neonatal, pediatric, geriatric, home health care and specially challenged patients, as well as incident command, ambulance services, rescue, hazardous materials, and crime scene operations.

LENGTH OF COURSE

The emphasis of paramedic education should be on the competence of the graduates, not the amount of education they receive. The time involved in educating a paramedic to an acceptable level of competence depends on many variables. Based on the experience in the pilot and field testing of the NSC, it is expected that the average program, with average students, will achieve average results in approximately 1,000 to 1,200 hours of instruction. This can be further broken down to 500 to 600 hours of classroom and practical lab time; 250 to 300 hours of clinical work; and 250 to 300 hours of field internship. Be sure to consult with your state agency for specific minimum times for these areas.

The length of this course will vary according to several factors, including, but not limited to:

- students' basic academic skills competence
- faculty-to-student ratio
- student motivation
- students' prior emergency/health care experience
- prior academic achievements
- clinical and academic resources available
- quality of the overall educational program

EMT-Basic is a prerequisite for the paramedic course. It helps to form a foundation for the paramedic student, and because the NSC module titles are the same, it will give the student a general overview on what topics to expect. In addition to the EMT-Basic prerequisite, the Paramedic curriculum has identified course work in anatomy and physiology as either a prerequisite or corequisite. A mastery of anatomy and physiology, beyond that covered in the anatomy and physiology review of each section of the program, is assumed throughout this curriculum. EMS educational programs have many options to address anatomy and physiology in paramedic education. For programs that have access to formal anatomy and physiology classes, an appropriate-level course can be identified as a prerequisite or corequisite to paramedic training. For other programs, anatomy and physiology can be "front loaded" in the paramedic course or presented throughout the course.

It has been a number of years since the U.S. DOT EMT-Paramedic National Standard Curriculum was revised, and changes have been made by most of the authorities that approve EMT-P courses. EMT-P instructors must ensure that they stay current with curriculum changes, because they affect their courses.

Educational Philosophy

Education standards are needed to guide program managers and instructors in making appropriate decisions about what material to cover in classroom instruction. Additionally, these standards are used as one component of program evaluation in the accreditation process and are used by publishers to develop instructional materials. In most allied health professions, education standards are developed by professional associations with broad community input. The complexity, interdisciplinary nature, and state government oversight of EMS necessitate a slightly different approach.

Where We Are

Currently the content of most EMS education programs is based on a national standard curriculum. The NSC is funded, developed, and updated periodically by the U.S. Department of Transportation, National Highway Traffic Safety Administration (NHTSA). The NSC has been developed for all nationally recognized levels of EMS education and consists of detailed, highly prescriptive objectives and declarative material. Since these documents are closely tied to scope of practice and because their revision is the only national venue for the discussion of scope of practice, the NSC revision process is time-consuming and expensive.

Many EMS education programs and faculty strictly follow the NSC in defining the content of their courses. A typical measure of quality for EMS programs has been their adherence to the current NSC. Although the use of the NSC has contributed to the standardization of EMS education, the quality and length of programs still vary nationally. The reliance on the NSC has decreased flexibility, limited creativity, and made the development of alternative delivery methods difficult. The strict focus on the NSC may result in the development of narrow technical and conceptual skills without consideration for the broad range of professional competencies expected of today's entry-level EMS providers.

Where We Want to Be

The National EMS Education Standards will be derived from the National EMS Scope of Practice Model. Each National EMS Education Standards document will provide the minimal terminal objectives necessary for successful program completion of a level of EMS provider identified in the *National EMS Scope of Practice Model*. All programs must adhere to these standards, but there will be significant flexibility in how to achieve the standards. The standards will be designed to encourage creativity in delivery methods such as problem-based learning, computer-aided instruction, distance learning, programmed self-instruction, and others. Without the constraint of an unduly prescriptive NSC, EMS educational institutions are held more accountable for the content and quality of their instruction. This would require institutions to, at a minimum, conduct evaluations of both educational process and outcome quality.

With less prescriptive curriculum standards, it will be much easier to modify curriculum content, both locally and nationally. Changes based on research, practice analysis, future direction of the profession, and experience are quickly reflected in education content, and these changes are communicated to programs through a variety of mechanisms. While all programs must meet national standards, they will be encouraged to continually improve and excel.

There will be a variety of outstanding instructional materials, including instructor lesson plans, available from publishers, educational institutions, and other interested parties to support local EMS instruction. EMS instructors will use published materials or develop their own for classroom use.

The scope of practice for EMS providers will not be defined by education standards or curriculum. National EMS Education Standards will be designed to prepare EMS providers who are competent to perform within a specific scope of practice. Education will support, rather than define, scope of practice. The scope of practice for EMS providers will be based on the National EMS Scope of Practice Model.

Further information may be found in the U.S. Department of Transportation's *EMS Education Agenda for the Future: A Systems Approach*.

Interventions

The goal of emergency medical services is to prevent or reduce morbidity and mortality from illness or injury. Toward that end result, the roles and responsibilities of the modern paramedics include the following:

- Having fulfilled prescribed requirements by a credentialing agency to practice the art and science of prehospital medicine in conjunction with medical direction
- Possessing the knowledge, skills, and attitudes consistent with the expectations of the public and the profession
- Recognizing that they are an essential component of the continuum of care and serve as linkages among health resources

xvi PARAMEDIC CARE *Special Considerations/Operations*

©2009 Pearson Education, Inc.
Paramedic Care: Principles & Practice, Vol. 5, 3rd. Ed.

- Striving to maintain high-quality, reasonable-cost health care by delivering patients directly to appropriate facilities
- Being proactive patient advocates in affecting long-term health care by working in conjunction with other provider agencies, networks, and organizations
- Participating in public education, health promotion, and injury and illness prevention programs
- Functioning as facilitators of access to care, as well as initial treatment providers
- Being accountable to medical direction, the public, and their peers
- Recognizing the importance of research and actively participating in the design, development, evaluation, and publication of research
- Seeking to take part in life-long professional development and peer evaluation and assuming an active role in professional and community organizations

INSTRUCTOR RESPONSIBILITIES

Many of us can remember a favorite teacher or instructor. Think back to what made that person special. Chances are the memorable instructor was a dynamic, knowledgeable person who took the job seriously yet was able to interject a sense of informality and fun that made learning the material easy and enjoyable.

Instructors who fit this description (and who probably became role models for many of their students) didn't get that way by accident. In addition to countless hours behind the desk or podium and in front of the keyboard learning about or presenting information on their chosen subjects, they also worked to develop a solid foundation of knowledge about the needs of student learners.

For the most part, students in paramedic programs are adult learners. This is significant, because adults learn differently than children do. They also have very different needs and motivational factors. Understanding these needs and motivations is the key to being a successful EMS instructor.

So what do adult learners require? Simply put, adult learners want to have a reason for being in the classroom. In other words, when adult learners sit down in the classroom, they expect to find out how the information being presented is pertinent to their needs.

Sometimes, the relevance of the learning is obvious and does not need to be clarified—for example, the idea that direct pressure stops most bleeding. The reasons for learning other things may take more explanation on the part of the instructor—for example, why learning and using correct terminology is important. The relevance of learning to student needs can sometimes be emphasized through textbook case studies or through the relation of personal experiences by the instructor.

This leads to another important aspect of adult learners. They have life experiences that are important to them. The life experiences that adult learners bring to the classroom can be a tremendous motivational tool for the student as well as the instructor. Perhaps a student is taking the EMT-Paramedic course because he or she was first on the scene of an accident and felt helpless at being unable to assist the victim. It is easy to see that this student will be highly motivated and will understand the reason for learning the material presented in class. For another example, a group of students might be in class because they plan to volunteer together with their local ambulance service. Their motivation will likely be quite high. Students such as the ones described above are some of the easiest for an instructor to teach.

Unfortunately, few paramedic classes will be so straightforward. Paramedic classes usually contain a mix of students with a wide variety of motivations and life experiences. Reaching out to, and making the class meaningful for, such a range of students is a real challenge for the instructor. To do so, the instructor must employ a variety of educational techniques. The following sections will be helpful to instructors in making the paramedic program a valuable experience.

Basic Course Coordination

The following section may be one of the most important for first-time instructors to read. Experienced instructors may also pick up some tips to help make teaching their paramedic courses a little easier.

Teaching a paramedic course involves much more than just preparing a lecture and presenting the material in class. Course coordination is the essential framework that holds the class together and can determine how successful the learning experience will be for students.

Depending on where the course is taught, much of the course coordination work may be done for the instructor. For example, an EMS instructor who teaches a program at a community college may have the schedule preset, books available at the campus bookstore, and access to audiovisual needs at a moment's notice. Other instructors may be asked to hold classes for a community agency and will be responsible for everything from site selection to equipment rental. Although the amount of work that goes into coordinating the course will vary, there are some basic components of course coordination that should be considered in any setting.

Regulations. The first area to look at when coordinating a paramedic program is the arena of state and local regulation. Many states have specific requirements that must be met before teaching of the course can begin. These requirements can range from applying for course approval to designating a physician sponsor for the course.

One of the easiest ways to get into serious trouble as an instructor is to ignore or not comply with applicable state and local regulations. Take the time to learn which regulations apply to teaching in your specific area.

Schedule. A great deal of time should be invested in developing a course schedule that works for the students as well as for the instructor. An EMT-P course contains a lot of information. Any course schedule should be paced to allow proper absorption and retention of the material. Generally, an 8-hour-a-day, 5-day-a-week course should not be considered. Exceptions can be made when a specific group of students being trained has a demonstrated history of EMS experience, but most adult learners have other obligations that would not permit them to take such a full-time course. Many instructors will schedule an EMT-P course for 3- to 4-hour blocks. These blocks for the most part work well in terms of teaching specific sections or chapters of the text. When scheduling the time for each class session, remember to build in enough time at the beginning of each class to give the quiz or to handle any administrative details.

The suggested amount of time it takes to teach a full EMT-Paramedic course is 1,000 to 1,200 hours. Given the amount of material to be covered, there is little to no extra time in the course. When setting the schedule, pay attention to the suggested teaching time listed in the front of each chapter of this manual.

Facility Selection. Forethought and planning in selecting the site where the course will be taught will save an instructor hours of headache. A comfortable, complete facility can have a profound effect on the students' ability to learn and on the instructor's ability to present the material. When selecting a facility for the course, several factors should be considered.

The site needs to be large enough to hold the number of students enrolled in the course comfortably. If the space available is limited, it can be maximized through proper arrangement of the tables and chairs or desks. Experiment with various setups to find the best placements for the size of the room. Keep in mind that the students need to be able to see the instructor and any audiovisual materials that are used.

The students need room to move around, as well as adequate space to sit comfortably. There also should be room for the instructor to move around in the front of the class. Some instructors are roamers and need a lot of space, while others are more "home oriented" and tend to stay at the podium or front table. Evaluate your own style and factor that into the site selection.

Remember also that an EMT-P course is very much skills-oriented. There must be plenty of room to break the students up into small groups to practice skills. A facility with access to more than one classroom is ideal. An appropriate facility is one that is relatively free from distractions. Trying to hold an entire EMT-P course in the kitchen of the fire station will more than likely prove a frustrating experience for the instructor. More importantly, an environment with too many distractions detracts from the learning process for the students.

Make sure the heating ventilation and air-conditioning systems for the facility are appropriate and working. If the classroom temperature is too hot or too cold, the students will pay more attention to trying to get comfortable and less attention to the instructor. Also avoid sites where the HVAC system is too noisy.

Other site selection factors to be considered include availability of restrooms, water fountains, and adequate parking for the students.

Course Materials and Resources. Not having required course materials in place for the class reflects poorly on the instructor. Planning far enough in advance can prevent most of the problems related to course materials. Some materials such as textbooks or workbooks can be ordered well ahead of time. Remember that it never hurts to order a few more texts than you think you'll need. It's more expensive to have to order just one or two books at a time.

Access to a copy machine is an absolute necessity. Everything from handouts to quizzes to CPR cards must be copied. It's probably best to do the copying of materials for the course every few class sessions instead of trying to make all the copies for the entire course in one sitting. Sometimes schedules and topics

 ©2009 Pearson Education, Inc. *Paramedic Care: Principles & Practice, Vol. 5, 3rd. Ed.*

change slightly, and smaller and more frequent copy jobs will prevent having to redo a quiz or handout. Leave yourself plenty of time to do the copying. It's inappropriate to take the first 30 minutes of the class time making copies.

Also, think about materials you'll need for skills demonstrations and practices and for role-playing scenarios. The lesson plans in this manual list the resources you'll need for such activities on the first page of each lesson.

If you are teaching in a dedicated classroom with equipment storage on site, equipment availability is generally not a problem. There may be times, however, when it is necessary to obtain extra pieces of equipment. Reserve such equipment far in advance to keep from being caught short when the equipment is actually needed.

Additional Instructors. There will be times at which another instructor may be invited to class, either to help with skills or to serve as guest lecturer. Guest lecturers can be valuable in several ways. They can give a new slant to required information and provide useful supplementary knowledge. They can spark student interest by providing a break in the routine. They can also give students the opportunity to observe different teaching styles and techniques, something that can be valuable for the regular instructor as well.

When a guest instructor is invited, he or she should be provided with both lesson objectives and a lesson plan. Plan on observing a first-time guest lecturer to get a sense of his or her instructional abilities and success in covering the objectives. Be alert for tendencies to deviate from the topic excessively. When additional instructors are used for skills practice sessions, a ratio of one instructor for every four to five students is probably most appropriate.

Final Considerations. In terms of coordinating a course, the instructor's best friend and worst enemy is time. If there is enough time, almost anything can be accomplished. If there isn't any time, nothing can be accomplished. The bottom line is that in order to make your course a truly successful one, take care of as many details as far in advance of the course as possible.

Preparation for State and/or National Certification. The successful end of an EMT-Paramedic course will be the completion by students of all requirements for state and/or national certification as EMT-Paramedics. Both students and instructors should have a very clear understanding of what those requirements are.

There are some other things that can be done to help increase the student's chances of passing the written and practical examinations for certification.

Written Exams. Most of the state certification exams as well as the National Registry written exam use the multiple-choice format. There are definite keys to successfully passing multiple-choice examinations. One of the best ways to prepare students for taking certification exams is to make multiple-choice examinations a part of the course from the very beginning. Doing so will hone students' test-taking skills and will prepare them for the format they are most likely to see. Each chapter in this manual contains a multiple-choice quiz to build student familiarity with the format, and the student workbook contains thousands of test questions. In addition, Prentice Hall TestGen for *Paramedic Care: Principles & Practice,* 3rd edition, allows you to easily prepare multiple-choice tests custom-tailored to your students' needs. The new online product, *EMT Achieve: Paramedic Test Preparation (www.prenhall.com/emtachieve)*, provides practice with immediate scoring and rationales and quizzes by module with immediate instructor access by students.

If multiple-choice testing reveals some deficiencies in student understanding of chapter material, you might assign some of the reinforcement handouts available with each lesson. The Chapter Review provides a fill-in-the-blank format, while other handouts offer a variety of approaches for reviewing chapter content. Yet other reinforcement materials can be found on the Student CD and Companion Website provided by Prentice Hall at *www.bradybooks.com/paramedic.*

Practical Exams. Students fear practical examinations from the first day of the paramedic course right up through test day. Nothing an instructor can do will completely eliminate this apprehension. The fear is generally of performance, not ability.

One of the best techniques to help relieve some of their anxiety is to have the students practice their skills at every opportunity. This will build their confidence and provide an opportunity for the instructor to stress some of the finer points of the more detailed skills.

It will be helpful to discuss the state and national examination process with the students at the first class session. Allow them to ask questions and give them frank answers. *Provide each of your students with the test-taking hints provided in this* Instructor's Resource Manual.

ABOUT LEARNING

Psychomotor Development

The work that paramedics do is very practical skills-oriented. These skills are based on a sound foundation of cognitive knowledge and the understanding of when and how to apply that knowledge in appropriate settings. At least 50 percent of the paramedic course will be spent teaching, demonstrating, and performing skills. The time, effort, and energy you put into the teaching of skills in the classroom will directly affect the future success of your students as competent EMT-Paramedics.

There are many ways of teaching the necessary skills in a paramedic course. No one way is correct for all instructors at all times. The appropriateness of methods used will depend on factors such as the number of students in the class, their motivations for being in the class, and the individual differences in learning styles among students in a particular class.

To be most effective at teaching skills in an EMT class, instructors must be competent in and fully aware of the skills criteria used locally. Some states or localities use a packet of skill sheets containing separate skill sheets for each discrete skill. Other areas may use the skill sheets developed by the National Registry of EMTs. Still other areas use both. Take the time to review and study such materials before the start of the course and before each class session in which skills will be taught.

Skill Demonstrations

Demonstrating a skill for paramedic students can be one of the most difficult and challenging responsibilities for an instructor. The pressure to perform is enormous because so much is riding on the outcome. Even an instructor who is very comfortable with his or her skills may suffer from intimidation or performance anxiety.

The first time a skill is demonstrated for the students is critical to the student's performance of that skill in the future. The first time most students see a skill performed leaves a strong impression; if a part of the skill was demonstrated incorrectly, the students are likely to repeat the mistake. It is easy to see why this first demonstration of a skill is so crucial and why it can produce anxiety for the instructor.

There are things that you as an instructor can do to help alleviate this anxiety. First and foremost, have faith in your ability. Many instructors have been paramedics for years and have the background and experience to support their textbook knowledge. Also, EMS instructors have been through the class before and, in many cases, have helped with skills training even before becoming instructors themselves. Have the confidence to realize that you know the skills and are more than capable of presenting them to the class.

It may be helpful for the instructor to practice certain skills before the class session. Review the skill sheet and the materials found in the textbook and this instructor's resource manual. It also may be helpful for the students to hear another instructor narrate the written steps of the skill as it is being demonstrated. Learning increases as the number of the students' senses are stimulated. You might also consider videotaping a demonstration of the skill before the class. This allows for greater control of any possible mistakes; the taped demonstration can also be used with other classes.

The disadvantage to videotaping is that, if the production quality is poor, it can distract students who will pay more attention to inadequacies of the lighting, script, or sound than the skill being demonstrated. Also, remember that the best way to become more comfortable with demonstrating skills in front of the class is demonstrating skills. As with public speaking, the only thing that makes it any easier is doing it often.

When demonstrating a skill to your students, remember that as adult learners they bring a multitude of life experiences with them. They may also have some experience with a particular skill and may offer comments, feedback, or suggestions. Do not discount such input. Instructors have a tendency to teach something the way they themselves were taught and too often fail to keep an open mind to other ways a skill might be performed or taught. The most important thing to remember is that a different technique is not necessarily wrong as long as the principles of the skill are correct. The best instructors are flexible and adapt to new information or circumstances and to the needs of their students.

Scenarios for Learning

One of the best ways for instructors to integrate cognitive knowledge with practical skills is through the use of scenarios. Throughout this *Instructor's Resource Manual*, there are You Make the Call scenarios pertinent to the chapters.

Scenarios are beneficial to the students in several ways. They can add a sense of realism to the course. They also can give students a hint of the pressures they will face in the real world. Scenarios promote interaction among the students and can go far in terms of enhancing student bonding and camaraderie/team building.

©2009 Pearson Education, Inc.
Paramedic Care: Principles & Practice, Vol. 5, 3rd. Ed.

Student performance in the scenarios will provide instructors with an opportunity to evaluate how well the students have grasped both the skill and the ideas in the textbook that are behind it.

There are some basic points that instructors should keep in mind when running patient care scenarios in the classroom setting:

- *The scenario has to be doable.* Giving students impossible scenarios sets them up for failure and can destroy their confidence.

- *The scenario has to be winnable.* A winnable scenario is one in which students have the opportunity to see an improvement in patient outcome based on their care.

- *Each scenario should be evaluated and feedback provided to the students.* Providing feedback on student performance will help reinforce positive performances and eliminate mistakes.

- *Keep the scenario simple.* The "busload of hypochondriacs that goes off the cliff into a toxic waste dump" scenario may be fun, but it's complicated, uses up too much precious time, and probably involves so many considerations that students actually learn very little.

- *Start using scenarios early in the course.* Even on the first night of class an appropriate scenario can be run. Consider a simple CPR call or a call for choking.

- *Use scenarios often.* Many instructors will use a scenario in every class session.

Like most things, scenarios work most effectively and smoothly when you take the time to plan them out in advance. There are detailed instructions for scenarios in this manual that make such planning easier. There are also collections of ready-to-go scenarios available from publishers. Your own experiences as a paramedic, however, may make the best, most effective scenarios for your class. There are many benefits to using personal experiences as a basis for scenarios. Real calls that you have been on have a different flavor from generic scripts borrowed from books. This heightens the sense of their realism. In addition, after the students have played out the scenario, you can tell them what actually happened and compare notes. By objectively evaluating your responses to the call with the students, you can demonstrate to them that there is no such thing as a "perfect" call. This will help remind them that there is always room for improvement, even for the instructor.

One key to running successful scenarios is the use of an appropriate evaluation tool. A proper evaluation tool need not be fancy—in fact, the simpler the better. An evaluation tool can consist of nothing more than a sheet of paper containing appropriate information about the call and room to write notes and comments about student performance. The evaluation tool can even be incorporated into the scenario planning sheet.

When developing your own classroom scenarios, always use a scenario planning sheet. A well-prepared planning sheet should ensure similar learning outcomes for students even if other instructors use the sheet to run the scenario. The planning sheet should contain the following:

- Description of the call
- Environmental factors that might affect the call
- Pertinent findings in the scene size-up, initial assessment, focused history and physical exam, and baseline and follow-up vital signs
- An area for information about such things as interventions performed and time they were done
- A list of the objectives for the call—what you are trying to teach the students with this scenario
- A list of equipment needed to run the call
- Moulage instructions, if pertinent
- Instructions to the "patient"
- A space for any additional comments in which you can evaluate student performance (Leaving enough space to write comments probably works better than trying to develop a complicated checklist of things the students should have done in the scenario.)

One of the easiest ways to incorporate scenarios into the classroom is to pair the students into responder teams and place a different team on call for each class session. This gives the students both a feel for what it's like to be on duty and an opportunity to apply their skills in a fairly realistic setting. The on-call crew should check at the beginning of the class to ensure that the jump kits to be used are complete and operational. It's also a good idea to assign a second crew as backup in case the first crew needs additional help.

There are many ways to make scenarios an everyday part of the class. Evaluate the characteristics of your facility and your students to determine the best way to use scenarios in your classes.

Assisting Student Learning

The type and amount of information covered in paramedic courses can be overwhelming for students if they are not prepared to study effectively. Unfortunately, many adult learners lack the tools and background for efficient study. For a large percentage of your students, the paramedic course represents a return to the classroom after many years. For some students the paramedic course may be their first formal experiences as adult learners. Much has changed in the way of educational methodology and technology since they were in school, and tools and resources taken for granted today were often unavailable then and are thus unfamiliar to these students. Anything that you can do as an instructor to help such students study more effectively is an investment that will pay off handsomely for both the students, in terms of their future employment prospects, and for your EMS system, in terms of better-trained, more capable EMT-Ps.

As adult learners, paramedic students must take responsibility for their own learning. It would be extremely difficult for most paramedic students to make it through the course without studying a substantial amount of time outside the classroom. It is not unusual for students to spend three to four hours studying for each hour spent in the classroom. To help students get the most from their study time, you might suggest some of the following strategies for success that have worked for others in the past:

- Encourage the formation of study groups. A study group can help students put pieces of information together in ways that "click" as they hadn't when students were studying on their own. Often a member of the study group can explain a concept in a way that allows another student to understand something that wasn't grasped in class. Some students will feel more comfortable asking that "stupid" question in a small group setting rather than the classroom. One problem with study groups, however, is that if students misunderstand something, the misinformation will be more widely circulated and it may take some time for the instructor to become aware that this has occurred. If your students do form study groups, pay attention to what your evaluation tools reveal about student understanding of key concepts and ideas.

- Use the student workbooks that are available with the basic textbook. Workbooks include many different types of activities that will reinforce what students have read in the text.

- Make yourself available for questions before and after class as well as during breaks. Some students are shy about classroom participation and will hesitate to bring up what they may see as "silly" questions.

- Use computer resources if available. There are some excellent computer programs that can enhance student understanding of key ideas, things like test banks for reviewing course knowledge or anatomy models for illustrating how the body works. If a classroom computer is available, consider purchasing one or more of these programs and make it (them) available for student use at appropriate times. (See "Classroom Tools" later in the introductory material.)

- Pace yourself when delivering lectures. Give students enough time to write their notes. Monitor the students' nonverbal cues that indicate they are ready to continue. When pencils stop moving, pick up the topic and carry on with the lecture.

- Consider giving students outlines of your lecture with plenty of spaces for them to write notes. Most of today's computer presentation software can generate such simplified outlines from the more detailed lecture preparations.

- Finally, encourage the students to seek to balance study, work, and play in their lives. Retention of course material will be enhanced if students are relatively relaxed and not overloading any one area of their lives. (The same will be true for their EMS careers.) This material should be covered during the "Well-being of the Paramedic" section of the course.

By applying some or all of the preceding ideas, you really can help students with their studies. Remember that instructors are responsible not just for lecturing and teaching skills but also for doing what it takes—within reason—to help students through the course.

CLASSROOM TOOLS

The instructional media an instructor will use in the classroom will vary with equipment and resource materials available. The instructor's comfort level with a particular medium also affects what resources are used in the classroom. Experimenting with different media is strongly encouraged; this will increase the instructor's familiarity with other media and enlarge the pool of resources he or she is likely to draw on.

Remember also that it is important to avoid saturating students with one type of audiovisual material. There may be an entire slide set for the course, but it may not be the soundest educational policy to use nothing but those slides as you teach the course. Students learn differently and different media will reach or interest different students.

Think of technology as critical to your classroom presentation. The following tips and techniques will guide you through the technology maze.

PowerPoint® Presentations

PowerPoint® presentations and slides are a wonderful tool to help teach topics in a paramedic course, and there are several advantages to using them. First, slides developed specifically for a particular textbook work extremely well with that text and other ancillary materials associated with it, such as the instructor's resource manual and the workbook. This instructor's resource manual tells you specifically which slides to use for which part of a lecture. The material presented in the slides is consistent with what students learn in their reading. Additionally, use of such slide programs can decrease preparation time for the instructor. The *Paramedic Care: Principles & Practice,* 3rd edition PowerPoint® Presentation is completely customizable if an instructor doesn't wish to be completely tied to a program prepared by someone else.

Disadvantages in the use of slides are usually related to equipment problems and a tendency to overuse the medium. For the slide presentation to be successful, the projector must be working and your computer must be in good working order so that there is no danger of the presentation freezing. Also remember that lighting conditions in the room must be appropriate for the projection of the slides. If there are no shades for the windows and class is held during daylight hours, students may have trouble seeing the images. Keep in mind, if this is the case, you can change the design colors on the presentation to make it easier to read.

Videotapes and DVD

The age of video has not left EMS instruction untouched. DVD has entered the training arena. The volume and range of subjects available in commercial training tapes today is tremendous. The many timely topics available in the format lend a state-of-the-art feel to the classroom. Also, students are extremely comfortable with the medium, probably more so than with any other.

Videotapes and DVD offer vivid, dynamic images and sounds that excite and stimulate most students and instructors. Real-life footage conveys the nature of EMS work in a way that other audiovisual aids cannot. Videos can be an excellent choice for dramatizing a specific point an instructor wants to make. Perhaps most important, difficult procedures can be shown on tape over and over until students understand the concept or skill.

The disadvantages of these media use include heavy reliance on the equipment. The TV has to be operating correctly, as do the VCR, videotape cassette, DVD player, and DVD. If any one component fails, the entire presentation fails. Initial outlay to purchase the equipment can be expensive. Also, in a large class setting it may be difficult to position the monitor so that all students have a good view of it. Finally, the fact that so many topics are available may tempt instructors to overuse this audiovisual aid in the classroom.

Tips for using video media include:

- Always preview the tape for quality and appropriateness of the material.
- Never put in a video and then leave the classroom. They should not be used to babysit the students.
- Have a backup plan in case of equipment failure.
- Preset the video for the appropriate starting point before class.
- Use short, pertinent video segments instead of always running entire tapes or DVDs. The shorter segments can have a more profound impact.
- Be prepared to pause the tape and ask or answer pertinent questions.
- Set up the TV/VCR/DVD player before class so that you can check to ensure sight and sound quality throughout the room.

Using media in the classroom can add a dynamic boost to your lectures. Sprinkle them liberally throughout the course and watch the impact they have on students.

Whiteboards

This modern-day relative of the chalkboard can be found in nearly every classroom setting. Students expect to see a writing surface of one type or another in a classroom, and the simplicity, spontaneity, and versatility that whiteboards make possible can hardly be matched.

The major limit on the use of the whiteboard is the instructor's imagination. Even if a lesson plan calls for a class to be lecture based, a particular point that needs to be emphasized or explained can be written on the board. The variety of colors available for use on the whiteboard enlivens presentations. Complicated or detailed drawings or formulas can be written on the board before class, allowing more time for discussion during the lesson. Finally, with no bulbs to burn out or other electronics to fail, whiteboards are extremely reliable.

The disadvantages of whiteboards are relatively few and often instructor related. Poor penmanship on the part of the instructor can leave students frustrated. The dry-erase markers used on whiteboards can dry up, leaving the instructor with few options. In very large classroom settings, it may be difficult for all students to see the board. Lastly, inadvertent use of a permanent marker may ruin a whiteboard.

Here are some tips for using whiteboards:

- Use blue or black for the main color, and use a bright color like red or green to highlight key words or concepts.
- Never use the yellow marker, as yellow will be nearly invisible to most students sitting any distance away.
- Don't talk to the board while you are writing—your listeners are in the seats.
- Draw complex images before the class starts.
- Print legibly.
- Use letters large enough for all to see.
- Do not allow permanent markers in the classroom, especially in the marker tray.
- Watch for spelling and grammatical errors.
- Give students ample time to write material in their notebooks before erasing it from the board.

Whiteboards are a wonderful visual aid that, when used appropriately can make the instructor's job easier, while providing students with a familiar and colorful visual stimulus.

Making It Real—Moulage Tips

Moulage is the application of materials to a volunteer "patient" to simulate injuries and other significant clinical signs. EMS instructors have used moulage techniques for years to enhance the realism of scenarios for their students. A well-done job of moulage creates an impressively real patient, while a poorly handled job detracts from the scenario and from student learning.

The application of makeup and other objects to simulate injuries has long been a staple in Hollywood films. However, EMS instructors do not need access to the movie industry's makeup artists to learn to create effects that are believable and accurate in "patients." Some great moulage techniques can be achieved with minimal amounts of material and training. Contrary to what some may think, applying good moulage does not have to be a time-consuming ordeal. The benefit of moulage is lost if it takes an hour to apply the makeup.

Basic Moulage Techniques. Injuries are not perfect, so it's difficult to make a "bad" injury. Here are some basic rules that will allow the instructor to create realistic injuries and signs simply:

- First and foremost, remember that "less is more." A light application of whites, blues, and grays will have a more profound impact than a heavily applied layer of clown white when simulating paleness or cyanosis.
- Simplicity is the key in creating realistic "injuries" in a short period of time. Most injuries can be simulated with a few commonly available items. A basic list of supplies for moulage can be found later in this section.
- Always apply a light application of cold cream under any injuries or skin signs that you apply. Cold cream helps the makeup stay on the skin and makes the removal of the makeup much easier for the "patient."
- Accuracy is important in creating believable injuries. Placing a giant bruise over the entire area of the chest to simulate a pneumothorax probably does more to detract from the scenario than illustrate it.
- To simulate cyanosis, try a light application of blue to the nail beds, ear lobes, and around the lips after applying a basic underlay of white or light gray.
- Use a mixture of water with a small amount of glycerin to simulate diaphoresis. Keep the mixture in a small spray bottle and apply immediately prior to the arrival of the "rescuers."
- To simulate burns, apply a layer of cold cream followed by a base coat of red to the entire area. Lay some tissue over the area and then apply some water-soluble lubricant such as K-Y® jelly over the tissue. Gently break the tissue by rolling it from the center of the "burned" area toward the edges. This will create a remarkably realistic looking second-degree burn.

©2009 Pearson Education, Inc.
Paramedic Care: Principles & Practice, Vol. 5, 3rd. Ed.

- Use activated charcoal applied with a cotton swab around the edges of the nares and the mouth and tongue to simulate a respiratory burn.
- Place a small amount of effervescent tablet in a simulated chest wound. Just prior to "rescuer" arrival, place a few drops of water on the tablet to help simulate a sucking chest wound. The bubbling action is usually quite impressive.
- Whenever there is a chance that the "patient" may "bleed" or "ooze," be sure to place a tarp under the patient to avoid staining the carpet or flooring underneath the patient.

The best way to become comfortable with moulage is to use it often. Experiment with different materials and household items. Remember that because real injuries are not perfect, it's difficult to go wrong if you keep it simple.

Resources for Moulage. Putting together a useful moulage kit does not have to be expensive or complicated. One of the biggest decisions to make is whether to build your own kit or purchase one of the commercially available injury simulation kits. There are advantages and disadvantages to each approach. Commercially available kits usually contain a variety of fake injuries made from rubber or plastic that can be either strapped on or held in place by spirit gum. They also contain a variety of colored makeup. The advantage to this type of moulage kit is its completeness.

The biggest drawback to such kits is the price. Some of the more elaborate kits can cost hundreds of dollars. Also, many of the injuries included are not very realistic, and the time that it takes an instructor to develop a level of expertise using the kits may be unreasonable for most EMS instructors.

Another drawback is that using a single source for moulage materials and techniques limits the development of the instructor's skill in using moulage as a resource. An instructor forced by circumstances to use a kit other than his or her own may have difficulty moulaging patients.

An alternative to purchasing a ready-made kit is putting together a kit of your own. Most of the materials are inexpensive, and this will also give you the flexibility to be creative. Experiment with different items and find the things that work the best for you. Some items that such a kit might contain include the following:

- Cold cream—for applying under makeup.
- Plumber's putty—to use as a modeling clay when building injuries.
- Eye shadow—a variety of shades of eye shadow to simulate cyanosis and bruises.
- Dirt—a container of dirt is handy to help make realistic road rashes and other injuries.
- Halloween makeup—haunt the costume aisles of your local store in October. A wide variety of makeup colors and simulated injuries are available. Hint: Shop the day after Halloween to get bargain prices.
- Chicken bones—for use in the simulation of open fractures. Place them in a bag and lightly crush them to obtain realistic bone fragments. Be sure to sanitize the bones before use.
- Clear plastic cups—crushed, they provide pieces of very real looking "glass" for use in an injury.
- Fake blood—one of those items that can be purchased commercially. Many instructors have also come up with their own recipes that work well. Try to avoid any red dyes that stain too easily.
- Knife handles—use just the handle of a knife and build putty around the knife end to simulate an impaled object.
- Effervescent tablets—to help simulate chest wounds.
- Condoms—filled with a little water or K-Y® jelly for creating simulated evisceration.
- Brushes—variety of makeup brushes for applying colors for cyanosis and bruising.
- Activated charcoal—for burn moulage.

INSTRUCTING LEARNING DISABLED STUDENTS

Each adult learner who enrolls in an EMS course possesses a unique personality and a unique ability to learn. Factors such as learning ability and style, preexisting knowledge, life experience, and motivation will contribute to the level of achievement of each student. Very few, if any, adult education classes will contain a truly homogeneous group of students. Competent educators realize this and use the strengths of each learner to achieve the desired educational outcomes. As a result, instructors have a responsibility to identify students who may be deficient in learning skills and to provide appropriate remediation and support.

Learning disabilities do not mean a lack of intelligence. Many famous people have overcome learning disabilities to contribute their talents to all walks of life—Albert Einstein, Winston Churchill, Cher, Walt Disney, Whoopi Goldberg, Bruce Jenner, and Woodrow Wilson, just to name a few. Although not all learning disabled people will achieve success, even in modest terms, many can complete training programs in a wide variety of fields such as EMS. The message is this: Learning disabled students of any age can learn.

In recent decades, state and federal governments have extended protection to learning disabled students through a wide variety of court decisions and laws such as the Americans With Disabilities Act (ADA) of 1990. Today educational institutions must have operational plans aimed at identifying and assisting learning disabled students. Adult learners who have benefited from these programs in their primary and secondary education are aware of these laws and are entering EMS programs in greater numbers than in the past. They will request—and rightly so—the educational accommodations and compensatory mechanisms that have helped them achieve prior learning success. EMS educators, therefore, will be asked to develop a wide variety of instructional strategies—diverse methods of presentation that will not only enrich the educational experience of learning disabled students, but of all the students in a class. Of the many types of learning disabilities, the ones that an EMS instructor can expect to encounter most frequently are "academic skills disorders." Of particular concern are developmental reading disorders, such as dyslexia. It may be necessary for a reading impaired student to go over a paragraph many times to reach an understanding. The assignment of a complex chapter on anatomy, for example, can seem like an impossible task.

If a student with a reading disorder (or any other learning disability) appears in a paramedic course, an instructor has a legal and/or an ethical responsibility to seek appropriate remediation. For example, assistance for a dyslexic student may include referral to a reading skills program or to a service that provides "audio books." In most cases, however, moderate assistance on the part of the instructor can help adult learners deficient in one or more skills, especially if they have received remediation during their earlier education.

In deciding upon a course of action for learning disabled students, an EMS educator must be careful not to confuse the educational process with certification. The educational component is designed to facilitate the acquisition of cognitive knowledge and psychomotor skills necessary to obtain a certificate or license to practice EMS. Although many EMS educational institutions work closely with the entities that certify and license EMS providers, the two processes—education and certification—must remain separate. The EMS educator's only concern should be that of preparing the student for the credentialing process. In the case of the learning disabled students, the educator should focus on strategies that will help each student accomplish the instructional objectives, while providing "reasonable" remediation and compensation measures.

Point out this distinction to learning disabled students. It would not be ethical to have learning disabled students—or any other students for that matter—assume that completion of an EMS course ensures success in the certification or licensure process. As a result, an EMS educator should urge learning disabled students to initiate early contact with the certifying or licensing agency to determine what accommodations will be accepted or made for them during the certification process.

All EMS instructors in the 21st century should investigate the programs, laws, and regulations related to learning disabilities specified by local, state, and federal governments. Some sources of information are listed in "Resources for Teaching Learning Disabled Students" at the end of the introductory material.

Most important, keep in mind that the majority of learning disabled adults function as normal, productive members of society. They aspire to the same educational goals as people without learning disabilities—and, in many cases, with a higher motivation. Far too often, however, they become frustrated by an inability to learn using the same method or at the same rate as other students.

An astute EMS educator must seek to create new opportunities for the learning disabled students. One of the best resources is a caring educator willing to take the time to recognize learning disabilities and then to provide the additional assistance—videos, audiotapes, and teamwork with other students—that can mean the difference between success and failure.

©2009 Pearson Education, Inc.
Paramedic Care: Principles & Practice, Vol. 5, 3rd. Ed.

WEBSITES AND OTHER RESOURCES

Below are lists of various types of resources that instructors might find valuable. The lists are not all inclusive, and instructors should add to them and create a file that suits their needs. Although all information has been checked and is current at time of publication, contact and website information may change.

Professional Organizations

(NOTE: Access to some areas of organizational websites may be limited to members only.)

American Ambulance Association
8201 Greensboro Drive Suite 300
McLean, VA 22102
800-523-4447
http://www.the-aaa.org

American College of Emergency Physicians
P.O. Box 619911
Dallas, TX 75261-9911
800-798-1822
http://www.acep.org

American Heart Association
7272 Greenville Avenue
Dallas, TX 75231
800-242-8721
http://www.americanheart.org

Association of Air Medical Services
526 King Street, Suite 415
Alexandria, Virginia 22314-3143
703-836-8732
http://www.aams.org

Citizen CPR Foundation
P.O. Box 15945-314
Lenexa, KS 66285-5945
913-495-9816
http://www.citizencpr.com

Emergency Nurses Association
915 Lee Street
Des Plaines, IL 60016-6569
800-900-9659
http://www.ena.org

National Association of EMS Educators
Foster Plaza 6
681 Andersen Drive
Pittsburgh, PA 15220-2766
412-920-4775
http://www.naemse.org

National Association of EMS Physicians
P.O. Box 15945-281
Lenexa, KS 66285-5945
800-228-3677
http://www.naemsp.org

National Association of EMTs
P.O. Box 1400
Clinton, MS 39060-1400
800-34-NAEMT
http://www.naemt.org

National Association for Search and Rescue
4500 Southgate Place, Suite 100
Chantilly, VA 20151-1714
703-222-6277
http://www.nasar.org

National Association of State EMS Directors
111 Park Place
Falls Church, VA 22046-4513
703-538-1799
http://www.nasemsd.org

National Council of State EMS Training
Coordinators
201 Park Washington Court
Falls Church, VA 22046-4513
703-538-1794
http://www.ncsemstc.org

National Emergency Medical Services Alliance
1947 Camino Vida Roble
Carlsbad, CA 92008
619-431-7054

National Registry of EMTs
6610 Busch Boulevard
P.O. Box 29233
Columbus, OH 43229
614-888-4484
http://www.nremt.org

EMS RESOURCES

One of the big advantages of owning a computer today is the availability of information through the Internet. To steer a course through this electronic maze, we've compiled a list of websites at which instructors can find information they can use in developing lectures or enhancing student knowledge of emergency medicine. These sites have the potential to provide access to a whole new realm of information and entertainment for you and your students.

Each of these EMS websites has been visited and reviewed for appropriateness and content. Remember to bookmark the sites for easy access to them the next time you are surfing.

News Groups

emsvillage.com
prehospitalperspective.net

These news groups are excellent places to learn about the latest trends in EMS. They also offer the opportunity to ask questions and gain insights into what other EMS providers across the country are doing.

In addition, many EMS organizations support list servers where members can ask questions and interact with other EMS professionals.

Websites

http://www.bennye.com
Makeup and kits for applying moulage.

http://www.bradybooks.com
The homepage of the publisher of *Paramedic Care: Principles and Practice*.

http://www.cdc.gov
The homepage for the Centers for Disease Control and Prevention. An excellent source of information on infectious diseases.

http://www.cpem.org
Teaching Resource for Instructors in Prehospital Pediatrics.

http://www.fire-ems.net
The fire and EMS information network. A site that features everything from chat areas to website development for fire and EMS services.

http://www.jems.com/
JEMS online. *The Journal of Emergency Medical Services* homepage.

http://www.LessStress.com
This site contains a prehospital care simulator.

http://www.lifeart.com
A source for medical clip art that can be useful for overheads and handouts.

http://www.meddean.luc.edu/lumen/index.html
Fantastic cross-sectional images of the human body.

http://www.merck.com
The famous Merck manual online.

http://www.ncemsf.org/
The National EMS Collegiate Foundation. This homepage contains information about EMS educational programs around the country.

http://www.nhtsa.gov/portal/site/nhtsa/menuitem
The homepage for the National Highway Traffic Safety Administration. Download curricula for all of the EMT levels.

http://www.osha.gov
The homepage for the Occupational Safety and Health Administration. Information from ergonomics to OSHA documents.

http://www.pcrf.mednet.ucla.edu/
The Prehospital Care Research Forum is dedicated to the promotion, education, and dissemination of prehospital research.

http://www.shrs.pitt.edu/emergency/index.html
The Center for Emergency Medicine's site with information about the revision of the EMT-Intermediate and EMT-Paramedic Curricula.

http://www.ptialaska.net/~bearmt/
Information on an inexpensive AED Trainer.

http://www.trauma.org/prehospital/ph-images.html
Prehospital images of accident scenes and the like.

Books

Brown, C. *Square Pegs and Round Holes*. Lake Worth, FL: EES Publications, 1990.

An easy-to-use text designed specifically for EMS instructors. Not quite as meaty as the McClincy text listed next, but it still contains some good information.

Hoff, R. *I Can See You Naked*. Kansas City, MO: Andrews and McMeel, 1992.

Once you get past the title, you will find a text that contains pertinent information on public speaking.

©2009 Pearson Education, Inc.
Paramedic Care: Principles & Practice, Vol. 5, 3rd. Ed.

Martini, F. H., Bartholomew, E. F., and Bledsoe, B. E. *Anatomy and Physiology for Emergency Care*. Upper Saddle River, NJ: Brady–Prentice Hall, 2002.

Anatomy and physiology text for students in emergency care and allied health programs requiring an overview of the human body's systems.

McClincy, W. *Instructional Methods in Emergency Services*. 2nd edition. Upper Saddle River, NJ: Brady–Prentice Hall, 2002.

This text is the most comprehensive manual to date on methods of instruction for EMS personnel. Experienced and new instructors alike will find this book to be a valuable source of information.

Nixon, R. G. *Communicable Diseases and Infection Control for EMS*. Upper Saddle River, NJ: Brady–Prentice Hall, 2000.

Oosterhof, A. *Classroom Applications of Educational Measurement*. Columbus, OH: Merrill, 2000.

This text is directed toward theory and makes a nice addition to the libraries of those instructors who want more information on evaluation tools.

Simmons, S. *How to Be the Life of the Podium*. New York: AMACOM, 1993.

This book contains quips, quotes, and stories that can be used to spice up almost any presentation.

U.S. Department of Transportation. *Paramedic and EMT-Intermediate National Standard Curricula*. Washington, D.C.: Government Printing Office, 1999.

Journals

ACLS Alert
3525 Piedmont Road NE
Six Piedmont Center
Suite 400
Atlanta, GA 30305

Annals of Emergency Medicine
P.O. Box 619911
Dallas, TX 75261

Emergency
6200 Yarrow Drive
P.O. Box 159
Carlsbad, CA 92008
800-854-6449

Emergency Medical Services
Creative Age Publications
7628 Densmore Ave.
Van Nuys, CA 91406
818-782-7328

Emergency Training
Miller Landing
Building 200
150 North Miller Road
Akron, OH 44333
216-836-0600

EMS Insider
Jems Communications
1947 Camino Vida Roble
Carlsbad, CA 92008
619-431-9797

Journal of Emergency Medical Services
P.O. Box 370
Escondido, CA 92033
800-334-8152

Journal of Emergency Medicine
Pergamon Press
660 White Plains Road
Tarrytown, NY 10591

911 Magazine
18201 Weston Place
Tustin, CA 92680
714-544-7776

Prehospital Emergency Care
Hanley & Belfus, Inc., Medical Publishers
210 South 13th Street, Philadelphia, PA 19107
800-962-1892
215-546-7293
Fax 215-790-9330
http://www.hanleybelfus.com

Rescue
Jems Communications
P.O. Box 370
Escondido, CA 92033
800-334-8152

Topics in Emergency Medicine
200 Orchard Ridge Drive
Gaithersburg, MD 20877
800-638-8437

Video Producers
Pulse/Emergency Medical Update
P.O. Box 11380
Winslow, WA 98110
800-327-3841

For Learning Disabled Students

This partial listing has been compiled from sources available at the time of the publication of the *Instructor's Resource Manual*. Changes in laws, regulations, and/or technology may have an affect on the resources available in the future.

Alliance for Technology Access (ATA)
2175 East Francisco Boulevard, Suite L
San Rafael, CA 94901
415-455-4575
Fax: 415-455-0491
http://www.atacess.org
> Provides access to supportive technology for people with disabilities.

Association on Higher Education and Disability (AHEAD)
P.O. Box 21192
Columbus, OH 43221
614-488-4972
Fax: 614-488-1174
http://www.ahead.org
> Provides information about full participation in higher education for people with disabilities.

Council for Learning Disabilities (CLD)
P.O. Box 40303
Overland Park, KS 66204
913-492-8755
Fax: 913-942-2546
*http://www.cldinternational.org/c/
@Oz8POnJZq6obU/Pages/home.html*
> Offers enhancement for the education and development of the learning disabled.

Division of Adult Education and Literacy Clearinghouse
U.S. Department of Education
Office of Vocational and Adult Education
400 Maryland Avenue, SW
Washington, DC 20202
202-205-9996
Fax: 202-205-8873
http://www.edu.gov
> Links the adult education community with existing resources in adult education available through the Adults in Education Act.

HEATH Resource Center
National Clearinghouse on Postsecondary Education for Individuals with Disabilities
American Council on Education
One Dupont Circle NW, Suite 800
Washington, DC 20036
202-939-9320
Fax: 202-833-4760
http://www.ACENET.edu
> Collects and disseminates information about postsecondary education for individuals with disabilities.

National Association for Adults with Special Learning Needs (NAASLN)
P.O. Box 716
Bryn Mawr, PA 19010
610-525-8336
Fax: 610-525-8337
http://www.naasln.org/
> Provides information for helping adults with special learning needs.

National Center for Learning Disabilities (NCDL)
381 Park Avenue South, Suite 1420
New York, NY 10016
212-545-7510
Fax: 212-545-9665
http://www.ncld.org
> Provides programs and services to promote a better understanding and acceptance of learning disabilities.

Rebus Institute
1499 Bayshore Boulevard, Suite 146
Burlingame, CA 94010
415-697-7424
Fax: 415-697-3734
> Disseminates information on adult issues related to specific learning disabilities and adult attention deficit disorders (AADD).

Recording for the Blind and Dyslexic (RFBD)
20 Roszel Road
Princeton, NY 20542
609-452-0606
800-221-4792
http://www.rfbd.org
> Offers free recordings and speech software versions of books for the blind and dyslexic.

U.S. Department of Education
National Library of Education
Office of Educational Resource and Improvement
Institute of Education Sciences
455 New Jersey Avenue, NW
Washington, DC 20208
202-219-2221
http://www.ed.gov
> Houses the Educational Resources Information Center (ERIC)—the source of a wide variety of educational literature and resources.

TEST-TAKING HINTS AND GUIDELINES FOR YOUR STUDENTS

The following list of helpful hints is probably most appropriate for the end-of-course examination, state certification, or National Registry written examination. Consider photocopying this section and giving it directly to your students.

- Study from your class notes and the workbook that accompanies the course text. Do not cram the night before, because cramming may hinder your efforts rather than help.

- Relax the evening before the examination and get a good night's sleep. You are usually in better mental shape if you are well rested. If you exercise regularly, consider doing your usual routine. A brisk walk before the exam can help you relax and it also reduces stress, especially if you worked during the day of the exam.

- Avoid anything that may over stimulate or tranquilize you. Too much coffee or caffeinated beverages will not be helpful.

- Eat a sensible meal about two hours before the exam. A large meal just before an examination may make you feel tired. Drink a small glass of water just before entering the exam room if you are thirsty. Too much to drink before a test may mean frequent restroom breaks. Most standardized tests do not give you extra time for breaks.

- Wear comfortable clothing that is appropriate for the climate and environment. It is a good idea to bring a light sweater or sweatshirt to the exam. Many exam rooms are large, and it is sometimes difficult to control the temperature in them.

- Plan to arrive early for the exam. You do not want to feel rushed, and you may need some extra time if you encounter unexpected delays en route.

- Make sure that you bring any exam supplies that you are responsible for. Make a list so you do not forget. It can be frustrating if you need to go home and get a photo ID card or ask to borrow a pencil.

- Carefully follow the instructions of the examination proctor. Do not begin the exam or make any entries on the answer form until you are instructed to do so. Ask questions if you do not understand any part of the instructions.

- Once the exam begins, pace yourself. Determine how many questions and how much time you are allowed. (A 100-question exam given over 3 hours allows an average of 3½ minutes per question.) Note the time the test starts, so you can keep track of how much time remains at any given time. If you spend too much time on one question, you may find yourself rushed in order to finish. It may be a good idea to bring your own watch in case a clock is not available and so you're not dependent on the proctors counting down the time. Calculator watches may not be allowed in the examination; the examination proctor can advise.

- After carefully reading the question, read all the answer choices before making a final decision as to the correct answer and marking the answer sheet. You may be sure you have figured out the correct response after reading only the first or second choice, but reading all the answers gives you some additional reinforcement that you are correct. Many times there are a few answers that you can eliminate almost immediately, making your final decision easier.

- Read each question carefully. Make sure you understand what is being asked. Does the question say all the following *EXCEPT* or which of the following is *NOT*. That means that they are looking for the one answer that doesn't fit. Take an extra few seconds to make sure you picked the correct answer.

- When presented with a scenario question with patient-specific or scenario-specific information consider reading the scenario, then reading the question and all answer choices, and then returning to the question to extract the relevant information and decide on the answer.

- Occasionally you may have a question that is very difficult or confusing. Consider skipping this question and moving to the next. Mark the question clearly. Do not write in the examination booklet if a separate answer sheet is provided, so you know you need to return and deal with it later. In addition, as most of these tests use a standardized testing sheet, make sure you skip to the next answer row. Obviously, misaligned answers will be read as wrong by a computer or answer key. This important detail needs the close attention of the test taker.

- If you have a question that you are struggling with, you should move on. Remember that there is a time limit, and you don't want to feel rushed as time is running out. If you know one or more of the answers are definitely wrong, mark them as such (do not write in the examination booklet if a separate answer sheet is provided), so when you return to the question you have fewer answers to consider. It is also possible to have your memory jogged by information in a later question.
- Once you make a decision and mark the answer sheet, be reluctant to change it. Unless you are sure the first answer marked is wrong, making a change may not be the right thing to do.
- If all else fails and you can't determine or remember what is the right answer, consider guessing. It is probably not to your advantage to leave any blank answers, because they will be scored as incorrect answers.
- Once you have answered all the questions, go back and check your work to ensure completeness. Make sure you have marked an answer for every question. Don't second-guess yourself. This is the time to make sure you have filled in all the answers according to the instructions and there are no stray marks on the answer sheet. Remember to completely erase any answer you want to change.

Good luck!

©2009 Pearson Education, Inc.
Paramedic Care: Principles & Practice, Vol. 5, 3rd. Ed.

Chapter 1 Neonatology

INTRODUCTION

Most deliveries in the out-of-hospital setting occur without complications. However, emergency deliveries can present a number of challenges to the paramedic. The risk of death or serious neurologic injury is much greater when a child is born after a spontaneous, out-of-hospital delivery compared to a controlled, in-hospital delivery. Care given in the first few minutes after birth may have a significant impact on future quality of life. A child born in the out-of-hospital setting also is more likely to be preterm, increasing the risk of complications. Finally, the presence of two patients—the mother and the newborn—adds to the challenges. This chapter discusses the assessment and management of the normal newborn, resuscitation of distressed neonates, and management of common problems encountered in infants during the first month of their lives.

CHAPTER OBJECTIVES

Knowledge Objectives

1. Define *newborn* and *neonate*. (p. 3)
2. Identify important antepartum factors that can affect childbirth. (p. 4)
3. Identify important intrapartum factors that can determine high-risk newborn patients. (p. 4)
4. Identify the factors that lead to premature birth and low-birth-weight newborns. (pp. 24, 29–30)
5. Distinguish between primary and secondary apnea. (p. 5)
6. Discuss pulmonary perfusion and asphyxia. (p. 5)
7. Identify the primary signs utilized for evaluating a newborn during resuscitation. (p. 11)
8. Identify the appropriate use of the APGAR scale. (p. 11)
9. Calculate the APGAR score given various newborn situations. (p. 11)
10. Formulate an appropriate treatment plan for providing initial care to a newborn. (pp. 11–14)
11. Describe the indications, equipment needed, application, and evaluation of the following management techniques for the newborn in distress:

    a. Blow-by oxygen (p. 20)
    b. Ventilatory assistance (pp. 20–22)
    c. Endotracheal intubation (pp. 21–22)
    d. Orogastric tube (p. 22)
    e. Chest compressions (p. 22)
    f. Vascular access (pp. 22–24)

TOTAL TEACHING TIME: 10.23 HOURS
The total teaching time is only a guideline based on the didactic and practical lab averages in the National Standard Curriculum. Instructors should take into consideration such factors as: the pace at which students learn, the size of the class, and breaks. The actual time devoted to teaching objectives is the responsibility of the instructor.

12. Discuss the routes of medication administration for a newborn. (pp. 22–24, 25)

13. Discuss the signs of hypovolemia in a newborn. (p. 31)

14. Discuss the initial steps in resuscitation of a newborn. (pp. 18–24)

15. Discuss the effects of maternal narcotic use on the newborn. (p. 24)

16. Determine the appropriate treatment for the newborn with narcotic depression. (p. 24)

17. Discuss appropriate transport guidelines for a newborn. (p. 26)

18. Determine appropriate receiving facilities for low- and high-risk newborns. (p. 26)

19. Describe the epidemiology, including the incidence, morbidity/mortality, risk factors and prevention strategies, pathophysiology, assessment findings, and management, of the following neonatal problems:

    a. Meconium aspiration (pp. 27–28)
    b. Apnea (p. 28)
    c. Diaphragmatic hernia (pp. 28–29)
    d. Bradycardia (p. 29)
    e. Prematurity (pp. 29–30)
    f. Respiratory distress/cyanosis (pp. 30–31)
    g. Seizures (pp. 31–32)
    h. Fever (pp. 32–33)
    i. Hypothermia (p. 33)
    j. Hypoglycemia (pp. 33–34)
    k. Vomiting (p. 34)
    l. Diarrhea (p. 35)
    m. Common birth injuries (pp. 35–36)
    n. Cardiac arrest (pp. 36–37)
    o. Postarrest management (p. 37)

Skill Objective

20. Given several neonatal emergencies, provide the appropriate procedures for assessment, management, and transport. (pp. 3–37)

FRAMING THE LESSON

Begin with a brief review of the important points from Chapter 14, "Obstetrics," in Volume 3. Discuss any material or information that students have not completely understood. Then proceed to the neonatology material in Chapter 1. Stress that though most out-of-hospital deliveries occur without complications, in situations where there are problems, immediate intervention can make a significant difference in a newborn's survival and future quality of life. Ask the class if anyone would be willing to share experiences they have had with their children or children of friends or relatives having to spend time in a neonatal intensive care unit. Ask the students to describe how they think they might feel in this situation.

CONSIDERING THE CASE STUDY

Ask a volunteer to read aloud the Case Study on text page 2. Suggest that students close their eyes as the scenario is read to help them mentally visualize the events described in it. You can use the following questions about the Case Study as a starting point for teaching the chapter—sort of a chapter preview in a

©2009 Pearson Education, Inc.
Paramedic Care: Principles & Practice, Vol. 5, 3rd. Ed.

functional setting. When the chapter is completed, you may wish to return to the Case Study and encourage further discussion aimed at answering the questions or solving the problems.

CASE STUDY DISCUSSION QUESTIONS (AND ANSWERS)

1. What is the most likely explanation for this neonate's being in distress?
    (The infant probably became asphyxiated during birth and now is hypoxic.)
2. What is the "inverted pyramid" approach to neonatal resuscitation?
    (The inverted pyramid is a stepwise approach to resuscitation that moves systematically through the following steps: (1) warming, positioning, drying, suctioning, and stimulating; (2) oxygen; (3) bag-mask ventilation; (4) chest compressions; (5) endotracheal intubation; and (6) use of medications. The inverted shape of the pyramid indicates that most infants respond to simple, noninvasive measures.)
4. Which of the vital signs is the most important indicator of neonatal distress?
    (Heart rate is the most important indicator of distress. Bradycardia in a newborn almost always is the result of hypoxia, and an increasing heart rate is an indicator that resuscitation efforts are effective.)
5. Why is it important to dry newborns thoroughly, wrap them in a blanket, and keep their heads covered?
    (Neonates lose heat rapidly because they have a much larger surface-to-volume ratio than adults. Allowing a newborn to remain wet accelerates heat loss through evaporation. Because they are prone to heat loss, neonates can rapidly become hypothermic at temperatures adults find comfortable.)

TEACHING STRATEGIES

People learn in a variety of ways. Some do better with the spoken word, while others prefer the written. Some prefer to work alone, whereas others profit from working in groups. Recognizing these different ways of acquiring knowledge, the authors of this *Instructor's Resource Manual* have provided a variety of teaching strategies for the different types of learners. These strategies are intended to foster higher-level cognitive skills and encourage creative learning and problem solving.

For greatest effectiveness, incorporate these strategies into your class lecture. Marginal notes in the Teaching Outline indicate the points at which various exercises might be most appropriate. Other strategies can be used to preview the lesson or to summarize it.

The following strategies are keyed to specific sections of the lesson:

1. In-the-Field Deliveries. Delivering a baby in the field is both frightening and exciting. Add meaning and interest to this lecture by inviting paramedics who have had the privilege of delivering a baby to speak to your class. Ask them to share their experiences, challenges, and feelings. If you cannot get them to come to class, at least interview these folks and videotape or audiotape or write down what they have to share. This activity is not only interesting but also covers objectives in the affective domain.

2. Identifying Risk Factors. Help students identify risk factors for delivery complications by placing the conditions in Table 1-1 and others discussed in the text on index cards. Have them sort by antepartum, intrapartum, and nonrisk factors for newborn complications. The students can do this in groups and compare piles when they are finished. Ask groups to justify or defend their decisions if any piles are different from those of the other groups. This activity promotes critical thinking by forcing students to discuss or defend their choices for placement of the cards. Additionally, students practice oral communication skills, cooperative learning skills, and acceptance of opinions and decisions different than their own.

3. NICU Field Trip. Neonatal resuscitation seems overwhelming because students often lack experience with this type of patient, situation, and even equipment. Improve the student's ability and desire to care for neonates by ensuring that they are very comfortable with the equipment involved in neonatal resuscitation. A field trip to the NICU or invitation for the neonatal transport team to visit your class would be beneficial here. Have the special care nursery staff cover the equipment used, noting the tiny sizes and differences in concentrations of medications and the like. This activity gets students out of the traditional classroom environment, provides a preview to the clinical experience, and can improve relations with the nursery staff and transport nurses whom your students will likely work with as practicing professionals.

4. Realistic Neonate Manikin. When practicing childbirth in class and lab situations, coat the neonate manikin in realistic material such as K-Y jelly mixed with powdered blood. Delivering a baby for the first time is often challenging because paramedics have never felt how slippery a newborn is and are surprised by the mess of fluids and blood. Give your students this experience in the classroom to improve their performance during the real thing. Adding realism to scenarios is a key element of problem-based learning.

5. Practice Determining APGAR. Use neonatal resuscitation case studies either in class on overheads or PowerPoint® or as a written assignment. Students need a great deal of practice determining APGAR scores and using the inverted triangle. Since this information is new and foreign, the amount of time available in classroom labs and simulations is not enough to reach mastery level, and this information will likely always seem frightening to your students. Give them the extra preparation needed by assigning case studies first, reinforcing with laboratory simulations, and, when possible, following up with clinical time in the NICU or with the neonatal transport team.

6. Mnemonic Memory Aid. Students often forget which should be suctioned first, the mouth or nose of a newborn. Help them remember to do this in alphabetical order: mouth first, then nose. Infants are obligate nose breathers, so as soon as the nostrils are stimulated, they will inhale everything in the upper airway, which includes the mouth and nose. Therefore, it is important to clear the mouth of any fluid or obstructions.

7. Resuscitation Reference Card. Make a pocket card of the resuscitation information in Table 1-4. Allow use of the reference card in simulations and classroom case studies. Following the American Heart Association's approach to PALS, encourage familiarity and understanding of equipment, drugs, and procedures rather than simple memorization. This improves the comfort level and therefore the ability to learn of most students.

The following strategy relates to Special Features in the student textbook and can be used to enhance the student's understanding:

Cultural Considerations: When Parents Request Baptism. Invite religious leaders from the various denominations in your area to speak to the students regarding their denomination's particular beliefs surrounding stillbirth. Ask them what, if anything, you can do to provide for the emotional transition. This could be baptism, last rights, and so on.

The following strategies can be used at various points throughout the lesson or to help summarize and demonstrate what students have learned:

Guest Speaker.   Consider inviting a neonatologist from the local or regional hospital to the class.

Clinical Rotations.   During labor and delivery rotations, encourage students to seek out opportunities to observe the management of patients with high-risk pregnancies. Students should observe and, if possible, assist with the management of distressed newborns in the delivery room. If possible, students should do clinical rotations in a neonatal intensive care unit.

TEACHING OUTLINE

Chapter 1 is the first lesson in Volume 5, *Special Considerations/Operations*. Distribute Handout 1-1 so that students can familiarize themselves with the learning goals for this chapter. If students have any questions about the objectives, answer them at this time.

Then present the chapter. One possible lecture outline follows. In the outline, the parenthetical references in regular type are references to text pages; those in bold type are to figures, tables, or procedures.

I. Introduction. This chapter concerns itself with babies 1 month old or younger. (p. 2)

A. Definitions (p. 2)
    1. Neonate
        a. Infant from birth to 1 month of age
    2. Newborn
        a. Baby in the first few hours of life (**Fig. 1-1**)
    3. Newborns also called *newly born infants*.
B. Considerations in unscheduled field deliveries (p. 3)
    1. Two patients, mother and infant
    2. Care of mother was discussed during obstetrics module.

II. General pathophysiology, assessment, and management. (pp. 3–11)

A. Epidemiology (p. 4)
    1. Risk of complications
        a. Approximately 6 percent of field deliveries require life support.
        b. About 80 percent of newborns weighing less than 1,500 grams (3 pounds, 5 ounces) at birth require resuscitation.
    2. Risk factors (**Table 1-1**)
        a. Antepartum factors
            i. Multiple gestation
            ii. Inadequate prenatal care
            iii. Mother's age <16 or >35
            iv. History of perinatal morbidity or mortality
            v. Postterm gestation
            vi. Drugs/medications
            vii. Toxemia, hypertension, diabetes
        b. Intrapartum factors
            i. Premature labor
            ii. Meconium-stained amniotic fluid

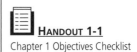
HANDOUT 1-1
Chapter 1 Objectives Checklist

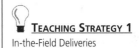
POWERPOINT PRESENTATION
Volume 5, Chapter 1, PowerPoint slides 1–4

TEACHING STRATEGY 1
In-the-Field Deliveries

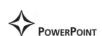
POWERPOINT PRESENTATION
Volume 5, Chapter 1, PowerPoint slides 5–27

POINT TO EMPHASIZE
For newborns who require additional care, your quick actions can make the difference between life and death.

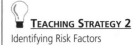
TEACHING STRATEGY 2
Identifying Risk Factors

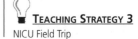
TEACHING STRATEGY 3
NICU Field Trip

READING/REFERENCE

Jaimovich, D. G., and D. Vidyasagar. *Handbook of Pediatric and Neonatal Transport Medicine*, 2nd ed. Philadelphia, PA: Hanley & Belfus, Inc. 2002.

      iii. Rupture of membranes more than 24 hours before delivery
      iv. Use of narcotics within 4 hours of delivery
      v. Abnormal presentation
      vi. Prolonged labor or precipitous delivery
      vii. Prolapsed cord
      viii. Bleeding

  3. Factors affecting successful resuscitation
    a. Training
    b. Practice
    c. Proper equipment
  4. Transport considerations

B. Pathophysiology (pp. 5–10)
  1. Dramatic changes at birth prepare the newborn for extrauterine life.
  2. The respiratory system must initiate and maintain oxygenation. (**Fig. 1-2**)
  3. Transition from fetal to neonatal circulation (**Fig. 1-2; Fig. 1-3**)
    a. *Ductus arteriosus* becomes the *ligamentum arteriosum*. *Foramen ovale* closes and becomes the *fossa ovalis*. *Ductus venosus* becomes the *ligamentus venosum*
    b. Umbilical vein becomes the *ligamentum teres*
    c. Umbilical arteries constrict although the proximal portions persist
  4. Remain alert to signs of respiratory distress
  5. Congenital anomalies
    a. May affect a single organ/structure or many organs/structures
    b. Recognized patterns or syndromes
    c. Few make resuscitation more difficult
    d. Causes are largely unknown
    e. Patent ductus arteriosus (also called a persistent ductus arteriosus) (**Fig. 1-4**)
      i. Ductus arteriosus fails to close
      ii. Increases pulmonary blood flow
    f. Septal defects
      i. Hole in the wall between the atria or the ventricles
      ii. Increases pulmonary blood flow
      iii. Atrial septal defect (**Fig. 1-5**)
        • Hole between the two atria
      iv. Ventricular septal defect (**Fig. 1-6**)
        • Hole between the two ventricles
    g. Tetralogy of fallot (**Fig. 1-7**)
      i. A combination of four congenital conditions
      ii. Decreases pulmonary blood flow
    h. Transposition of the great vessels (**Fig. 1-8**)
      i. Normal outflow tracts of the right and left ventricles are switched
      ii. Decreases pulmonary blood flow
    i. Coarctation of the aorta (**Fig. 1-9**)
      i. Narrowing in the arch of the aorta
      ii. Obstructs blood flow
    j. Aortic, mitral, or pulmonary stenosis (**Fig. 1-10; Fig. 1-11**)
      i. Problems with either the mitral, pulmonary, or aortic valve
      ii. Can cause blood flow obstruction
    k. Hypoplastic left heart syndrome
      i. The left side of the heart is underdeveloped.
      ii. Usually fatal by 1 month of age if untreated
    l. Diaphragmatic hernia
      i. Defect that allows some of the abdominal contents to enter the chest cavity

  ii. If you suspect a diaphragmatic hernia, do not treat the infant with bag-valve-mask (BVM) ventilation.

- BVM or other positive-pressure ventilation will cause the stomach to distend and protrude into the chest cavity, thus decreasing ventilation capacity.
- Immediately intubate the infant.

 m. Meningomyelocele
  i. Defect in the area of the spine
  ii. In some cases, spinal canal contents may protrude.
  iii. Place infant in prone or laterally recumbent position and cover spinal defect with sterile gauze pads soaked in warm sterile saline and covered with an occlusive dressing.

 n. Omphalocele
  i. Defect in the area of the umbilicus
  ii. In some cases, the abdominal contents will fill this defect.
  iii. If you encounter a newborn with an omphalocele, cover the defect with an occlusive dressing.

 o. Choanal atresia
  i. Most common birth defect involving the nose
  ii. Presence of a bony or membranous septum between the nasal cavity and the pharynx
  iii. Suspect this condition if you are unable to pass a catheter through either nare into the oropharynx.
  iv. An oral airway will usually bypass the obstruction

 p. Cleft palate
  i. Fairly common congenital anomaly
  ii. Failure of the palate to completely close during fetal development
  iii. Requires endotracheal intubation if prolonged ventilation needed

 q. Cleft lip
  i. Failure of the upper lip to close
  ii. Requires endotracheal intubation if prolonged ventilation is needed

 r. Pierre Robin syndrome
  i. Small jaw and large tongue in conjunction with a cleft palate
  ii. Use nasal or oral airway to bypass obstruction; if bypass is unsuccessful, endotracheal intubation may be necessary

C. Assessment (pp. 10–11)
 1. General considerations
  a. Note time of birth.
  b. Remember, newborns are slippery.
  c. Someone needs to be caring for, watching mother
 2. Respirations
  a. Should be 40 to 60/min
  b. Ventilate if inadequate.
 3. Heart rate
  a. Should be 150 to 180/min at birth, soon slowing to 130 to 140
  b. Less than 100 requires emergency intervention.
 4. Skin color
  a. Cyanosis of extremities is common immediately after birth, but central cyanosis or persistent peripheral cyanosis is abnormal
  b. Give 100 percent oxygen until cause determined or condition corrected
 5. The APGAR Scale (**Table 1-2**)
  a. Appearance (skin color)
   i. Completely pink—2

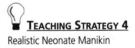

TEACHING STRATEGY 4
Realistic Neonate Manikin

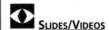

SLIDES/VIDEOS
"Newborn Assessment," *Pulse: Emergency Medical Update,* Feb. 1997.

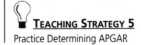

TEACHING STRATEGY 5
Practice Determining APGAR

      ii. Body pink, extremities blue—1

      iii. Blue, pale—0

   b. Pulse rate

      i. Above 100—2

      ii. Below 100—1

      iii. Absent—0

   c. Grimace (Irritability)

      i. Cries—2

      ii. Grimaces—1

      iii. No response—0

   d. Activity (Muscle tone)

      i. Active motion—2

      ii. Some flexion of extremities—1

      iii. Limp—0

   e. Respiratory effort

      i. Strong cry—2

      ii. Slow and irregular—1

      iii. Absent—0

   f. Significance of scores

      i. 7–10
- Active
- Vigorous newborn requiring only routine care

      ii. 4–6
- Moderately distressed newborn requiring oxygenation and ventilation

      iii. 0–4
- Severely distressed newborn requiring immediate resuscitation

      iv. If infant not breathing or otherwise obviously distressed, do not delay resuscitation to obtain APGAR scores.

III. Treatment. (pp. 11–14)

A. Establishing the airway (pp. 11–12)
1. One of the most critical steps in newborn care
2. As soon as head delivers, suction mouth then nose so there is nothing to aspirate if infant gasps when nose is suctioned.
3. If meconium is present or the amniotic fluid is meconium stained, nasopharyngeal and orophraryngeal suctioning should not be performed.
4. After delivery, position infant at level of vagina with head 15° below torso. **(Fig. 1-12)**
5. If large amount of secretions is present, use DeLee suction trap attached to suction source.

B. Breathing (pp. 11–12)
1. Stimulate by drying and suctioning.
2. If additional stimulation needed, flick soles of feet or rub back **(Fig. 1-13)**
3. Do NOT vigorously rub newborn.
4. Do NOT slap newborn on buttocks.

C. Prevention of heat loss (pp. 12–13)
1. Cold infants quickly become distressed infants.
2. Heat loss
   a. Evaporation
   b. Convection
   c. Conduction
   d. Radiation

POINT TO EMPHASIZE

If a newborn is not breathing, DO NOT withhold resuscitation until determining the APGAR score.

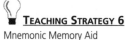

POINT TO EMPHASIZE

Severely distressed newborns, those with APGAR scores of less than 4, require immediate resuscitation.

TEACHING STRATEGY 6

Mnemonic Memory Aid

POINT TO EMPHASIZE

Airway management is one of the most critical steps in caring for the newborn.

POINT TO EMPHASIZE

Always suction the mouth first so that there is nothing for the infant to aspirate if he or she gasps when the nose is suctioned.

POINT TO EMPHASIZE

If the newborn does not cry immediately, stimulate it by gently rubbing its back or flicking the soles of its feet. Do not spank or vigorously rub a newborn baby.

3. To prevent heat loss **(Fig. 1-14)**
   a. Dry
   b. Maintain ambient temperature at 23 to 24°C (74 to 76°F)
   c. Close all windows and doors.
   d. Swaddle infant in warm, dry receiving blanket or other suitable material
   e. Cover infant's head.
   f. Place well-insulated containers of warm water (40°C/104°F) around (but not against) infant.
D. Cutting umbilical cord (pp. 13–14) **(Fig. 1-15)**
   1. After airway is stabilized and heat loss minimized
   2. Maintain infant at same level as vagina to prevent under- or overtransfusion.
   3. Do not "milk" or strip cord.
      a. Causes polycythemia and increased blood viscosity
      b. Polycythemia can lead to excess red cell destruction and to hyperbilirubinemia.
   4. Clamp cord within 30 to 45 seconds of birth.
   5. Place first clamp about 10 cm (4 inches) from newborn.
   6. Place second clamp about 4 cm (2 inches) away from first.
   7. Cut cord between clamps.
   8. Inspect cord periodically for additional bleeding.

IV. The distressed newborn. (pp. 14–26)

A. Resuscitation (p. 14) **(Proc. 1-1)**
   1. The vast majority of newborns require no resuscitation beyond stimulation, airway maintenance, and body temperature maintenance.
   2. Predicting which newborns will require resuscitation is difficult.
   3. A neonatal resuscitation kit should be available in the unit.
B. Inverted pyramid resuscitation steps (pp. 15–24) **(Fig. 1-16; Fig. 1-17; Proc. 1-1)**
   1. Step 1: Drying, warming, positioning, suctioning, tactile stimulation
      a. Dry newborn to minimize heat loss
      b. Place in warm, dry blanket
      c. Position on back with head slightly lower than body, neck slightly extended. **(Fig. 1-18)**
      d. Place small blanket folded to 2-cm (3/4-inch) thickness under shoulders.
      e. Suction using bulb syringe or DeLee suction trap **(Proc. 1-2)**
      f. If meconium is present, and the infant is vigorous (strong respiratory efforts, good muscle tone, and heart rate > 100 per minute)
         i. Tracheal intubation and suctioning is not recommended.
      g. If the infant is not vigorous
         i. Endotracheal intubation and suctioning should be immediately carried out. **(Proc. 1-2)**
         ii. Stimulate by flicking soles of feet or rubbing back.
      h. Neonatal assessment parameters
         i. Respiratory effort
         ii. Heart rate
         iii. Color
         iv. APGAR score
   2. Step 2: Supplemental oxygen
      a. For central cyanosis or inadequate ventilation, give warmed, humidified supplemental oxygen by blow-by. **(Fig. 1-19)**
      b. Continue oxygen until color has improved.
      c. Blow-by oxygen in the prehospital setting will NOT cause oxygen toxicity.

POINT TO EMPHASIZE
Cold infants quickly become distressed infants.

POINT TO EMPHASIZE
Do not "milk" or strip the umbilical cord.

POWERPOINT PRESENTATION
Volume 2, Chapter 1, PowerPoint slides 28–51

POINT TO EMPHASIZE
Of the vital signs, fetal heart rate is the most important indicator of neonatal distress.

TEACHING TIP
Problems caused by overextension and underextension of the neck can be illustrated with plastic soda straws simulating the flexible neonatal trachea. Students can see how over- or underextension of a small, flexible tube can result in obstruction and decrease air entry.

POINT TO EMPHASIZE
Suctioning of the newborn should take no longer than 10 seconds.

POINT TO EMPHASIZE
Never deprive a newborn of oxygen in the prehospital setting for fear of oxygen toxicity.

TEACHING TIP
Students frequently have difficulty understanding why they do chest compressions on bradycardic infants and small children with pulses, but not on adults. Explain the underlying physiology by reviewing the fact that cardiac output equals heart rate times stroke volume. As hearts become smaller they are less able to vary their stroke volume to compensate for a decreased rate. In infants and small children, cardiac output becomes almost entirely rate-dependent. Therefore, chest compressions become necessary to support cardiac output in the presence of a slow heart rate.

POINT TO EMPHASIZE
In an infant, vascular access for the administration of fluids and drugs can most readily be managed by using the umbilical vein.

POINT TO EMPHASIZE
Keep in mind that naloxone may induce a withdrawal reaction in an infant born to a narcotic-addicted mother.

POWERPOINT PRESENTATION
Volume 5, Chapter 1, PowerPoint slides 52–85

3. Step 3: Ventilation (**Fig. 1-20**)
   a. Begin positive-pressure ventilation if:
      i. Heart rate is less than 100 beats per minute.
      ii. Apnea is present.
      iii. Central cyanosis is present after oxygen is given.
   b. Ventilate at rate of 40 to 60 breaths per minute.
   c. Use BVM.
4. Step 4: Chest compressions (**Fig. 1-21**)
   a. Begin chest compressions if the heart rate is
      i. Less than 60 beats/min
      ii. Encircle the newborn's chest, placing both of your thumbs on the lower one third of the sternum. If the newborn is very small, you may need to overlap your thumbs. If the newborn is very large, you may need to place the ring and middle fingers of one hand just below the nipple line and perform two-finger compression (**Fig. 1-21**)
      iii. Compress the lower half of the sternum at a rate of 100 times per minute. Accompany compressions with positive-pressure ventilation. Maintain a ratio of 30 compressions to 2 breaths (one rescuer) or 15 compressions to 2 breaths (two rescuers).
      iv. Reassess heart rate, respiration, and color every 30 seconds. Coordinate with chest compressions and ventilation.
      v. Discontinue compressions if the spontaneous heart rate exceeds 60 per minute.
5. Step 5: Medications and fluids
   a. Most newborn cardiopulmonary arrests result from hypoxia and respond to oxygenation and ventilation.
   b. Vascular access is most readily obtained through the umbilical vein. (**Fig. 1-22**)
   c. If umbilical vein catheter cannot be placed, lidocaine, atropine, naloxone, and epinephrine can be given via the endotracheal tube.
   d. Other options for vascular access include peripheral veins or the intraosseous route.
   e. Fluid therapy should consist of 10 mL/kg of saline or lactated Ringer's solution as a slow IV push.
6. Maternal narcotic use
   a. Naloxone (Narcan) is treatment of choice for respiratory depression caused by maternal narcotic use within 4 hours of delivery.
   b. Narcan may induce withdrawal reactions in infants born to narcotic-addicted mothers.
   c. Dosage is 0.1 mg/kg, may be repeated every 2–3 minutes as needed.
7. Neonatal transport (**Fig. 1-23**)

V. Specific neonatal situations. (pp. 26–37)

A. Meconium-stained amniotic fluid (pp. 27–28)
   1. Meconium is a dark green substance found in the digestive tract of full-term newborns indicative of fetal distress.
   2. Hypoxia can cause meconium to be passed into amniotic fluid.
   3. Infant born through thin meconium may not require treatment if the infant is vigorous (strong respiratory efforts, good muscle tone, and heart rate >100 per minute).
   4. Nonvigorous infants born through thick, particulate (pea-soup) meconium-stained fluid should be intubated immediately, prior to the first ventilation (**Fig. 1-24**)

B. Apnea (p. 28)

    1. Absence of spontaneous ventilation with stimulation or respiratory pauses of greater than 20 seconds

    2. Assessment findings

        a. Failure to breathe spontaneously after stimulation

        b. Respiratory pauses greater than 20 seconds

    3. Management

        a. Stimulate baby by flicking soles of feet or rubbing back.

        b. Ventilate with BVM.

        c. Suction as needed.

        d. Intubate if apnea is prolonged or heart rate is less than 60 with adequate ventilation and chest compressions.

        e. Gain circulatory access.

        f. Monitor heart rate continuously.

        g. If apnea is due to narcotics given in previous 4 hours, consider naloxone.

        h. Prevent hypothermia.

C. Diaphragmatic hernia (pp. 28–29)

    1. Abdominal contents displaced into thorax to varying degrees.

    2. Can make the lung on affected side compressed and may displace the heart.

    3. Assessment findings

        a. Little to severe distress

        b. Dyspnea and cyanosis unresponsive to ventilations

        c. Scaphoid (flat) abdomen

        d. Bowel sounds heard in chest

        e. Heart sounds displaced to right

    4. Management

        a. Position infant with head and thorax higher than abdomen and feet. (**Fig. 1-25**)

        b. Place nasogastric tube and apply low, intermittent suction.

        c. Do NOT use BVM.

        d. Endotracheal intubation may be necessary.

        e. Explain need for possible surgery to parents.

D. Bradycardia (p. 29)

    1. Management

        a. Follow procedures in inverted pyramid.

        b. Avoid temptation to treat with pharmacological measures alone.

        c. Avoid prolonged suctioning or airway instrumentation.

        d. Keep newborn warm.

E. Premature infants (pp. 29–30) (**Fig. 1-26**)

    1. Epidemiology

        a. Born before 37 weeks gestation or with weight from 0.6 to 2.2 kg (1 lb, 5 oz to 4 lb, 13 oz)

        b. Healthy premature infants weighing greater than 1,700 g (3 lb, 12 oz) have survivability and outcomes approximating those of full-term infants

        c. Mortality decreases weekly with gestation beyond the onset of viability (currently around 23 to 24 weeks of gestation)

    2. Assessment findings

        a. Degree of immaturity determines the physical characteristics

        b. Larger head relative to body size

        c. Generally a large trunk and short extremities

        d. Skin transparent with fewer wrinkles

        e. Less subcutaneous fat

    3. Management

        a. Attempt resuscitation if the infant has any sign of life

POINT TO EMPHASIZE

Do not discuss "chances of survival" with a newborn's family or caregivers.

TEACHING TIP

Communication with family members is important during care of neonates. However, paramedics (and other health care providers) frequently have trouble explaining disease processes and their management to laypeople. Try having your students develop verbal or written explanations of disease processes or treatments that a person without specialized training can understand.

POINT TO EMPHASIZE

Do not use narcotic antagonists if the mother is a drug abuser.

POINT TO EMPHASIZE

If you suspect a diaphragmatic hernia, do not use bag-valve mask ventilation, which can worsen the condition by causing gastric distension.

POINT TO EMPHASIZE

When administering to a newborn, resist the temptation to treat bradycardia with pharmacological measures alone.

POINT TO EMPHASIZE

Prematurity should not be a factor in short-term management. Resuscitation should be attempted if there is any sign of life.

      b. Follow same procedures as those for newborns of normal maturity and weight

      c. Maintain patent airway

      d. Avoid potential aspiration of gastric contents

      e. Consider use of epinephrine

      f. Maintain body temperature

      g. Transport to facility with services for low-birth-weight newborns.

F. Respiratory distress/cyanosis (pp. 30–31)

  1. Prematurity is the single most common factor

  2. Assessment findings

      a. Tachypnea

      b. Paradoxical breathing

      c. Periodic breathing

      d. Intercostal retractions

      e. Nasal flaring

      f. Expiratory grunt

  3. Management (**Fig. 1-16**)

      a. Follow inverted pyramid of treatment, paying particular attention to airway and ventilation

      b. Suction as needed

      c. Provide high concentration of oxygen

      d. Ventilate as needed with BVM

      e. Consider endotracheal intubation if prolonged ventilation is needed

      f. Perform chest compressions if indicated

      g. Sodium bicarbonate may be helpful in prolonged resuscitation

      h. Consider dextrose if newborn is hypoglycemic

      i. Maintain body temperature

G. Hypovolemia (p. 31)

  1. Leading causes of shock in newborns: dehydration, hemorrhage, third-spacing of fluids

  2. Assessment findings

      a. Pale color

      b. Cool skin

      c. Diminished peripheral pulses

      d. Delayed capillary refill, despite normal ambient temperature

      e. Mental status changes

      f. Diminished urination (oliguria)

  3. Management

      a. Provide fluid bolus resuscitation with isotonic crystalloid (LR or NS)

      b. Give 10 mL/kg over 5 to 10 minutes

      c. Assess response

      d. If signs of shock continue, give second bolus

      e. Hypovolemic infants may require 40 to 60 mL/kg in first hour

      f. Avoid giving volume expanders too rapidly, as rapid infusion of large volumes of fluid has been associated with brain (intraventricular) hemorrhage

H. Seizures (pp. 31–32)

  1. Occur in a very small percentage of all newborns, but represent relative medical emergencies because they are usually a sign of an underlying abnormality

  2. Prolonged and frequent multiple seizures may result in metabolic changes and cardiopulmonary difficulties

  3. Pathophysiology

      a. Generalized tonic-clonic convulsions normally do not occur in the first month of life

      b. Subtle seizure

        i. Chewing motions

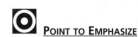
POINT TO EMPHASIZE

In treating hypovolemia in a newborn, do not use solutions containing dextrose, as they can produce hypokalemia or worsen ischemic brain injury.

©2009 Pearson Education, Inc.
Paramedic Care: Principles & Practice, Vol. 5, 3rd. Ed.

        ii. Excessive salivation

        iii. Blinking

        iv. Sucking

        v. Swimming movements of arms

        vi. Pedaling movements of legs

        vii. Apnea

        viii. Color changes

    c. Tonic seizure

        i. Rigid posturing of extremities and trunk

        ii. Sometimes fixed deviation of eyes

        iii. More common in premature infants, especially in those with intraventricular hemorrhage

    d. Focal clonic seizure

        i. Rhythmic twitching of muscle groups, particularly extremities and face

        ii. Occurs in both full-term and premature infants

    e. Multifocal seizure

        i. Similar to focal clonic seizures

        ii. Involves multiple muscle groups

        iii. Randomly migrates to another area of the body

        iv. Occurs primarily in full-term infants

    f. Myoclonic seizure

        i. Brief jerks of the upper or lower extremities

        ii. May occur singly or in a series of repetitive jerks

4. Assessment findings

    a. Decreased level of consciousness

    b. Seizure activity

5. Management considerations

    a. Manage airway and ventilation

    b. Maintain oxygen saturation

    c. Consider $D_{10}W$ or $D_{25}W$ for hypoglycemia

    d. Consider benzodiazepine (lorazepam) for status epilepticus

    e. Maintain normal body temperature

I. Fever (pp. 32–33)

1. Epidemiology

    a. Average normal newborn's temperature is 99.5°F (37.5°C)

    b. Rectal temperature greater than 100.4°F (38.0°C) is considered fever

    c. Neonates do not develop fever as easily as older children

    d. Fever in a neonate may indicate a life-threatening condition and requires extensive evaluation

    e. Any neonate with a fever should be considered to have meningitis until proven otherwise

2. Assessment findings

    a. Mental status changes (irritability/somnolence)

    b. Decreased intake

    c. Caretaker history

    d. Feels warm

    e. Observe patient for rashes, petechiae

    f. Term newborns will produce beads of sweat on their brow but not over the rest of their body

    g. Premature infants will have no visible sweat

3. Management

    a. Ensure adequate oxygenation and ventilation

    b. Avoid use of cold packs

    c. Perform chest compressions if bradycardia develops

    d. Administration of antipyretic agent is questionable in the prehospital setting

POINT TO EMPHASIZE

Any neonate with a fever should be considered to have meningitis until proven otherwise.

POINT TO EMPHASIZE

In assessing a neonate with a fever, remember that infants have a limited ability to control their body temperature. As a result, fever can be a serious condition.

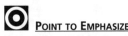

J. Hypothermia (p. 33)
  1. Pathophysiology
     a. Increased surface-to-volume ratio makes newborns extremely sensitive to environmental conditions, especially when they are wet after delivery
     b. Can be an indicator of sepsis in the neonate
     c. Increased metabolic demand can cause metabolic acidosis, pulmonary hypertension, and hypoxemia
  2. Assessment findings
     a. Pale color
     b. Cool to touch, particularly in extremities
     c. Acrocyanosis
     d. Respiratory distress
     e. Apnea
     f. Bradycardia
     g. Central cyanosis
     h. Initial irritability
     i. Lethargy in later stage
     j. Generally do not shiver
  3. Management
     a. Ensure adequate oxygenation and ventilation
     b. Perform chest compressions if indicated
     c. Warm IV fluids via IV fluid warmer
     d. $D_{10}W$ or $D_{25}W$ if hypoglycemic
     e. Environmental conditions should be 24 to 26.5°C (75.2 to 78.8°F)
     f. Warm hands before touching patient

K. Hypoglycemia (pp. 33–34)
  1. Epidemiology
     a. Newborns are the only age group that can develop severe hypoglycemia without having diabetes mellitus
     b. May be due to inadequate glucose intake or increased utilization of glucose
     c. Persistent low blood glucose levels may have catastrophic effects on the brain
  2. Pathophysiology
     a. Glycogen stores are sufficient to meet glucose requirements for 8 to 12 hours
     b. Time frame is decreased in infants with decreased glycogen stores or with problems that increase glucose utilization
     c. Body responds to hypoglycemia by releasing counterregulatory hormones including glucagon, epinephrine, cortisol, and growth hormone
     d. Hormones may cause symptoms of hyperglycemia that last for several hours
     e. Blood glucose concentration should be determined on all sick infants
     f. Blood glucose screening test below 45 mg/dL indicates hypoglycemia
  3. Assessment findings
     a. Twitching or seizures
     b. Limpness
     c. Lethargy
     d. Eye-rolling
     e. High-pitched cry
     f. Apnea
     g. Irregular respirations
     h. Possible cyanosis

4. Management
      a. Ensure adequate oxygenation and ventilation
      b. Perform chest compressions if indicated
      c. Administer dextrose ($D_{10}W$ or $D_{25}W$)
      d. Maintain normal body temperature
L. Vomiting (p. 34)
   1. Epidemiology
      a. Vomiting mucus, occasionally blood-streaked, in the first few hours of life is not uncommon
      b. Persistent vomiting is a warning sign
      c. Vomiting in the first 24 hours of life suggests obstruction in the upper digestive tract or increased intracranial pressure
      d. Vomitus containing dark blood is usually a sign of a life-threatening illness
      e. Aspiration of vomitus can cause respiratory insufficiencies or obstruction of the airway
   2. Assessment findings
      a. Distended stomach
      b. Infection
      c. Increased ICP
      d. Drug withdrawal
   3. Management considerations
      a. Maintain a patent airway
      b. Suction/clear vomitus from airway
      c. Ensure adequate oxygenation
      d. Fluid administration may be required
      e. Bradycardia may be caused by vagal stimulus of vomiting
M. Diarrhea (p. 35)
   1. Five to six stools per day is normal, especially if infant is breast-feeding, but severe diarrhea can cause dehydration and electrolyte imbalance
   2. Causes
      a. Bacterial or viral infections
      b. Gastroenteritis
      c. Lactose intolerance
      d. Phototherapy
      e. Neonatal abstinence syndrome
      f. Thyrotoxicosis
      g. Cystic fibrosis
   3. Assessment findings
      a. Loose stools
      b. Decreased urinary output
      c. Signs of dehydration
   4. Management
      a. Take proper standard precautions
      b. Ensure adequate oxygenation and ventilation
      c. Perform chest compressions if indicated
      d. Fluid therapy may be indicated
N. Common birth injuries (pp. 35–36)
   1. Avoidable and unavoidable mechanical and anoxic trauma incurred by the infant during labor and delivery
   2. Pathophysiology
      a. Cranial injuries
      b. Intracranial hemorrhage
      c. Spine and spinal cord injury from strong traction exerted when the spine is hyperextended or pull is lateral
      d. Peripheral nerve injury
      e. Liver injury

 POINT TO EMPHASIZE

In treating distressed neonates who have birth injuries or other critical conditions, provide professional and compassionate communication to the parents or caregivers.

     f. Rupture of spleen

     g. Adrenal hemorrhage

     h. Clavicle and extremity fractures

     i. Hypoxia-ischemia

  3. Assessment findings

     a. Diffuse, sometimes ecchymotic, edematous swelling of the soft tissues of the scalp

     b. Paralysis below the level of spinal cord injury

     c. Paralysis of the upper arm with or without paralysis of the forearm

     d. Diaphragmatic paralysis

     e. Movement on only one side of the face when newborn cries

     f. Inability to move arm freely on side of fractured clavicle

     g. Lack of spontaneous movement of the affected extremity

     h. Hypoxia

     i. Shock

  4. Management

     a. Ensure adequate oxygenation and ventilation

     b. Perform chest compressions if indicated

     c. Transport to facility capable of providing specialized care

     d. Provide professional, compassionate communication to parents or caregivers

O. Cardiac resuscitation, postresuscitation, and stabilization (pp. 36–37)

  1. Risk factors

     a. Bradycardia

     b. Intrauterine asphyxia

     c. Prematurity

     d. Drugs administered to or taken by the mother

     e. Congenital neuromuscular diseases

     f. Congenital malformations

     g. Intrapartum hypoxemia

  2. Pathophysiology

     a. Primary apnea

     b. Secondary apnea

     c. Bradycardia

     d. Persistent fetal circulation

     e. Pulmonary hypertension

  3. Assessment findings

     a. Peripheral cyanosis

     b. Inadequate respiratory effort

     c. Ineffective or absent heart rate

  4. Management

     a. Follow inverted pyramid

     b. Consult medical direction and follow its instructions

     c. Maintain normal body temperature

VI. Summary (p. 37)

A. After a delivery you must care for two patients.

B. Newborn's special needs include:

  1. Protection of airway

  2. Support of ventilations

  3. Maintenance of body temperature

C. Distressed newborns should receive:

  1. Stimulation

  2. Support of oxygenation and ventilation

  3. CPR, as needed

TEACHING TIP

Since caring for a sick neonate includes communicating with and supporting the parents or other caregivers, patient-care simulations should include "parent" role-players. Students should be expected to communicate with the "parents" appropriately during the role-play.

TEACHING STRATEGY 7

Resuscitation Reference Card

POWERPOINT PRESENTATION

Volume 5, Chapter 1, PowerPoint slide 86

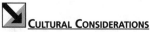

CULTURAL CONSIDERATIONS

When Parents Request Baptism, p. 36.

D. If possible, transport should be to a facility with a NICU

E. Communication must be maintained with family members and other caregivers

SKILLS DEMONSTRATION AND PRACTICE

Students can practice skills discussed in this chapter in the following Skills Lab activities.

Skills Lab: Provide students with Handouts 1-5 and 1-6. Demonstrate umbilical vein catheterization and infant resuscitation techniques. Make the following key points:

- The majority of newborns can be resuscitated with drying, warming, positioning, suctioning, and stimulating.
- Bradycardia in a newborn is a result of hypoxia.
- Drug therapy is rarely needed in the resuscitation of the newborn.
- Hypothermia in the newborn must be avoided by rapid drying and warming.
- Meconium aspiration is a potentially lethal complication of delivery. Particulate meconium must be suctioned from the oro-/nasopharynx and from the trachea before the baby takes its first breath.

After your demonstration, have students circulate through the stations, making sure that each station is equipped as detailed below. Monitor the students to be sure each has a chance to practice each of the skills. You may wish to have other instructors or qualified paramedics assist in these activities.

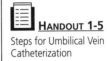
HANDOUT 1-5
Steps for Umbilical Vein Catheterization

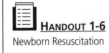
HANDOUT 1-6
Newborn Resuscitation

Station	Equipment and Personnel Needed	Activities
Umbilical vein catheterization	Disposable gloves, latex and nonlatex Protective eyewear Umbilical cords, kept in sterile saline Baby bottles, 4 oz Nipples Umbilical catheter, 5 French Syringe, 10 mL Umbilical tape Gauze Saline Red food coloring Scalpel blade, #10 1 instructor	Have students cannulate the umbilical vein of a newborn, following the steps in Handout 1-5. Ensure that all participants wear goggles and protective eyewear during this procedure.
Resuscitation of the normal newborn	Infant manikin Infant intubation manikin Bulb syringe DeLee suction trap Meconium aspirator Endotracheal tubes: 2.5, 3.0, and 3.5 Suction catheters:	Have students practice resuscitating a normal newborn as described in Handout 1-6, Scenario One. Choose a team leader or allow students to self-select their roles. Follow an interactive format by presenting the initial

Station	Equipment and Personnel Needed	Activities
	5, 6, and 8 French 20-mL syringe and 8-French feeding tube for gastric suction Towels Cord clamp Sterile scissors or scalpel IV catheters: 22- and 24-gauge over-the needle; 23- and 25-gauge butterfly Tape Bag-valve-mask device with infant-sized mask Stethoscope Blood glucose testing materials Laryngoscope handle Laryngoscope blades: 0, 1 straight 1 instructor	scenario, and then provide additional historical and physical exam information in response to participants' questions. Advance students to the next case when their actions are acceptable. If a student is having difficulty managing a case, other participants may give suggestions. Continued inappropriate management is better handled by stopping the scenario and discussing key points than by continuing to have the patient's condition deteriorate. When the case is completed, use the suggested steps in the Answer Key to review its management with the students, acknowledging correct treatment decisions and critiquing errors. Any content points not made during the course of the scenario should be addressed in a short didactic session or discussion at this time. Instructor information to be given upon request:

1. What number pregnancy is this? *First*

2. Do you feel like you need to push? *Yes*

3. Baby's head is crowning

4. Meconium present? *No*

5. Twins? *No*

6. Term delivery? *Yes*

7. First ABC assessment: *Beginning to make strong, effective breathing efforts; heart rate is 80 and rising.*

8. Reassessment of ABCs: *Breathing is becoming faster and easier; heart rate is 40.* |
| Resuscitation of the distressed newborn | Infant manikin Infant intubation manikin Bulb syringe DeLee suction trap | Have students practice resuscitating a distressed newborn as described in Handout 1-6, Scenario Two. |

Station	Equipment and Personnel Needed	Activities
	Meconium aspirator Endotracheal tubes: 2.5, 3.0, and 3.5 Suction catheters: 5, 6, and 8 French 20-mL syringe and 8-French feeding tube for gastric suction Towels Cord clamp Sterile scissors or scalpel IV catheters: 22- and 24-gauge over-the-needle; 23- and 25-gauge butterfly Tape Bag-valve-mask device with infant-sized mask Stethoscope Blood glucose testing materials Laryngoscope handle Laryngoscope blades: 0, 1 straight 1 instructor	Choose a team leader or allow students to self-select their roles. Follow an interactive format by presenting the initial scenario, and then provide additional historical and physical exam information in response to participants' questions. Advance students to the next case when their actions are acceptable. If a student is having difficulty managing a case, other participants may give suggestions. Continued inappropriate management is better handled by stopping the scenario and discussing key points than by continuing to have the patient's condition deteriorate. When the case is completed, use the suggested steps in the Answer Key to review its management with the students, acknowledging correct treatment decisions and critiquing errors. Any content points not made during the course of the scenario should be addressed in a short didactic session or discussion at this time. Instructor information given upon request:

1. What number pregnancy is this? *Third*

2. Do you feel like you need to push? *Yes*

3. Baby's head is crowning

4. Meconium present? *Yes*

5. Twins? *No*

6. Term delivery? *Yes*

7. First ABC assessment: *Gasping without air movement; heart rate is 40.*

8. Reassessment of ABCs: *Good chest rise with BMV; heart rate is 55.*

YOU MAKE THE CALL

Review student responses to the You Make the Call scenario on text page 37. Suggested responses to the questions that follow the scenario are given below. Point out to students that these are acceptable answers but not necessarily the only ones. Discuss with students pros and cons of points where their responses differ from these.

1. Should you stimulate this baby to breathe as soon as it is delivered? Why or why not?
   (You should not stimulate this baby to breathe, either while on the perineum or immediately following delivery, because of the presence of thick meconium. Quickly prepare equipment and visualize the airway with a laryngoscope. Suction the airway with a catheter or, preferably, insert an appropriately sized uncuffed endotracheal tube. Apply suction to the endotracheal tube with a suction adaptor. After a few seconds, the majority of the meconium should be removed from the airway. Discard the soiled tube and place a new one. This whole procedure should take no longer than 30 to 45 seconds. After securing the airway, stimulate the infant. The infant may require a brief trial of mechanical ventilation. Always administer 100 percent supplemental oxygen. Be sure to report the presence of thick meconium to the receiving staff.)

2. What is the major danger associated with this type of problem?
   (Meconium aspiration syndrome is a very serious problem in which the infant aspirates meconium. This often results in pulmonary infections and extended mechanical ventilation and NICU time. Taking time to aspirate the airway results in much better outcomes in neonates exposed to meconium in utero.)

3. Once you have stabilized this infant, where should it be transported?
   (The infant should be transported to a hospital with an NICU with an available bed and mechanical ventilation.)

ASSIGNMENTS

Assign students to complete Chapter 1, "Neonatology," of the Workbook. Also assign them to read Chapter 2, "Pediatrics," before the next class.

Chapter Quiz and Scenario   Distribute copies of the Chapter Quiz provided in Handout 1-3 to evaluate student understanding of this chapter. Make sure each student reads the scenario (Handout 1-4) to reinforce critical thinking on the scene. Remind students not to use their notes or textbooks while taking the quiz.

Student CD   Quizzes for every chapter are contained on the dynamic and highly visual in-text student CD.

Companion Website   Additional quizzes for every chapter are contained on this exciting website.

TestGen   You may wish to create a custom-tailored test using *Prentice Hall TestGen for Paramedic Care: Principles & Practice*, 3rd edition, to evaluate student understanding of this chapter.

Online Test Preparation (for students and instructors)   Additional test preparation is available through Brady's new online product, EMT Achieve: Paramedic Test Preparation, at *http://www.prehall.com/emtachieve*. Instructors can also monitor student mastery online

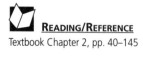

READING/REFERENCE
Textbook Chapter 2, pp. 40–145

WORKBOOK
Chapter 1 Activities

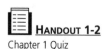

HANDOUT 1-2
Chapter 1 Quiz

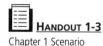

HANDOUT 1-3
Chapter 1 Scenario

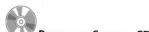

PARAMEDIC STUDENT CD
Student Activities Evaluation

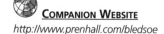

COMPANION WEBSITE
http://www.prenhall.com/bledsoe

TESTGEN
Volume 5, Chapter 1

EMT ACHIEVE:
PARAMEDIC TEST PREPARATION
Mistovich & Beasley. *EMT Achieve: Paramedic Test Preparation,* http://www.prenhall.com/emtachieve.

Success! for the Paramedic   Keyed to *Paramedic Care: Principles & Practice* and *Essentials of Paramedic Care*, this comprehensive exam review contains hundreds of test questions and rationales.

REINFORCEMENT

Handouts   If classroom discussion or performance on the quiz indicates that some students have not fully mastered the chapter content, you may wish to assign some or all of the Reinforcement Handouts for this chapter.

Student CD (for students)   A wide variety of material on this CD-ROM will reinforce and also expand student knowledge and skills.

PowerPoint Presentation (for instructors)   The PowerPoint material developed for this chapter offers useful reinforcement of chapter content.

Companion Website (for students)   Additional review quizzes and links to EMS resources will contribute to further reinforcement of the chapter.

OneKey   Online support is offered for this course on one of three platforms: CourseCompass, Blackboard, or WebCT. Includes the IRM, PowerPoints, Test Manager, and Companion Website for instruction. Ask your local sales representative for more information.

Brady Skills Series: Advanced Life Skills (Video or CD)   Have your students watch the skills come to life on VHS or CD-ROM, or they can purchase the highly visual, full-color text with step-by-step procedures with rationales.

Paramedic National Standards Self-Test   Another comprehensive review manual containing hundreds of review questions with page references keyed to several Brady texts.

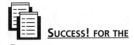

SUCCESS! FOR THE PARAMEDIC

Cherry. *SUCCESS! for the Paramedic*, 4th edition.

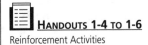

HANDOUTS 1-4 TO 1-6

Reinforcement Activities

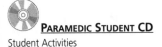

PARAMEDIC STUDENT CD

Student Activities

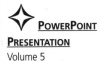

POWERPOINT PRESENTATION

Volume 5

COMPANION WEBSITE

http://www.prenhall.com/bledsoe

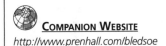

ONEKEY

Volume 5, Chapter 1

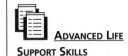

ADVANCED LIFE SUPPORT SKILLS

Larmon & Davis. *Advanced Life Support Skills.*

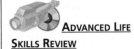

ADVANCED LIFE SKILLS REVIEW

Larmon & Davis. *Advanced Life Skills Review.*

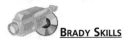

BRADY SKILLS SERIES: ALS

Larmon & Davis. *Brady Skills Series: ALS.*

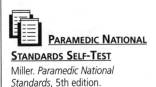

PARAMEDIC NATIONAL STANDARDS SELF-TEST

Miller. *Paramedic National Standards*, 5th edition.

OBJECTIVES

Student's Name _____

CHAPTER 1 OBJECTIVES CHECKLIST

Knowledge Objective	Date Mastered
1. Define *newborn* and *neonate*.	
2. Identify important antepartum factors that can affect childbirth.	
3. Identify important intrapartum factors that can determine high-risk newborn patients.	
4. Identify the factors that lead to premature birth and low-birth-weight newborns.	
5. Distinguish between primary and secondary apnea.	
6. Discuss pulmonary perfusion and asphyxia.	
7. Identify the primary signs utilized for evaluating a newborn during resuscitation.	
8. Identify the appropriate use of the APGAR scale.	
9. Calculate the APGAR score given various newborn situations.	
10. Formulate an appropriate treatment plan for providing initial care to a newborn.	
11. Describe the indications, equipment needed, application, and evaluation of the following management techniques for the newborn in distress:	
a. Blow-by oxygen	
b. Ventilatory assistance	
c. Endotracheal intubation	
d. Orogastric tube	
e. Chest compressions	
f. Vascular access	
12. Discuss the routes of medication administration for a newborn.	
13. Discuss the signs of hypovolemia in a newborn.	
14. Discuss the initial steps in resuscitation of a newborn.	

Knowledge Objective	Date Mastered
15. Discuss the effects of maternal narcotic use on the newborn.	
16. Determine the appropriate treatment for the newborn with narcotic depression.	
17. Discuss appropriate transport guidelines for a newborn.	
18. Determine appropriate receiving facilities for low- and high-risk newborns.	
19. Describe the epidemiology, including the incidence, morbidity/mortality, risk factors and prevention strategies, pathophysiology, assessment findings, and management, of the following neonatal problems:	
a. Meconium aspiration	
b. Apnea	
c. Diaphragmatic hernia	
d. Bradycardia	
e. Prematurity	
f. Respiratory distress/cyanosis	
g. Seizures	
h. Fever	
i. Hypothermia	
j. Hypoglycemia	
k. Vomiting	
l. Diarrhea	
m. Common birth injuries	
n. Cardiac arrest	
o. Post-arrest management	
Skill Objective	**Date Mastered**
20. Given several neonatal emergencies, provide the appropriate procedures for assessment, management, and transport.	

Student's Name _____

CHAPTER 1 QUIZ

Write the letter of the best answer in the space provided.

_____ **1.** A neonate is an infant from the time of birth to:
    A. 1 week of age.   **C.** 1 month of age.
    B. 2 weeks of age.   **D.** 3 months of age.

_____ **2.** The term *newborn* or *newly born infant* is used to describe a neonate:
    A. until the umbilical cord is cut.
    B. during the time it spends in the delivery room.
    C. until it is discharged from the hospital.
    D. during the first few hours of life.

_____ **3.** The difference between primary apnea and secondary apnea in a newborn is that:
    A. infants with primary apnea typically will respond to simple stimulation and oxygen while those in secondary apnea will not.
    B. bradycardia is present in primary apnea but not in secondary apnea.
    C. infants with secondary apnea typically will respond to simple stimulation and oxygen whereas those in primary apnea will not.
    D. bradycardia is present in secondary apnea but not in primary apnea.

_____ **4.** A normal newborn's respiratory rate should average:
    A. 12 to 20 breaths per minute.
    B. 20 to 30 breaths per minute.
    C. 40 to 60 breaths per minute.
    D. 60 to 80 breaths per minute.

_____ **5.** A newborn's heart rate should normally be:
    A. 80 to 100 at birth, speeding to 140 to 160 thereafter.
    B. 150 to 180 at birth, slowing to 130 to 140 thereafter.
    C. 170 to 190 at birth, slowing to 80 to 100 thereafter.
    D. 60 to 80 at birth, speeding to 150 to 180 thereafter.

_____ **6.** Which of the following statements about skin color in the newborn immediately after birth is correct?
    A. Cyanosis of the extremities is common, but central cyanosis is abnormal.
    B. Central cyanosis is common, but cyanosis of the extremities is abnormal.
    C. Both cyanosis of the extremities and central cyanosis are common and normal.
    D. Both central cyanosis and cyanosis of the extremities are abnormal.

_____ **7.** An infant is in distress and requires emergency intervention if its pulse rate is less than:
    A. 60.   **C.** 100.
    B. 80.   **D.** 120.

_____ **8.** Determine the APGAR score for the following infant:
    Appearance—completely pink
    Pulse—over 100
    Grimace—crying
    Activity—some flexion, slowly
    Respiration—strong cry
    A. 5   **C.** 9
    B. 7   **D.** 10

_____ **9.** Determine the APGAR score for the following infant:
Appearance—completely cyanotic
Pulse—below 100
Grimace—frowns when stimulated
Activity—limp
Respiration—slow, irregular
  A. 1   **C.** 5
  B. 3   **D.** 7

_____ **10.** You have just delivered an infant. The baby is limp with central cyanosis. There is no apparent respiratory effort. You should:
  A. begin resuscitation immediately.
  B. withhold resuscitation for 1 minute so the APGAR score can be used to guide your efforts.
  C. give oxygen by blow-by, but withhold other resuscitative measures until a 1-minute APGAR score can be determined.
  D. position, dry, warm, suction, and stimulate the infant, but withhold other resuscitation until a 1-minute APGAR score can be determined.

_____ **11.** An infant is considered to be in severe distress and in need of immediate resuscitation if its APGAR score is less than:
  A. 2.   **C.** 6.
  B. 4.   **D.** 8.

_____ **12.** When you suction a newborn's airway, you should:
  A. suction the mouth first so there is nothing there to aspirate if the infant gasps when its nose is suctioned.
  B. suction the nose first so there is nothing there to aspirate if the infant gasps when its mouth is suctioned.
  C. suction either the nose or the mouth first depending on which you can reach most easily.
  D. squeeze the suction bulb only after placing it into the infant's mouth.

_____ **13.** Appropriate methods of stimulating a newborn include:
  A. flicking the soles of its feet; slapping its buttocks.
  B. flicking the soles of its feet; gently rubbing its back.
  C. vigorous rubbing; flicking the soles of the feet.
  D. vigorous rubbing; slapping the buttocks.

_____ **14.** "Milking" or stripping the umbilical cord is:
  A. contraindicated because it increases blood viscosity and produces polycythemia.
  B. indicated because it increases the newborn's red cell mass and improves oxygenation.
  C. contraindicated because it decreases blood viscosity and causes hypovolemia.
  D. indicated because it helps reverse hypovolemia that may have developed during birth.

_____ **15.** The first priority following the birth of a baby is to:
  A. clamp and cut the umbilical cord.
  B. deliver the placenta.
  C. ensure that the infant's airway and breathing are adequate.
  D. control maternal blood loss.

_____ **16.** Acceptable techniques for checking the heart rate of an infant include all of the following, EXCEPT:
  A. listening over the cardiac apex with a stethoscope.
  B. lightly grasping the stump of the umbilical cord.
  C. palpating the femoral or brachial pulses.
  D. attaching the infant to an ECG monitor and watching the heart-rate meter.

_____ **17.** At 1540 hours you respond to a call in a maternity store at a shopping mall where you find a woman in labor. Exam reveals that the baby's head is crowning, and the mother says she needs to push. When you deliver the infant, it is covered with a greenish-black material. The infant's respirations are gasping and are not moving air. You should:
  A. position the infant head down and rub its back to stimulate breathing.
  B. begin immediate ventilation with oxygen using the bag-valve mask.
  C. intubate the trachea and apply suction to the ET tube to remove any foreign material from the lower airway.
  D. give blow-by oxygen and transport immediately.

_____ **18.** A newborn should receive positive-pressure ventilations with a bag-valve mask if its heart rate is not at least:
  A. 60.
  B. 80.
  C. 100.
  D. 120.

_____ **19.** A newborn has a heart rate of 140 and regular, unlabored respirations at 42. Cyanosis of the chest and abdomen are present. You should:
  A. withhold oxygen since central cyanosis is common in the first few minutes after birth.
  B. withhold oxygen since high-concentration oxygen has been linked with blindness in newborn infants.
  C. give oxygen immediately using a bag-valve mask.
  D. give oxygen by blowing oxygen across the newborn's face.

_____ **20.** A newborn has a heart rate of 86 and regular, unlabored respirations at 40. Cyanosis of the extremities is present. You should:
  A. blow oxygen across the newborn's face.
  B. wait for 1 minute, then reassess the pulse to see if it is increasing.
  C. begin chest compressions immediately.
  D. immediately begin positive-pressure ventilation with a bag-valve mask.

_____ **21.** A newborn initially presented with a heart rate of 152 and regular, unlabored respirations at 46. Since central cyanosis was present, oxygen was given by blow-by. After about a minute, the cyanosis was still present. You should:
  A. discontinue the oxygen since the cause is probably not respiratory in nature.
  B. begin positive-pressure ventilation with a bag-valve mask.
  C. immediately intubate the newborn's trachea, then ventilate with a bag-valve mask.
  D. begin chest compressions.

_____ **22.** Chest compressions should be initiated in a newborn if the heart rate is:
  A. less than 60 beats/min.
  B. between 60 and 80 beats/min, but does not increase with 30 seconds of oxygenation and ventilation.
  C. between 80 and 100 beats/min and central cyanosis is present.
  D. either A or B.

_____ **23.** Which of the following best describes the correct technique for two rescuer chest compressions and ventilations to a newborn?
  A. Rate 120/min; 30 compressions to 2 ventilations
  B. Rate 100/min; 30 compressions to 2 ventilations
  C. Rate 120/min; 15 compressions to 2 ventilations
  D. Rate 100/min; 15 compressions to 2 ventilations

_____ 24. You are delivering the infant of a 17-year-old female who has been living in a shelter for the homeless. During your assessment of the mother, you notice needle tracks on her arms. Her speech is slurred, and she appears to be drowsy and apathetic. When you question her about drug abuse, she admits to "shooting up" with heroin about 2 hours ago to relieve the pain of labor. Which of the following statements best describes your considerations in this situation?
   A. The infant will probably suffer respiratory depression following delivery and should receive naloxone as quickly as possible to reverse this problem.
   B. The infant will probably not suffer significant problems since narcotics do not cross the placental barrier easily.
   C. The infant will probably suffer respiratory depression following delivery but should not be given naloxone since a withdrawal reaction might occur.
   D. Naloxone should be given by IV push to the mother immediately to avoid serious respiratory depression in her newborn.

_____ 25. An infant you have just delivered is in severe respiratory distress. Central cyanosis unresponsive to bag-valve-mask ventilation is present. Physical exam reveals a small, flat abdomen, absent breath sounds over the left lung field, and displacement of the heart sounds to the right. What problem do you suspect?
   A. meconium aspiration   C. diaphragmatic hernia
   B. omphalocele   D. meningomyelocele

_____ 26. Appropriate management of the infant in question 25 would include positioning her head and thorax:
   A. higher than the abdomen and feet; placing a nasogastric or orogastric tube; ventilating with a bag-valve mask while preparing to intubate.
   B. higher than her abdomen and feet; placing a nasogastric or orogastric tube; withholding further bag-valve-mask ventilation until an endotracheal tube is placed.
   C. lower than her abdomen and feet; placing a nasogastric or orogastric tube; withholding further bag-valve-mask ventilation until an endotracheal tube is placed.
   D. higher than her abdomen and feet; avoiding placement of a nasogastric or orogastric tube; ventilating with a bag-valve mask while preparing to intubate.

_____ 27. The most common cause of bradycardia in the newborn is:
   A. increased intracranial pressure.   C. hypoxia.
   B. acidosis.   D. hypothyroidism.

_____ 28. The most effective initial treatment for bradycardia in the newborn is to give:
   A. atropine.   C. epinephrine.
   B. oxygen.   D. $D_{10}W$.

_____ 29. A premature newborn is an infant born before:
   A. 40 weeks gestation or with a weight less than 2.2 kg.
   B. 37 weeks gestation or with a weight less than 2.2 kg.
   C. 32 weeks gestation or with a weight less than 0.6 kg.
   D. 28 weeks gestation or with a weight less than 0.6 kg.

_____ 30. Premature infants are susceptible to hypothermia because:
   A. they have a large surface-to-volume ratio.
   B. they have small stores of subcutaneous fat and therefore less insulation.
   C. they are unable to shiver.
   D. all of the above.

_____ 31. The most common factor causing respiratory distress and cyanosis in the newborn is:
   A. meconium aspiration.   C. diaphragmatic hernia.
   B. prematurity.   D. aspiration pneumonitis.

_____ **32.** The leading cause of shock in newborns is:
  A. sepsis.
  B. cardiac failure secondary to hypoxia.
  C. hypovolemia.
  D. hypoglycemia.

_____ **33.** A newborn suspected of being hypovolemic should be given a bolus of:
  A. 10 mL/kg of Ringer's lactate or normal saline.
  B. 10 mL/kg of D_5LR or D_5NS.
  C. 40 mL/kg of Ringer's lactate or normal saline.
  D. 40 mL/kg of D_5LR or D_5NS.

_____ **34.** Fever in a neonate:
  A. is not a cause for concern since their immune systems are immature and they frequently develop mild infections.
  B. is not a cause for concern unless the infant is sweating heavily.
  C. should be treated with application of cold packs to lower the core temperature.
  D. should be considered a sign of meningitis or another life-threatening infection until proven otherwise.

_____ **35.** Infants of diabetic mothers should have their blood glucose levels checked about 30 minutes after birth because:
  A. they will frequently develop hypoglycemia.
  B. an elevated blood glucose at this time will help predict whether the infant also will be diabetic.
  C. they will frequently develop hyperglycemia.
  D. a decreased blood glucose at this time will help predict whether the infant also will be diabetic.

©2009 Pearson Education, Inc.
Paramedic Care: Principles & Practice, Vol. 5, 3rd. Ed.

CHAPTER 1 SCENARIO

Review the following real-life situation. Then answer the questions that follow.

At 2230 hours on a snowy winter evening, you are dispatched for a woman in preterm labor. Weather and traffic conditions slow your response, and a trip that normally would have taken 5 minutes requires 15. When you finally reach the location of the call, a suburban home, you discover that a 28-year-old female, assisted by her husband, has just delivered a 30-week-gestation boy.

The infant is flaccid with no spontaneous movement. He has no apparent respiratory effort. The pulse, felt at the base of the umbilical cord, is 44 beats/min and weak. Central cyanosis is present. You estimate the infant's weight at 1 kg. There are no obvious congenital abnormalities.

1. What is this newborn's status and the most likely cause of this situation?

2. What should you do?

3. Thirty seconds after beginning ventilation, the baby's heart rate is still 44 beats/min. What should you do now?

4. After 30 seconds of CPR, the baby's heart rate rises to 88 beats/min. What should you do now?

CHAPTER 1 REVIEW

Write the word or words that best complete the following sentences in the space(s) provided.

1. An infant from the time of birth to 1 month of age is a(n) _____.

2. A baby in the first few hours of life is referred to as a(n) _____. These infants also are sometimes called _____ _____ _____.

3. After an unscheduled delivery in the field, you have _____ patients to manage, the _____ and the _____.

4. Factors present before onset of labor that indicate possible complications in newborns are called _____ factors.

5. Factors occurring during childbirth that indicate possible complications in newborns are called _____ factors.

6. The channel between the main pulmonary artery and the aorta in the fetus is the _____ _____.

7. A condition in the newborn in which blood continues to bypass the fetal respiratory system resulting in ongoing hypoxia is _____ _____ _____.

8. The initial period of apnea in a hypoxic newborn that can be reversed with simple stimulation and exposure to oxygen is _____ apnea.

9. _____ apnea is a condition characterized by falling heart rate, blood pressure, and oxygen saturation that is not responsive to stimulation and that will not spontaneously reverse.

10. Apnea in a newborn should always be assumed to be _____ apnea.

11. Protrusion of abdominal contents into the thoracic cavity through an opening in the diaphragm is a(n) _____ _____.

12. Herniation of the spinal cord and membranes through a defect in the spinal column is a(n) _____.

13. A defect in the area of the umbilicus that results in herniation of the abdominal contents is a(n) _____.

14. The most common birth defect of the nose, which is due to the presence of a bony or membranous septum between the nasal cavity and the pharynx, is _____ _____.

15. A numerical system for distinguishing newborns who need only routine care from those who need greater assistance is the _____ _____, which has five parameters: _____, _____ _____, _____, _____, and _____ _____.

16. As soon as you deliver a newborn's head, suction the _____ first, then the _____.

17. The dark green material that can be expelled from the intestine into the amniotic fluid during periods of distress is _____.

18. Two acceptable methods of stimulating a newborn who does not cry immediately are _____ _____ _____ and _____ _____ _____.

19. Heat loss from the newborn can result from _____, _____, _____, and _____.

©2009 Pearson Education, Inc.
Paramedic Care: Principles & Practice, Vol. 5, 3rd. Ed.

20. "Milking" or stripping the umbilical cord can cause _____ _____ _____ and _____.

21. The most important indicator of neonatal distress is the _____ _____.

22. The first steps on the "inverted pyramid" of neonatal resuscitation are _____, _____, _____, _____, and _____ _____.

23. If a newborn has central cyanosis and a heart rate greater than 100, you should administer _____.

24. An infant should receive positive-pressure ventilation if it has a heart rate less than _____, _____, or persistence of _____ _____ after administration of oxygen.

25. An infant who needs positive-pressure ventilation should be ventilated at a rate of _____ to _____ breaths per minute.

26. Chest compressions should be initiated in a newborn if the heart rate is less than _____.

27. Chest compressions in the newborn should be performed at a rate of _____ per minute.

28. Vascular access in the newborn can be most readily obtained by using the _____ _____.

29. If naloxone is given to an infant born to a narcotic-addicted mother, it may induce a _____ _____.

30. If you suspect a diaphragmatic hernia, DO NOT use _____-_____ _____, which can worsen the condition by causing gastric distention.

31. Bradycardia in the newborn is most commonly caused by _____.

32. A premature newborn is an infant born before _____ weeks or who weighs less than _____ kg.

33. The single most common factor causing respiratory distress and cyanosis in the newborn is _____.

34. The most common cause of shock in the newborn is _____.

35. Fluid bolus resuscitation in the newborn consists of _____ mL/kg of isotonic crystalloid.

36. Any neonate with a fever should be considered to have _____ until proven otherwise.

37. Newborns are extremely sensitive to environmental temperatures because of their increased _____ to _____ relationship.

38. Newborns of diabetic mothers have an increased risk of developing _____.

39. Hypoglycemia in the newborn is indicated by a blood glucose of less than _____.

40. Hypoglycemia in the newborn can be corrected by giving _____ or _____.

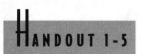
REINFORCEMENT

Student's Name _____

STEPS FOR UMBILICAL VEIN CATHETERIZATION

1. Fill baby bottle with saline (food coloring may be added to simulate blood).

2. Make two cross-slits in the nipple of the bottle.

3. Pull the umbilical cord through the nipple and attach the nipple to the bottle.

4. Cut the umbilical cord horizontally until the two arteries and the vein are easily seen.

5. Place umbilical tape at the base of the cord.

6. Fill a syringe and the umbilical catheter with saline.

7. Locate the orifice of the umbilical vein and insert the catheter.

8. Advance the catheter slowly until a fluid return is obtained.

   (*Note:* When this procedure is performed on a newborn, the catheter should be advanced only a short distance to avoid entering the hepatic venous system.)

9. When there is good blood return, tighten the tape in a purse string.

   (*Note:* This step should be demonstrated by your instructor but not practiced.)

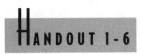

Student's Name _____

NEWBORN RESUSCITATION

SCENARIO ONE: RESUSCITATION OF THE NORMAL NEWBORN

At 2245 hours, you respond to a report of "abdominal pain" in a small community that is about 30 minutes from the closest emergency room. The patient is a 15-year-old female who is screaming as she lies on a couch in the living room of her home. The girl's mother is standing by perplexed. After a quick exam, you determine that the patient is pregnant and is in active labor. What do you do?

_____

_____

_____

_____

_____

_____

_____

_____

_____

_____

_____

_____

_____

_____

_____

_____

_____

_____

_____

REINFORCEMENT

SCENARIO TWO: RESUSCITATION OF THE DISTRESSED NEWBORN

At 1415 hours, you are dispatched to a report of a "woman in labor" at a shopping mall. When you arrive, mall security quickly escorts you to a maternity store where you find a 28-year-old female in active labor. What do you do?

_____

_____

_____

_____

_____

_____

_____

_____

_____

_____

_____

_____

_____

_____

_____

_____

_____

_____

_____

_____

_____

_____

_____

Chapter 1 Answer Key

Handout 1-2: Chapter 1 Quiz

1.	C	10.	A	19.	D	28.	B
2.	D	11.	B	20.	D	29.	B
3.	A	12.	A	21.	B	30.	D
4.	C	13.	B	22.	A	31.	B
5.	B	14.	A	23.	D	32.	C
6.	A	15.	C	24.	C	33.	A
7.	C	16.	D	25.	C	34.	D
8.	C	17.	C	26.	B	35.	A
9.	B	18.	C	27.	C		

Handout 1-3: Chapter 1 Scenario

1. He is in cardiopulmonary failure, probably as a result of hypoxia.
2. Clamp and cut the umbilical cord. Dry, warm, position, suction, and stimulate the newborn. Reassess for breathing. Then begin bag-valve-mask ventilations at 40 to 60 breaths/min with high-concentration oxygen. After 30 seconds, recheck the heart rate.
3. Check for adequate chest rise and air entry with bag-valve-mask ventilation. Continue to ventilate while your partner begins chest compressions at a rate of 120/min. Reassess heart rate in 30 seconds.
4. Stop chest compressions. Continue to ventilate with the bag-valve-mask. Reassess heart rate after 30 seconds. Check for spontaneous respirations and for central cyanosis. Make preparations to transport, including maximizing heat in the patient compartment of the ambulance.

Handout 1-4: Chapter 1 Review

1. neonate
2. newborn, newly born infants
3. two, mother, baby
4. antepartum
5. intrapartum
6. ductus arteriosus
7. persistent fetal circulation
8. primary
9. Secondary
10. secondary
11. diaphragmatic hernia
12. meningomyelocele
13. omphalocele
14. choanal atresia
15. APGAR scale, Appearance, Pulse rate, Grimace, Activity, Respiratory effort
16. mouth, nose
17. meconium
18. rubbing its back, flicking its soles
19. conduction, evaporation, convection, radiation
20. increased blood viscosity, polycythemia
21. heart rate
22. drying, warming, positioning, suction, tactile stimulation
23. oxygen
24. 100, apnea, central cyanosis
25. 40, 60
26. 60
27. 120

28. umbilical vein
29. withdrawal reaction
30. bag-mask ventilation
31. hypoxia
32. 37, 2.2
33. prematurity
34. hypovolemia
35. 10
36. meningitis
37. surface, volume
38. hypoglycemia
39. 45 mg/dL
40. $D_{10}W$, $D_{25}W$

Handout 1-6: Newborn Resuscitation

Scenario 1: Resuscitation of the Normal Newborn

Expected sequence of interventions

1. Obtained and opened OB kit.
2. Questioned mother about length of gestation and twins.
3. Observed for presence of meconium.
4. Assisted with delivery.
   a. Delivered infant's head.
   b. Suctioned mouth, then nose with bulb syringe.
   c. Allowed mother to push on next contraction to complete delivery.
5. Received baby in sterile towel, warmed if possible.
6. At the perineum, positioned the infant's head in a dependent position.
7. Suctioned mouth, then nose again.
8. Stimulated respirations by drying infant with towel.
9. Assessed ABCs.
10. Continued stimulation/drying.
11. Reassessed breathing and circulation.
12. Applied cord clamps.
13. Cut umbilical cord.
14. Placed infant in new dry towel, dried thoroughly while observing.
15. Wrapped infant to prevent hypothermia.
16. Prepared for transport.

Scenario 2: Resuscitation of the Distressed Newborn

Expected sequence of interventions

1. Obtained and opened OB kit.
2. Prepared suction and intubation equipment.
3. Questioned mother about length of gestation and twins.
4. Assisted with delivery.
   a. Delivered infant's head.
   b. Suctioned mouth, pharynx, nose thoroughly.
   c. Allowed mother to push on next contraction to complete delivery.
5. Received baby in sterile towel, warmed if possible.
6. Clamped and cut the umbilical cord.
7. Positioned infant with head in slightly dependent position.
8. Intubated trachea; observed for presence of meconium on vocal cords during procedure.

9. Withdrew endotracheal tube while applying direct suction to endotracheal tube, using meconium aspiration adaptor.
10. Repeated intubation and suctioning until meconium was no longer returned.
11. Stimulated respirations by drying infant with towel.
12. Assessed ABCs.
13. Administered bag-valve-mask ventilation at 40 to 60 breaths/minute with 100 percent oxygen.
14. Reassessed heart rate after 30 seconds of oxygenation and ventilation.
    a. Breathing (good chest rise with bag-valve-mask ventilation)
    b. Circulation (heart rate is 140)

15. Began chest compressions if heart rate was below 60, at a rate of 100 compressions per minute and a ratio of either 30 compressions to 2 ventilations for one rescuer or 15 compressions to 2 ventilations for two rescuers.
16. Reassessed heart rate after 30 seconds of oxygenation and ventilation.
17. Performed endotracheal intubation.
18. Wrapped infant to prevent hypothermia.
19. Prepared for transport.

Chapter 2 Pediatrics

INTRODUCTION

Management of sick or injured children requires knowledge of common pediatric emergencies, strong patient assessment skills, and a well-organized approach. Children are not little adults. The etiologies that lead to catastrophic events, such as cardiopulmonary arrest, are different from those in adults. Because children typically have healthy cardiovascular and respiratory systems, they tend to compensate well when they are stressed physiologically. Accordingly, the signs and symptoms of distress may be subtle. Paramedics must recognize that although children make up a relatively small portion of the patients cared for by the EMS system, their unique needs require specialized preparation and responses.

CHAPTER OBJECTIVES

Knowledge Objectives

1. Discuss the paramedic's role in the reduction of infant and childhood morbidity and mortality from acute illness and injury. (pp. 43–45)
2. Identify methods/mechanisms that prevent injuries to infants and children. (p. 44)
3. Describe Emergency Medical Services for Children (EMSC) and how it can affect patient outcome. (p. 44)
4. Identify the common family responses to acute illness and injury of an infant or child. (pp. 46–47)
5. Describe techniques for successful interaction with families of acutely ill or injured infants and children. (pp. 46–47)
6. Identify key anatomical, physiological, growth, and developmental characteristics of infants and children and their implications. (pp. 47–51)
7. Outline differences in adult and childhood anatomy, physiology, and "normal" age-group-related vital signs. (pp. 51–56)
8. Describe techniques for successful assessment and treatment of infants and children. (pp. 56–70)
9. Discuss the appropriate equipment utilized to obtain pediatric vital signs. (pp. 68–70)
10. Determine appropriate airway adjuncts, ventilation devices, and endotracheal intubation equipment; their proper use; and complications of use with infants and children. (pp. 70–84)
11. List the indications and methods of gastric decompression for infants and children. (pp. 84–85, 86)
12. Define pediatric respiratory distress, failure, and arrest. (pp. 94–95)

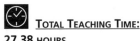

**TOTAL TEACHING TIME:
27.38 HOURS**
The total teaching time is only a guideline based on the didactic and practical lab averages in the National Standard Curriculum. Instructors should take into consideration such factors as: the pace at which students learn, the size of the class, and breaks. The actual time devoted to teaching objectives is the responsibility of the instructor.

13. Differentiate between upper airway obstruction and lower airway disease. (pp. 96–103)
14. Describe the general approach to the treatment of children with respiratory distress, failure, or arrest from upper airway obstruction or lower airway disease. (pp. 96–103)
15. Discuss the common causes and relative severity of hypoperfusion in infants and children. (pp. 103–107)
16. Identify the major classifications of pediatric cardiac rhythms. (pp. 107–110)
17. Discuss the primary etiologies of cardiopulmonary arrest in infants and children. (pp. 85, 94–95, 103)
18. Discuss age-appropriate sites, equipment, techniques, and complications of vascular access sites for infants and children. (pp. 85, 87)
19. Describe the primary etiologies of altered level of consciousness in infants and children. (pp. 93–121, 126–127, 138)
20. Identify common lethal mechanisms of injury in infants and children. (pp. 121–124)
21. Discuss anatomical features of children that predispose or protect them from certain injuries. (pp. 127–130)
22. Describe aspects of infant and child airway management that are affected by potential cervical spine injury. (pp. 124–125)
23. Identify infant and child trauma patients who require spinal immobilization. (pp. 88, 90)
24. Discuss fluid management and shock treatment for infant and child trauma patients. (pp. 103–104, 126)
25. Determine when pain management and sedation are appropriate for infants and children. (p. 126)
26. Define sudden infant death syndrome (SIDS), child abuse, and child neglect. (pp. 130–134)
27. Discuss the parent/caregiver responses to the death of an infant or child. (p. 131)
28. Define children with special health care needs and technology-assisted children. (pp. 134–138)
29. Discuss basic cardiac life support (CPR) guidelines for infants and children. (pp. 70–77)
30. Integrate advanced life support skills with basic cardiac life support for infants and children. (pp. 77–78, 108–112)
31. Discuss the indications, dosage, route of administration, and special considerations for medication administration in infants and children. (pp. 90–93)
32. Discuss appropriate transport guidelines for low- and high-risk infants and children. (pp. 90–93)
33. Describe the epidemiology, including the incidence, morbidity/mortality, risk factors, prevention strategies, pathophysiology, assessment, and treatment of infants and children with:

   a. Respiratory distress/failure (pp. 94–103)
   b. Hypoperfusion (pp. 103–108)
   c. Cardiac dysrhythmias (pp. 108–112)
   d. Neurologic emergencies (pp. 110, 113–115)
   e. Trauma (pp. 121–130)
   f. Abuse and neglect (pp. 131–134)
   g. Special health care needs, including technology-assisted children (pp. 134–138)
   h. SIDS (pp. 130–131)

©2009 Pearson Education, Inc.
Paramedic Care: Principles & Practice, Vol. 5, 3rd. Ed.

34. Given several preprogrammed simulated pediatric patients, provide the appropriate assessment, treatment, and transport. (pp. 43–141)

FRAMING THE LESSON

Begin the session by asking the students to imagine and list the feelings of an acutely ill or injured child entering the emergency health care system. Next ask them to imagine and list the feelings they might experience in the role of the child's parent or other caregiver. Finally, ask the students to imagine and list the feelings they would have if they were the paramedic responding to provide care to this child. List the feelings and emotions of each person involved in a pediatric emergency on a flip chart or board and compare them. Emphasize that pediatric emergencies frequently are emotionally charged, highly stressful situations that require not only knowledge and skill but also a high level of professionalism and mental discipline to manage. Because EMS responses to pediatric patients are relatively infrequent, study, practice, and planning are critical to maintaining the knowledge, skill, and discipline necessary for good outcomes.

CONSIDERING THE CASE STUDY

Ask a volunteer to read aloud the Case Study that begins on text page 42. Suggest that students close their eyes as the scenario is read to help them mentally visualize the events described in it. You can use the following questions as a starting point for teaching the chapter—a sort of chapter preview in a functional setting.

When the chapter is completed, you may wish to return to the Case Study to encourage further discussion aimed at answering the questions or solving the problems.

CASE STUDY DISCUSSION QUESTIONS (AND ANSWERS)

1. From what problem does the patient appear to be suffering?
   (The patient appears to be suffering from volume depletion [dehydration] and hypovolemic shock secondary to prolonged vomiting.)
2. What is the significance of the child's pale, cool, clammy skin?
   (Children usually have healthy cardiovascular systems. When their intravascular volume decreases, they compensate by constricting the peripheral blood vessels and shifting the remaining volume to the core organs. The pale, cool, clammy skin indicates that this child is compensating for volume depletion.)
3. What is the significance of the absence of tears when the child cries?
   (Absence of tears in a child suffering from volume depletion indicates severe dehydration.)
4. Why did the paramedic give fluid to the child using 20 mL/kg boluses?
   (Because children are small they are more easily placed in a state of volume overload by overly aggressive fluid resuscitation. Giving volume in controlled boluses followed by a reassessment of perfusion allows the paramedic to correct hypovolemia without causing volume overload, heart failure, or pulmonary edema.)

TEACHING STRATEGIES

People learn in a variety of ways. Some do better with the spoken word, while others prefer the written. Some prefer to work alone, whereas others profit from working in groups. Recognizing these different ways of acquiring knowledge, the authors of this *Instructor's Resource Manual* have provided a variety of teaching strategies for the different types of learners. These strategies are intended to foster higher-level cognitive skills and encourage creative learning and problem solving.

For greatest effectiveness, incorporate these strategies into your class lecture. Marginal notes in the Teaching Outline indicate the points at which various exercises might be most appropriate. Other strategies can be used to preview the lesson or to summarize it.

The following strategies are keyed to specific sections of the lesson:

1. *National and Local Agencies.* Identify national and local agencies that promote the education of pediatric clinical skills and education, such as the American Heart Association, American Academy of Pediatrics, Children's Hospital, and Maternal and Child Health Services. Help students to understand the courses and materials offered by each of these organizations and their roles in the care and prevention of childhood illness and injuries. Be sure to have brochures and contact information in your classroom to promote lifelong learning and the importance of continuing education.

2. *Pediatric Health Fair.* Volunteer your students at a local pediatric health fair. If one does not exist in your area, have students organize such an event. Include blood pressure screening, height and weight measurements, blood glucose checks, and even immunizations if possible. Volunteerism teaches valuable life lessons about being a public servant and giving to others. In addition, this activity can substitute for clinical time in a pediatric health clinic, which is sometimes hard to secure. This event will expose your students to many children of various ages and backgrounds, giving them practice communicating with and assessing children in a noncrisis situation, which is often easier than during an ambulance call.

3. *Child Observation Exercise.* The differences in development, behavior, and communication abilities of children may seem like a mystery to students, especially those without children of their own. A simple observation exercise can help. Have students, either individually or in small groups, observe children and parents in a public setting, such as the mall, the zoo, a playground, or a park. Have your students record the behaviors and language used by children and their parents, along with an estimation of their age and size. When students come back to class, ask the entire group to share behaviors or characteristics of children in several different developmental stages, such as infant, toddler, preschool, adolescent, and so on. You will likely prepare a list that is remarkably similar to those listed in the text, and the students will have actual behavioral observations to improve their understanding of the material. The skill of observation is important to the paramedic, who often must communicate with and assess a patient while being aware of his or her total environment. This is a social psychology exercise that reaches both the cognitive and affective domains. The assignment should be given before the class session on this material to provide a context for discussion.

4. *Elementary School Health Clinic.* Many elementary schools, especially in urban areas, have health clinics or at least a school nurse's office. Arrange for students to spend time in these clinics, where they are likely to encounter basically healthy children with a single complaint. This allows students to gain comfort communicating with and assessing pediatric patients in the absence of a major crisis that usually accompanies a 911 call. In addition, the staff in these

©2009 Pearson Education, Inc.
Paramedic Care: Principles & Practice, Vol. 5, 3rd. Ed.

clinics are usually overworked and often appreciate the assistance. This activity improves the quality of clinical time, covers all three educational domains, and improves relationships with community health servants whom your students are likely to encounter as professional paramedics.

5. *Researching an EMSC Project.* Several years ago, emphasis in EMS was placed on pediatrics. Significant funds were allocated to EMS for Children (EMSC) projects all over the country. Many of these projects were wildly successful, improving the care to children and placing an emphasis on prevention. Have students research an EMSC project and share with the class the project's goals and successes. Have them discuss how their project could be extrapolated to your community, considering and solving any barriers to the project's success. This activity emphasizes research, oral communication, and problem-solving skills. Additionally, it encourages students to look outside their own community or EMS system for solutions to problems.

The following strategy relates to Special Features in the student textbook and can be used to enhance the student's understanding:

Legal Notes: When Is a Child No Longer a Child? Provide students with information from your state's legal statutes identifying when children are no longer children. This may include being 18 years of age or if they are pregnant or a mother. Some states may also recognize that a patient is no longer a minor if he is under 18 years old and a father. Be sure to check with legal counsel for specifics in your state.

The following strategies can be used at various points throughout the lesson or to help summarize and demonstrate what students have learned:

Guest Speaker: Developmental or Child Psychologist. Invite a developmental or child psychologist to class to share techniques for interviewing and communicating with children. This person will likely have many tips and tricks to build rapport quickly with children of all ages. He should also be able to explain why certain approaches work with children of various ages. Any hospital with a pediatric wing is likely to have a child psychologist on staff. Many even employ psychologists who specialize in working with sick children or those in need of special health care. A psychologist with expertise in these areas could be an even greater asset to your classroom. In some cases, use of a subject matter expert is your best bet for an interesting and informative lecture.

Guest Speaker. Consider inviting a pediatrician, pediatric intensivist, pediatric surgeon, or pediatric anesthesiologist from the local or regional hospital to the class to discuss topics related to his specialty.

Clinical Rotations. Pediatric clinical rotations should be designed so students can see a wide range of pediatric patients and illnesses. Opportunities include:
- **Day care centers**—to allow students to see and interact with healthy young children.
- **Immunization clinics**—to allow students to obtain practice giving IM and subcutaneous injections to pediatric patients and interacting with healthy children who are under stress.
- **Pediatric clinics and pediatricians' offices**—to allow students to interact with children who are presenting with common injuries and illnesses of minor to moderate severity in a primary care setting.
- **Pediatric emergency departments**—to allow students to interact with children presenting with minor to critical injuries and illnesses.

- **Pediatric intensive care units**—to allow students to interact with and care for critically ill or injured children.
- **Pediatric long-term care facilities**—to allow students to interact with and care for chronically ill children, including those who are technology-assisted or dependent.

HANDOUT 2-1
Chapter 2 Objectives Checklist

POWERPOINT
PRESENTATION
Volume 5, Chapter 2, PowerPoint slides 1–3

READING/REFERENCE
Perkin, R., and D. van Stralen. "20 Things You May Not Know about Pediatrics," *JEMS*, Mar. 2000.

POWERPOINT
PRESENTATION
Volume 5, Chapter 2, PowerPoint slides 4–14

TEACHING STRATEGY 1
National and Local Agencies

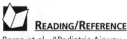
TEACHING STRATEGY 2
Pediatric Health Fair

TEACHING OUTLINE

Chapter 2 is the second lesson in Volume 5, *Special Considerations/Operations.* Distribute Handout 2-1 so that students can familiarize themselves with the learning goals for this chapter. If the students have any questions about the objectives, answer them at this time.

Then present the chapter. One possible lecture outline follows. In the outline, the parenthetical references in regular type are references to text pages; those in bold type are to figures, tables, or procedures.

I. Introduction. (p. 43)

A. More than 20,000 pediatric deaths occur each year in the United States (p. 43)

B. Top causes of pediatric deaths (p. 43)
1. Motor vehicle accidents
2. Burns
3. Drownings
4. Suicides
5. Homicides

II. Role of paramedics in pediatric care. (pp. 43–45)

A. Continuing education and training programs (pp. 43–44)
1. Pediatric Advanced Life Support (PALS)
2. Pediatric Basic Trauma Life Support (PBTLS) Pediatric Education for Paramedic Professionals (PEPP)
3. Advanced Pediatric Life Support (APLS)
4. Prehospital Pediatric Care (OOC)
5. Regional conferences and seminars
6. Pediatric education sites on the Internet
7. Center for Pediatric Medicine (CPEM) at NYU and Bellevue Hospital
8. Textbooks and journals
9. Teaching Resource for Instructors of Prehospital Pediatrics (TRIPP)

B. Improved health care and injury prevention (pp. 44–45)
1. Emergency Medical Services for Children (EMSC)
2. Coordinated national effort
3. Identification of specific areas of pediatric health care concern (**Fig. 2-1**)
4. Advanced life support skills in pediatrics
   a. Up to 85 percent need only BLS skills

III. General approach to pediatric emergencies. (pp. 45–47)

A. Communication and psychological support (pp. 46–47)

B. Responding to patient needs (p. 46)
1. Common fears of children include:
   a. Separation from parents, caregivers
   b. Removal from home and never returning
   c. Injury
   d. Mutilation or disfigurement
   e. The unknown

READING/REFERENCE
Baren et al., "Pediatric Airway Management," *JEMS*, Jun. 2004.

Garza, M. A. "Smart Pediatric Transport," *JEMS*, Mar. 2000.

Losavio, K. "EMS for Kids," *JEMS*, Dec. 2000.

2. Be honest with children about what is being done to them and about discomfort and pain associated with procedures.

3. Use language appropriate for the age of the child.

C. Responding to parents and caregivers (pp. 46–47)

    1. Caregivers' responses may include

      a. Shock

      b. Grief

      c. Denial

      d. Anger

      e. Guilt

      f. Fear

      g. Complete loss of control

    2. Designate one paramedic to deal with adults on the scene to avoid conflicts in information.

    3. Paramedic confidence and professionalism help parents regain control.

IV. Growth and development. (pp. 47–51)

A. Newborns (first hours after birth) (p. 47)

    1. Assessed with APGAR scoring system

    2. Resuscitation follows inverted pyramid and NeoNatal Resuscitation (NNR) guidelines.

B. Neonates (birth to 1 month) (pp. 47–48)

    1. Physical development

      a. Initially loses up to 10 percent of birth weight

      b. Lost weight normally recovered within 10 days

      c. Premature neonates are not as neurologically or physically developed as their term counterparts.

    2. Cognitive and emotional development

      a. Development centers on reflexes.

      b. Personality begins to form.

      c. May stare at faces and smile

      d. Mother, and occasionally father, can comfort and quiet

    3. Common illnesses

      a. Jaundice

      b. Vomiting

      c. Respiratory distress

C. Infants (1 to 5 months) (p. 48)

    1. Physical development

      a. Should have doubled birth weight

      b. Should be able to follow movements of others with their eyes

      c. Development of muscle tone moves from head to trunk and from trunk to extremities.

    2. Cognitive and emotional development centers closely on parents and caregivers.

    3. Common illnesses and accidents

      a. SIDS

      b. Vomiting

      c. Dehydration

      d. Meningitis

      e. Child abuse

      f. Household accidents

    4. Paramedic considerations

D. Infants (6 to 12 months) (p. 48)

    1. Physical development

      a. May stand or walk without assistance

      b. Active

POINT TO EMPHASIZE

Because you will encounter pediatric patients less frequently than adult patients, you have a professional responsibility to maintain and improve your pediatric knowledge, particularly your clinical skills.

POWERPOINT PRESENTATION

Volume 5, Chapter 2, PowerPoint slides 15–44

TEACHING STRATEGY 3

Child Observation Exercise

POINT TO EMPHASIZE

Tragedies involving children account for some of the most stressful incidents that you will encounter in EMS practice.

POINT TO EMPHASIZE

Examine infants and toddlers in a toe-to-head direction.

      c. Enjoy exploring world with their mouths, causing serious risk for foreign body airway obstruction

  2. Cognitive and emotional development (**Fig. 2-2**)
      a. Have more fully formed personalities; express themselves readily
      b. Have anxiety toward strangers
      c. Don't like lying on backs
      d. Tend to cling to mother

  3. Common illnesses and accidents
      a. Febrile seizures
      b. Vomiting
      c. Diarrhea
      d. Dehydration
      e. Bronchiolitis
      f. Motor vehicle collisions
      g. Croup
      h. Child abuse
      i. Poisonings
      j. Falls
      k. Airway obstruction
      l. Meningitis

  4. Paramedic considerations

E. Toddlers (1 to 3 years) (pp. 48–49)
  1. Physical development
      a. Great strides in motor development, mobility
      b. Always on the move

  2. Cognitive and emotional development
      a. Begin to stray away from parents, caregivers more frequently
      b. Will cling to parents, caregivers if frightened
      c. Understand better than they can speak
      d. Can answer simple, specific questions

  3. Common illnesses and accidents
      a. Motor vehicle collisions
      b. Homicide
      c. Burn injuries
      d. Drowning
      e. Vehicle vs. pedestrian collisions
      f. Vomiting
      g. Diarrhea
      h. Febrile seizures
      i. Poisonings
      j. Falls
      k. Child abuse
      l. Croup
      m. Meningitis
      n. Foreign body airway obstruction

  4. Paramedic considerations

F. Preschoolers (3 to 5 years) (p. 49)
  1. Physical development
      a. Tremendous increase in fine and gross motor development
      b. Know how to talk, but may refuse to speak, especially to strangers

  2. Cognitive and emotional development
      a. Vivid imaginations
      b. May see monsters as part of their world
      c. Have tempers and will express them
      d. Fear mutilation; may feel threatened by treatment

POINT TO EMPHASIZE
Do not trick or lie to the child and always explain what you are going to do.

©2009 Pearson Education, Inc.
Paramedic Care: Principles & Practice, Vol. 5, 3rd. Ed.

      e. Often run to a particular parent or caregiver

      f. Are openly affectionate; seek support and comfort from within home

  3. Common illnesses and accidents

      a. Croup

      b. Asthma

      c. Poisonings

      d. Motor vehicle collisions

      e. Burns

      f. Child abuse

      g. Ingestion of foreign bodies

      h. Drownings

      i. Epiglottitis

      j. Febrile seizures

      k. Meningitis

  4. Paramedic considerations

G. School-age children (6 to 12 years) (pp. 49–50)

  1. Physical development

      a. Tend to be active and carefree

      b. Growth spurts may lead to clumsiness.

  2. Cognitive and emotional development

      a. Protective and proud of parents or caregivers

      b. Seek attention of parents, caregivers

      c. Value peers, but also need home support

  3. Common illnesses and accidents

      a. Drownings

      b. Motor vehicle collisions

      c. Bicycle collisions

      d. Falls

      e. Fractures

      f. Sports injuries

      g. Child abuse

      h. Burns

  4. Paramedic considerations (**Fig. 2-3; Fig. 2-4**)

H. Adolescents (13 to 18 years) (pp. 50–51)

  1. Usually defined as end of childhood and beginning of puberty

      a. Highly child-specific

      b. Male, average 13 years

      c. Female, average 11 years

  2. Physical development

      a. Significant variation among children

      b. Tend to be body conscious and concerned about physical image

  3. Cognitive and emotional development

      a. Most consider themselves to be grown up

      b. Take offense at the use of the word "child"

      c. Relationships with peers are very important.

      d. Relationships with parents may be strained by growing need for independence.

  4. Common illnesses and accidents

      a. Mononucleosis

      b. Asthma

      c. Motor vehicle collisions

      d. Sports injuries

      e. Drug and alcohol problems

      f. Suicide gestures

      g. Sexual abuse

      h. Pregnancy

  5. Paramedic implications

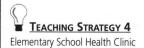

TEACHING STRATEGY 4

Elementary School Health Clinic

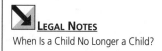

LEGAL NOTES

When Is a Child No Longer a Child?

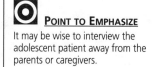

POINT TO EMPHASIZE

It may be wise to interview the adolescent patient away from the parents or caregivers.

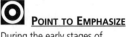
V. Anatomy and physiology. (pp. 51–56) (Fig. 2-5; Table 2-1)

  A. Head (pp. 52–53) (Fig. 2-6)

    1. Larger size

    2. Larger occipital region

    3. Fontanelles open in infancy

    4. Face small in comparison to size of head

    5. Paramedic implications

      a. Higher proportion of blunt trauma involves the head.

      b. Different airway positioning techniques

      c. Examine fontanelles in infants.

        i. Bulging fontanelles suggest increased intracranial pressure.

        ii. Sunken fontanelles suggest dehydration.

  B. Airway (pp. 53–54)

    1. Narrower at all levels

    2. Infants are obligate nose breathers.

    3. Tongue takes up more space in mouth.

    4. Jaw is proportionally smaller in young children.

    5. Larynx is higher (C-3 to C-4) and more anterior.

    6. Cricoid ring is narrowest part of airway in young children.

    7. Tracheal cartilage softer

    8. Trachea smaller in both length and diameter and more flexible

    9. Epiglottis

   10. Paramedic implications

      a. Keep nares clear in infants <6 months.

      b. Keep in mind that narrower upper airways are more easily obstructed.

      c. Differences in intubation technique

  C. Chest and lungs (p. 54)

    1. Ribs positioned horizontally

    2. Ribs more pliable than adults' ribs and offer less protection to organs

    3. Chest muscles are immature and fatigue easily.

    4. Lung tissue more fragile than adults'

    5. Mediastinum more mobile than adults'

    6. Thin chest wall easily transmits breath sounds

    7. Paramedic implications

      a. Infants and children are diaphragmatic breathers.

      b. Infants and children are prone to gastric distention.

      c. Rib fractures less frequent, but not uncommon in child abuse and trauma

      d. Following trauma, children can have significant internal injury without external signs.

      e. Pulmonary contusions more common in major trauma

      f. Lungs prone to pneumothorax following barotraumas

      g. Mediastinum has greater shift with tension pneumothorax

      h. Easy to miss pneumothorax or misplaced intubation due to transmitted breath sounds

  D. Abdomen (p. 54)

    1. Immature abdominal muscles offer less protection.

    2. Abdominal organs closer together

    3. Liver and spleen proportionally larger and more vascular

    4. Paramedic implications

      a. Liver and spleen more frequently injured

      b. Multiple organ injuries more common

  E. Extremities (p. 54)

    1. Bones softer and more porous until adolescence

    2. Growth plate injuries may disrupt bone growth.

3. Paramedic implications
   a. Immobilize any "sprain" or "strain," because it is likely a fracture.
   b. Avoid piercing growth plate during intraosseous needle insertion.
F. Skin and body surface area (BSA) (pp. 54–55)
   1. Thinner and more elastic
   2. Thermal exposure results in deeper burn.
   3. Less subcutaneous fat
   4. Larger surface area relative to body mass
   5. Paramedic implications
      a. Children are more easily and deeply burned.
      b. They suffer larger losses of fluid and heat.
G. Respiratory system (infants and children) (p. 55)
   1. Tidal volume proportionally similar to adolescents' and adults', but children require double metabolic oxygen
   2. Have smaller oxygen reserves
   3. Are susceptible to hypoxia
H. Cardiovascular system (p. 55)
   1. Cardiac output is rate dependent in infants and small children.
   2. Vigorous but limited cardiovascular reserves
   3. Bradycardia in response to hypoxia
   4. Can maintain blood pressure longer than an adult
   5. Circulating blood volume proportionally larger than adults'
   6. Absolute blood volume smaller than adults'
   7. Paramedic implications
      a. Smaller absolute volume of fluid/blood loss needed to cause shock
      b. Larger proportional volume of fluid/blood loss needed to cause shock
      c. Hypotension is a late sign of shock.
      d. A child may be in shock despite normal blood pressure.
      e. Shock assessment is based on clinical signs of tissue perfusion.
      f. Carefully assess for shock if tachycardia is present.
      g. Monitor carefully for development of hypotension.
I. Nervous system (p. 55)
   1. Develops throughout childhood
   2. Developing neural tissue is fragile.
   3. Brain and spinal cord less well protected by skull and spinal column
   4. Paramedic implications
      a. Brain injuries more devastating in young children
      b. Greater force transmitted to underlying brain of young children
      c. Spinal cord injury can occur without spinal column injury.
J. Metabolic differences (pp. 55–56)
   1. Infants and children have limited glycogen and glucose stores.
   2. Significant volume loss can result from vomiting and diarrhea.
   3. Prone to hypothermia due to increased BSA
   4. Newborns and neonates unable to shiver to maintain body temperature
   5. Paramedic implications
      a. Keep child warm during treatment and transport.
      b. Cover the head to minimize heat loss.

VI. General approach to pediatric assessment. (pp. 56–70)

A. Basic considerations (pp. 56–57)
   1. Use "assessment from doorway" patient observation.
   2. Involve parent/caregiver.
   3. Observe parental/caregiver interaction with patient.

POINT TO EMPHASIZE

Infants and children increase their cardiac output by increasing their heart rate. They have very limited capacity to increase their stroke volume.

POINT TO EMPHASIZE

Bleeding that would not be dangerous in an adult may be life-threatening in an infant or child.

TEACHING TIP

See if students reason from the fact that infants and small children lose heat more rapidly to the fact that they must have higher metabolic rates, and therefore higher respiratory rates and heart rates.

POWERPOINT PRESENTATION

Volume 5, Chapter 2, PowerPoint slides 45–64

B. Scene size-up (p. 57)
   1. Observe scene for hazards or potential hazards.
   2. Observe scene for mechanism of injury/illness.
   3. Observe the parent/guardian/caregiver interaction with the child.
C. Initial assessment (pp. 57–58) (**Fig. 2-7**)
   1. General impression
      a. Appearance
      b. Breathing
      c. Circulation
   2. Vital functions (**Table 2-2**)
      a. Level of consciousness
   3. Airway (**Figs. 2-8; Fig. 2-11**)
   4. Breathing (**Fig. 2-12; Table 2-2; Table 2-3**)
   5. Circulation (**Table 2-2**)
   6. Anticipating cardiopulmonary arrest (**Fig. 2-13**)
   7. Transport priority (**Table 2-4**)
      a. Urgent
      b. Nonurgent
      c. Pediatric trauma and Glasgow coma scales
   8. Transitional phase
      a. Allows the infant or child to become familiar with you and your equipment
      b. Use depends on the seriousness of the patient's condition
      c. Skip transition phase and proceed directly to treatment and transport for unconscious or acutely ill child.
D. Focused history and physical exam (pp. 65–70) (**Fig. 2-7**)
   1. History
      a. For infant, toddler, and preschool-age patient, obtain from parent/guardian.
      b. For school-age and adolescent patient, most information may be obtained from patient.
      c. For older adolescent patient, question patient in private regarding sexual activity, pregnancy, illicit drug and alcohol use.
   2. Physical exam
      a. Focused exam
         i. Head-to-toe in older child
         ii. Toe-to-head in younger child
      b. Glasgow coma scale (**Table 2-4**)
         i. Mild: 13–15
         ii. Moderate: 9–12
         iii. Severe: ≤8
      c. Vital signs (**Fig. 2-14**) (**Table 2-2; Table 2-5**)
      d. Noninvasive monitoring (**Fig. 2-15**)
         i. Pulse oximeter
         ii. Automated blood pressure devices
         iii. Self-registering thermometers
         iv. ECGs
E. Ongoing assessment (p. 70)
   1. Stable patient: every 15 minutes
   2. Critical patient: every 5 minutes

VII. General management of pediatric patients (pp. 70–93)

A. Basic airway management (pp. 70–77) (**Table 2-6**)
   1. Manual positioning
   2. Foreign body airway obstruction (FBAO)
      a. Mild obstruction
         i. Place in position of comfort; transport

  b. Severe airway obstruction
   i. Infants
    • Five back blows, five chest thrusts (**Proc. 2-1**)
    • If unconscious, begin CPR.
   ii. Children
    • Abdominal thrusts until the item is expelled (**Fig. 2-16**)
    • If unconscious, begin CPR.
 3. Suctioning (**Fig. 2-17**) (**Table 2-7**)
 4. Oxygenation
  a. Nonrebreather mask (**Fig. 2-18**)
  b. Blow-by oxygen if mask is not tolerated
 5. Oropharyngeal airway
  a. Size by measuring from corner of mouth to front of earlobe.
  b. Use the tongue blade to depress tongue and jaw for insertion. (**Fig. 2-19; Fig. 2-20; Table 2-8**)
 6. Nasopharyngeal airway
  a. Use for children who have a gag reflex but require prolonged ventilation.
  b. DO NOT use in patients with head or midface trauma.
 7. Ventilation
  a. Avoid excessive bag pressure and volume.
  b. Use proper-sized mask. (**Fig. 2-21**)
  c. Obtain chest rise with each breath.
  d. Allow adequate time for full chest recoil and exhalation.
  e. Provide 100 percent oxygen by using bag-value-mask (BVM) device reservoir.
  f. Do not use flow-restricted, oxygen-powered ventilation devices in pediatric resuscitation.
  g. Do not use BVMs with pop-off valves unless they can be readily occluded.
  h. Use Sellick maneuver to apply cricoid pressure. (**Fig. 2-22**)
  i. Position to avoid hyperextension of neck.
B. Advanced airway and ventilation management (pp. 77–85)
 1. Foreign-body clearing methods
 2. Needle cricothyrotomy
 3. Endotracheal intubation
  a. Anatomical and physiological concerns
   i. Creation of a visual plane from mouth to pharynx to glottis is difficult.
   ii. Selection of proper-sized tubes is critical.
   iii. Depth of insertion can be estimated based on age. (**Table 2-9**)
   iv. Either cuffed or uncuffed endotracheal tubes can be used in children, although in certain conditions a cuffed tube may be superior, but cuff pressure should be limited to 20 cm H_2O.
   v. Laryngoscopy and passage of an endotracheal tube are likely to cause a vagal response, slowing the heart rate.
  b. Indications
   i. Need for prolonged artificial ventilation
   ii. Inadequate ventilations with a BVM
   iii. Cardiac or respiratory arrest
   iv. Control of airway in a patient without cough or gag reflex
   v. To obtain a route for drug administration
   vi. Access to the airway for suctioning
  c. Technique (**Fig. 2-23**) (**Proc. 2-2**)
   i. Tube placement verification, preferably with end-tidal CO_2 detector

TEACHING STRATEGY 5
Researching an EMSC Project

TEACHING TIP
See if students can explain why younger children require support under the torso to maintain their airway. What is the anatomical difference?

POINT TO EMPHASIZE
Never use blind finger sweeps in a pediatric patient. DO NOT use nasal airways on a child with midface or head trauma.

TEACHING TIP
Ask students, What is the problem with using these devices on children?

POINT TO EMPHASIZE
Alternative airways (EOA, PTL, ETC) cannot be used in children. A proper-sized laryngeal mask (LMA) can be used in the pediatric patient. However, you should remember that LMAs do not protect the airway from aspiration.

ii. DOPE pneumonic
  - Displacement
  - Obstruction
  - Pneumothorax
  - Equipment failure
4. Rapid sequence intubation
  a. Indications
    i. Advanced airway management required
    ii. Patient has significant level of consciousness or gag reflex.
  b. Medications used are succinylcholine (Anectine) and a sedative agent such as midazolam, diazepam, thiopental, or fentanyl.
5. Rescue airways
  a. Laryngeal Mask Airway (LMA) (**Fig. 2-24**)
6. Nasogastric intubation
  a. Indications
    i. Inability to achieve adequate tidal volume during ventilation due to gastric distention
    ii. Presence of gastric distention in unresponsive patient
  b. Contraindicated with head trauma and midface trauma
  c. Technique (**Proc. 2-3**)
C. Circulation (pp. 86–88)
  1. Vascular access
    a. Techniques are basically same as in adults.
    b. Additional veins accessible in infants include neck and scalp veins.
  2. Intraosseous infusion (**Fig. 2-25a**)
    a. Used for fluids and medications
    b. Indications
      i. Existence of shock and cardiac arrest
      ii. Unresponsive patient
      iii. Unsuccessful attempts at peripheral IV insertion
    c. Contraindicated in the presence of fracture in extremity to be used or fracture of pelvis or bone proximal to chosen site
    d. Technique (**Fig. 2-25b; Fig. 2-26**)
  3. Fluid therapy
    a. Administer initial dosage of 20 mL/kg of lactated Ringer's or normal saline titrated to perfusion for hypovolemic shock.
    b. Monitor IV infusions closely.
  4. Medication objectives
    a. Correction of hypovolemia
    b. Increased perfusion pressure during chest compressions
    c. Stimulation of spontaneous or more forceful cardiac contractions
    d. Acceleration of heart rate
    e. Correction of metabolic acidosis
    f. Suppression of ventricular ectopy
    g. Maintenance of renal perfusion
  5. Dosages (**Table 2-10; Table 2-11**)
D. Electrical therapy (p. 88)
  1. Used less frequently in pediatric patients than in adults.
  2. Use initial dose of 4 J/kg.
  3. If unsuccessful, focus attention on correcting hypoxia and acidosis.
  4. Transport to a pediatric critical care unit, if possible.
E. C-spine immobilization (pp. 88–90)
  1. Special considerations
    a. Spinal injury less common in children than adults
    b. Larger head makes cervical spine more vulnerable

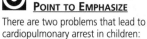

POINT TO EMPHASIZE

There are two problems that lead to cardiopulmonary arrest in children: shock and respiratory failure.

POINT TO EMPHASIZE

Any time an infant or child sustains a head injury, assume that a neck injury may also be present.

      c. Spinal cord injury can occur without injury to vertebral column.

      d. Children with positive mechanism should be immobilized until evaluated by hospital personnel.

  2. Techniques (**Proc. 2-4; Proc. 2-5**)

F. Transport guidelines (pp. 90–93) (**Fig. 2-27**)

  1. Time of transport

  2. Specialized facilities

  3. Specialized personnel

VIII. Specific medical emergencies. (pp. 93–121)

A. Infections (pp. 93–94)

  1. Account for majority of pediatric illnesses

  2. Varied signs and symptoms, depending on agent and extent of infection

  3. Management

      a. Take all standard precautions.

      b. Be familiar with common infections in your area.

      c. Be aware of status of your own immunity.

      d. Limit exposure to diseases to which you are not immune.

B. Respiratory emergencies (distress, failure, arrest) (pp. 94–96)

  1. Respiratory distress

      a. Signs and symptoms

         i. Normal mental status deteriorating to irritability and anxiety

         ii. Tachypnea

         iii. Retractions

         iv. Nasal flaring in infants

         v. Poor muscle tone

         vi. Tachycardia

         vii. Head bobbing

         viii. Grunting

         ix. Cyanosis that improves with supplemental oxygen

         x. If uncorrected, leads to respiratory failure

  2. Respiratory failure

      a. Assessment

         i. Irritability or anxiety deteriorating to lethargy

         ii. Marked tachypnea later deteriorating to bradypnea

         iii. Poor muscle tone

         iv. Marked tachycardia later deteriorating to bradycardia

         v. Central cyanosis

         vi. Ominous condition; patient is on verge of respiratory arrest

  3. Respiratory arrest

      a. Assessment

         i. Unresponsiveness deteriorating to coma

         ii. Bradypnea deteriorating to apnea

         iii. Absent chest wall motion

         iv. Bradycardia deteriorating to asystole

         v. Profound cyanosis

  4. Management of respiratory compromise

      a. Use graded approach to treatment based on severity of problem.

      b. Manage upper airway obstructions as needed.

      c. Insert airway adjunct if needed.

      d. Early respiratory failure: administer high-flow oxygen.

      e. Late respiratory failure/respiratory arrest

         i. Establishment of an airway

         ii. High-flow, high-concentration, supplemental oxygen administration

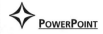

POWERPOINT PRESENTATION

Volume 5, Chapter 2, PowerPoint slides 112–195

POINT TO EMPHASIZE

Carefully count the pediatric patient's respiratory rate for at least 30 seconds, preferably for 1 minute.

iii. Mechanical ventilation with a BVM device attached to a reservoir delivering 100 percent oxygen

iv. Endotracheal intubation (or another acceptable airway) if mechanical ventilation does not rapidly improve the patient's condition

v. Consideration of gastric decompression with an orogastric or nasogastric tube if abdominal distention is impeding ventilation

vi. Consideration of needle decompression of the chest if a tension pneumothorax is thought to be present

vii. Consideration of cricothyrotomy if complete airway obstruction is present and the airway cannot be obtained by any other method

f. Obtain venous access.

g. Transport to appropriate facility.

h. Provide emotional, psychological support to parents

C. Specific respiratory emergencies (upper airway obstruction) (pp. 96–100)

1. Croup

a. Assessment (**Table 2-12; Fig. 2-28**)

i. Signs and symptoms of respiratory distress or failure, depending on severity

ii. Appears sick

iii. Stridor

iv. Barking (seal- or dog-like) or brassy cough

v. Hoarseness

vi. Low-grade fever

vii. Usually with history of upper respiratory infection in classic croup (1 to 2 days)

b. Management

i. Maintain airway.

ii. Administer cool mist oxygen at 4 to 6 L/min.

iii. Administer nebulized racemic epinephrine or albuterol.

iv. Keep child in position of comfort.

v. Do not agitate patient (no IVs, no BP, and so on).

vi. Keep parent/caregiver with infant or child if appropriate.

2. Epiglottitis

a. Assessment (**Table 2-12; Fig. 2-29**)

i. Signs and symptoms of respiratory distress or failure, depending on severity

ii. Appears agitated, sick

iii. Stridor

iv. Muffled voice

v. Drooling

vi. Sore throat and pain on swallowing

vii. High fever

viii. Usually no previous history but a rapid onset of symptoms (6 to 8 hours)

ix. Can quickly progress to respiratory arrest

b. Management (**Fig. 2-30**)

i. Allow parent to administer oxygen.

ii. Use two-rescuer ventilation with BVM if airway becomes obstructed.

iii. Attempt intubation with stylet in place if BVM not effective.

iv. Do not attempt intubation in settings with short transport times.

v. Know that performing chest compression upon glottic visualization during intubation may produce a bubble at the tracheal opening.

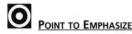

POINT TO EMPHASIZE

Whenever you find an infant, toddler, or young child in respiratory or cardiac arrest, assume complete upper airway obstruction until proven otherwise.

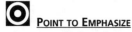

POINT TO EMPHASIZE

Never attempt to visualize the airway in patients with epiglottitis.

TEACHING TIP

Have students compare and contrast croup and epiglottitis.

©2009 Pearson Education, Inc.
Paramedic Care: Principles & Practice, Vol. 5, 3rd. Ed.

      vi. Consider needle cricothyrotomy per medical direction as a last resort if complete upper airway obstruction is present.

     vii. Allow patient to assume position of comfort.

   viii. Notify hospital of patient status early.

      ix. Do not agitate the patient—no IVs, no BP, do not look in patient's mouth.

       x. Keep the caregiver with the child if appropriate.

3. Bacterial tracheitis

 a. Assessment

       i. Respiratory distress or failure, depending on severity

      ii. Appears agitated, sick

    iii. High-grade fever

     iv. Inspiratory and expiratory stridor

      v. Coughing up pus/mucus

     vi. Hoarse voice

    vii. Pain in throat

  viii. Usually a history of croup in preceding few days

     ix. May progress to respiratory failure or arrest

 b. Management

       i. Ensure airway and ventilation.

      ii. Administer oxygen (possibly by blow-by).

    iii. With complete obstruction or respiratory failure/arrest: use BVM ventilation, intubation, endotracheal suctioning.

     iv. Use high pressure as required to adequately ventilate.

      v. Do not agitate the patient—no IVs, no BP. Do not look in patient's mouth.

     vi. Keep caregiver with child if appropriate.

4. Foreign body aspiration—upper airway

 a. Assessment—mild obstruction

       i. Signs and symptoms of respiratory distress or failure, depending on severity

      ii. Appears irritable or anxious, but not toxic

    iii. Inspiratory stridor

     iv. Muffled or hoarse voice

      v. Drooling

     vi. Pain in throat

    vii. Usually a history of choking if observed by adult

 b. Management—mild obstruction

       i. Place patient in sitting position.

      ii. Deliver oxygen by nonrebreather mask or blow-by.

    iii. Do not attempt to look in mouth.

     iv. Interventions other than oxygen and transport may precipitate complete obstruction.

 c. Assessment—severe obstruction

       i. Signs and symptoms of respiratory failure or arrest, depending on severity

      ii. Appears agitated or lethargic

    iii. No or minimal air movement

     iv. History often lacking

      v. Inability to ventilate despite proper airway positioning

 d. Management—severe obstruction

       i. Open airway and attempt to visualize the obstruction.

      ii. Sweep *visible* obstructions with your finger; do NOT perform blind finger sweeps.

    iii. Perform BLS FBAO maneuvers.

     iv. Attempt BVM ventilations.

      v. Perform laryngoscopy if BVM is unsuccessful.

      vi. Remove object if possible with pediatric Magill forceps.

      vii. Intubate if possible.

      viii. Continue BLS FBAO maneuvers if ALS is unsuccessful.

      ix. Consider needle cricothyrotomy as last resort.

      x. Notify hospital of patient status.

      xi. Keep caregiver with child, if appropriate.

D. Specific respiratory diseases (lower airway distress) (pp. 100–103)

  1. Asthma

    a. Assessment

      i. Respiratory distress or failure, depending on severity

      ii. Anxiety

      iii. Wheezing

      iv. Prolonged expiratory phase

      v. Symptoms usually began following exposure to known trigger.

    b. Management

      i. Administer oxygen by tolerated method.

      ii. Use BVM ventilations for respiratory failure/arrest (progressive lethargy, poor muscle tone, shallow respiratory effort).

      iii. Use endotracheal intubation for respiratory failure/arrest with prolonged BVM ventilations or inadequate response to BVM.

      iv. Administer nebulized beta agonists. (**Fig. 2-31**)

      v. Give steroids, particularly if transport times are long.

      vi. Use subcutaneous epinephrine 1:1000 or terbutaline with severe respiratory distress or failure.

      vii. Allow patient to assume position of comfort.

      viii. Keep caregiver with child if appropriate.

  2. Bronchiolitis

    a. Assessment

      i. Signs and symptoms of respiratory distress or failure, depending on severity

      ii. Anxiety

      iii. Wheezing

      iv. Diffuse crackles (rales)

      v. Usually history of upper respiratory infection symptoms

      vi. Bronchiolitis and asthma may present very similarly.

    b. Management

      i. Administer oxygen by tolerated method.

      ii. Use BVM ventilations for respiratory failure/arrest (progressive lethargy, poor muscle tone, shallow respiratory effort).

      iii. Use endotracheal intubation for respiratory failure/arrest with prolonged BVM ventilations or inadequate response to BVM ventilations.

      iv. Administer nebulized bronchodilators.

      v. Monitor cardiac rhythm and oxygen saturation.

      vi. Keep caregiver with child if appropriate.

  3. Pneumonia

    a. Assessment

      i. Signs and symptoms of respiratory distress or failure, depending on severity

      ii. Anxiety

      iii. Decreased breath sounds

      iv. Crackles (rales)

      v. Rhonchi (diffuse or localized)

      vi. Pain in chest

©2009 Pearson Education, Inc.
Paramedic Care: Principles & Practice, Vol. 5, 3rd. Ed.

   vii. Fever

   viii. Usually a history of lower airway respiratory tract infection

  b. Management

   i. Administer oxygen by tolerated method.

   ii. Use BVM ventilations for respiratory failure/arrest (progressive lethargy, poor muscle tone, shallow respiratory effort).

   iii. Use endotracheal intubation for respiratory failure with prolonged BVM ventilations or inadequate response to BVM ventilations.

   iv. Allow patient to assume position of comfort.

   v. Provide emotional, psychological support to parents.

   vi. Keep caregiver with child if appropriate.

 4. Foreign body lower airway obstruction—lower airway

  a. Assessment

   i. Signs and symptoms or respiratory distress or failure, depending on severity

   ii. Anxiety

   iii. Decreased breath sounds

   iv. Crackles (rales)

   v. Rhonchi (localized or diffuse)

   vi. Pain in chest

   vii. May be a history of choking if witnessed by an adult

  b. Management

   i. Administer oxygen by tolerated method.

   ii. Use BVM ventilations for respiratory failure/arrest (progressive lethargy, poor muscle tone, shallow respiratory effort).

   iii. Use endotracheal intubation for respiratory failure/arrest with prolonged BVM ventilations or inadequate response to BVM ventilations.

   iv. Do not attempt to retrieve foreign body, because it is beyond the reach of Magill forceps.

   v. Allow patient to assume position of comfort.

E. Shock (hypoperfusion) (pp. 103–110)

 1. Types of shock

  a. Compensated (early) shock—signs and symptoms

   i. Irritability or anxiety

   ii. Tachycardia

   iii. Tachypnea

   iv. Weak peripheral pulses, full central pulses

   v. Delayed capillary refill

   vi. Cool, pale extremities

   vii. Systolic blood pressure within normal limits

   viii. Decreased urinary output

  b. Decompensated shock—signs and symptoms (**Fig. 2-32**)

   i. Lethargy or coma

   ii. Marked tachycardia or bradycardia

   iii. Marked tachypnea or bradypnea

   iv. Absent peripheral pulses, weak central pulses

   v. Markedly delayed capillary refill

   vi. Cool, pale, dusky, mottled extremities

   vii. Hypotension

   viii. Markedly decreased urinary output

   ix. Absence of tears

  c. Irreversible shock

   i. Occurs when treatment is inadequate or is begun too late to prevent significant tissue damage and death.

POINT TO EMPHASIZE
A slight increase in the heart rate is one of the earliest signs of shock.

POINT TO EMPHASIZE
The hallmark of decompensated shock is a fall in blood pressure (an ominous sign in children).

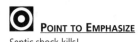
2. Hypovolemic noncardiogenic shock results from loss of extracellular fluid secondary to vomiting, diarrhea, blood loss, and/or burns. Treatment involves giving supplemental oxygen, obtaining vascular access, and giving fluid in 20 mL/kg boluses until perfusion is restored.

3. Distributive shock
   a. Distributive shock (septic shock) is caused by infection of bloodstream by a pathogen (usually bacterial).
   b. Distributive shock (anaphylaxis) is caused by exposure to an antigen to which the patient previously has been sensitized.
   c. Distributive shock (neurogenic shock) is caused by sudden peripheral vasodilation resulting from interruption of nervous control of the peripheral nervous system.

4. Cardiogenic shock in children usually occurs secondary to another problem, such as drowning or toxic ingestion.

5. Congenital heart disease
   a. Primary cause of heart disease in children
   b. Most cases detected at birth, but some problems not discovered until later in childhood
   c. Common symptom is cyanosis resulting from mixing of oxygenated and unoxygenated blood via openings in cardiac septum or between great vessels.

6. Cardiomyopathy
   a. Disease or dysfunction of the heart muscle
   b. Management
      i. Supplemental oxygen
      ii. Vascular access
      iii. Restriction of IV fluids
      iv. Diuretics
      v. Use of pressor agents

7. Dysrhythmias
   a. Generally uncommon in children
   b. Tachydysrhythmias
      i. Rate is greater than estimated maximum normal heart rate for child.
      ii. Can result from primary heart disease or secondary causes
   c. Supraventricular tachycardia
   d. Ventricular tachycardia with a pulse (**Fig. 2-33**)
   e. Bradydysrhythmias (**Fig. 2-34**)
      i. Most common type of dysrhythmia
   f. Asystole (**Fig. 2-35**)
   g. Ventricular fibrillation/pulseless ventricular tachycardia
   h. Pulseless electrical activity

F. Neurologic emergencies (pp. 110–115)
   1. Seizures
      a. Common reason for EMS being summoned for pediatric patients
      b. Results from abnormal firing of neurons in brain
      c. Assessment—generalized seizure
         i. Sudden jerking of both sides of the body followed by tenseness and relaxation of the body
         ii. Loss of consciousness
      d. Assessment—focal seizure
         i. Sudden jerking of a part of the body (arm, leg)
         ii. Lip smacking
         iii. Eye blinking
         iv. Staring
         v. Confusion
         vi. Lethargy

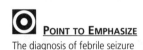

e. Management
  i. Evaluate
    • Adequacy of respirations
    • Level of consciousness
    • Neurologic signs
    • Evidence of injury
    • Status of hydration
  ii. Maintain patent airway.
  iii. Place patient on side.
  iv. Do not place anything in mouth.
  v. Prevent injury.
  vi. Administer high-flow oxygen.
  vii. If patient is febrile, remove excess clothing but avoid extreme cooling.
  viii. Check blood glucose levels. Give dextrose if hypoglycemic.
  ix. If status epilepticus, give diazepam or lorazepam.
  x. If seizure appears to be due to fever and a long transport time is anticipated, consider acetaminophen elixir or suppositories.

2. Meningitis
  a. Infection of the meninges, the lining of the brain and spinal cord
  b. Types
    i. Viral
      • Aseptic meningitis
    ii. Bacterial
      • *Streptococcus pneumoniae*
      • *Haemophilus influenzae*
      • *Neisseria meningitides*
  c. Assessment (**Fig. 2-36**)
    i. History of recent ear or respiratory tract infection
    ii. High fever
    iii. Lethargy or irritability
    iv. Severe headache
    v. Stiff neck
    vi. Infants may not develop stiff neck, but will become lethargic, will not feed well, and may have a bulging anterior fontanelle.
  d. Management
    i. Supportive care
    ii. Rapid transport to hospital
    iii. 20 mL/kg fluid boluses if shock present

G. Gastrointestinal emergencies (pp. 115–116)
  1. Nausea and vomiting
    a. Not diseases in themselves, but symptoms of other diseases
    b. Assessment (**Table 2-13**)
    c. Management
      i. Supportive care
      ii. Vascular access if patient unable to keep fluids down
      iii. For severe dehydration, 20 mL/kg boluses of lactated Ringer's or normal saline
  2. Diarrhea
    a. Common occurrence in childhood
    b. Generally considered to be 10 or more stools a day
    c. Usually a result of viral gastroenteritis or secondary to infection elsewhere in body
    d. Management
      i. Supportive care
      ii. Vascular access if dehydration present

POINT TO EMPHASIZE

Some medical directors prefer lorazepam (Ativan) as the anticonvulsant of choice for pediatric patients with febrile seizures.

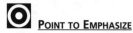
       iii. For severe dehydration, 20 mL/kg boluses of lactated Ringer's or normal saline

H. Metabolic emergencies (pp. 116–119)

  1. Hypoglycemia

    a. Usually seen in newborn infants and in children with type I diabetes

    b. Assessment (**Table 2-14**)

    c. Measure blood glucose. (**Fig. 2-37**)

    d. Management

      i. Monitor ABCs.

      ii. Determine if caregivers have given any glucose-containing material before EMS arrived.

      iii. Check blood glucose level.

      iv. If patient is conscious and alert, give oral glucose or glucose-containing fluids.

      v. If no response or if patient has altered mental status:
- Administer $D_{25}W$ intravenously.
- Administer glucagon IM if IV access is not possible.
- Repeat blood glucose test 10 to 15 minutes after dextrose infusion.

      vi. Provide emotional, psychological support to caregivers and patient.

      vii. Avoid labeling test results as "good" or "bad."

  2. Hyperglycemia

    a. Abnormally high concentration of blood glucose

    b. Most common finding in new-onset diabetics

    c. Early assessment (**Table 2-15**)

      i. Increased thirst

      ii. Increased urination

      iii. Weight loss

    d. Late assessment (dehydration and early ketoacidosis)

      i. Weakness

      ii. Abdominal pain

      iii. Generalized aches

      iv. Loss of appetite

      v. Nausea

      vi. Vomiting

    e. Measure blood glucose

      i. >200 mg/dL indicates hyperglycemia

    f. Management

      i. Monitor ABCs and vital signs.

      ii. Establish vascular access.

      iii. Give 20 mL/kg boluses of IV fluid titrated to vital signs and mental status.

      iv. Be prepared to intubate if patient's respirations decrease.

      v. If patient's blood glucose level cannot be determined reliably and there is uncertainty as to whether patient is hypoglycemic or hyperglycemic, give glucose.

I. Poisoning and toxic exposure (pp. 119–121)

  1. Common substances of pediatric poisonings (**Fig. 2-38**)

  2. Assessment (**Fig. 2-39**)

    a. Signs and symptoms vary depending upon both the poisoning/toxic substance and the time since the child was exposed.

    b. Respiratory system depression

    c. Circulatory system depression

    d. Central nervous system stimulation or depression

    e. Alterations of thought or behavior

    f. Gastrointestinal system irritation

  3. Management—responsive patient

    a. Give oxygen.

    b. Contact medical direction and/or poison center.

    c. Consider need for activated charcoal.

    d. Transport patient and product.

    e. Monitor patient continuously.

  4. Management—unresponsive patient

    a. Ensure patent airway, suction as needed.

    b. Give oxygen.

    c. Be prepared to assist ventilations.

    d. Contact medical direction and/or poison center.

    e. Transport.

    f. Monitor patient continuously.

    g. Rule out trauma as cause of altered mental status.

IX. Trauma emergencies. (pp. 121–130)

A. Mechanisms of injury (pp. 121–124)

  1. Falls

    a. Single most common cause of injury in children (**Fig. 2-40**)

    b. Serious injury or death resulting from truly accidental falls is relatively uncommon unless from a significant height.

  2. Motor vehicle collisions (**Fig. 2-41**)

    a. Leading cause of permanent brain injury and new cases of epilepsy

    b. Leading cause of death and serious injury in children

  3. Car vs. pedestrian injuries

  4. Drownings and near-drownings

    a. Third leading cause of injury or death in children between birth and 4 years old

  5. Penetrating injuries

    a. Stab wounds and firearm injuries account for approximately 10 to 15 percent of all pediatric trauma admissions.

  6. Burns

    a. Leading cause of accidental death in the home for children under 14 years old

  7. Physical abuse

    a. Factors influencing

      i. Increased poverty

      ii. Domestic disturbance

      iii. Younger-aged parents

      iv. Substance abuse

      v. Community violence

    b. All cases must be thoroughly documented

B. Special considerations (pp. 124–127)

  1. Airway control (**Fig. 2-42**)

    a. Maintain in-line stabilization in neutral, not sniffing, position.

    b. Administer 100 percent oxygen to all trauma patients.

    c. Maintain patent airway via suctioning and jaw thrust.

    d. Be prepared to assist ineffective respirations.

    e. Perform intubation when airway remains inadequate. (**Fig. 2-43**)

    f. Place gastric tube after intubation.

    g. Know that needle cricothyrotomy is rarely indicated for traumatic upper airway obstruction.

POWERPOINT PRESENTATION
Volume 5, Chapter 2, PowerPoint slides 196–220

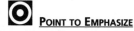

POINT TO EMPHASIZE
Trauma is the number one cause of death in children.

2. Immobilization
   a. Use appropriate-sized pediatric immobilization equipment.
   b. Maintain supine neutral in-line position for infants, toddlers, and preschoolers by placing padding from shoulders to hips.
3. Fluid management
   a. Management of the airway and breathing take priority over management of circulation because circulatory compromise is less common in children than adults.
   b. Vascular access
      i. Insert large-bore intravenous catheter into a large peripheral vein.
      ii. Do not delay transport to gain access.
      iii. Use intraosseous access in children <6 years of age if intravenous access fails.
      iv. Administer initial fluid bolus of 20 mL/kg of lactated Ringer's or NS.
      v. Reassess vital signs and bolus with 20 mL/kg if no improvement.
      vi. If improvement does not occur after the second bolus, there is likely to be significant blood loss and the need for rapid surgical intervention.
4. Pediatric analgesia and sedation
   a. Frequently overlooked aspect of care
   b. Indications for analgesia include burns, long bone fractures, and dislocations.
   c. Morphine and fentanyl are common choices.
   d. Butorphanol and nalbuphine have unpredictable effects on children.
   e. Indications for sedation include penetrating eye injuries, prolonged rescues, cardioversion, and painful procedures.
   f. Intranasal administration of fentanyl is an effective route of administering analgesia in the prehospital setting without first obtaining IV access.
5. Traumatic brain injury
   a. Glasgow coma scale
      i. Mild: 13–15
      ii. Moderate: 9–12
      iii. Severe: ≤ 8
   b. Early recognition and aggressive management can reduce mortality and morbidity.
   c. Signs of increased ICP
      i. Elevated blood pressure
      ii. Bradycardia
      iii. Rapid, deep respirations (Kussmaul) progressing to slow, deep respirations alternating with rapid, deep respirations (Cheyne-Stokes)
      iv. Bulging fontanelle (infant)
   d. Specific management
      i. Administer high-concentration oxygen for mild to moderate head injuries (GCS 9 to 15).
      ii. Intubate and ventilate at normal breathing rate with 100 percent oxygen for severe head injuries (GCS 3 to 8).
         • Use of lidocaine may blunt rise in ICP (controversial).
         • Consider RSI per medical direction.

 ©2009 Pearson Education, Inc. *Paramedic Care: Principles & Practice, Vol. 5, 3rd. Ed.*

C. Specific injuries (pp. 127–130)
   1. Head, face, and neck injury
      a. Larger relative mass of the head and lack of neck muscle strength contribute to increased momentum in acceleration-deceleration injuries and a greater stress to the cervical spine region.
      b. Sixty to 70 percent of pediatric fractures occur in C-1 or C-2.
      c. Head injury is the most common cause of death in pediatric trauma victims.
      d. Soft tissues, skull, and brain are more compliant in children than in adults.
      e. Due to open fontanelles and sutures, infants up to an average age of 16 months may be more tolerant of an increase in intracranial pressure and can have delayed signs.
      f. Subdural bleeds in an infant can produce hypotension (extremely rare).
      g. Significant blood loss can occur through scalp lacerations and should be controlled immediately.
      h. The modified Glasgow coma scale should be used for infants and young children.
   2. Chest injury
      a. Chest injuries in children under 14 years of age are usually the result of blunt trauma.
      b. Due to the compliance of the chest wall, severe intrathoracic injury can be present without signs of external injury.
      c. Tension pneumothorax is poorly tolerated and is an immediate threat to life.
      d. Flail segment is an uncommon injury in children; when noted without a significant mechanism of injury, suspect child abuse.
      e. Many children with cardiac tamponade will have no physical signs of tamponade other than hypotension.
   3. Abdominal injury
      a. Musculature is minimal and poorly protects the viscera.
      b. Organs most commonly injured are liver, kidney, and spleen.
      c. Onset of symptoms may be rapid or gradual.
      d. Due to the small size of the abdomen, be certain to palpate only one quadrant at a time.
      e. Any child who is hemodynamically unstable without evidence of obvious source of blood loss should be considered as having an abdominal injury until proven otherwise.
   4. Extremity injury (**Fig. 2-44**)
      a. Relatively more common in children than adults.
      b. Flexible bones tend to result in incomplete breaks (bend, buckle, and greenstick fractures).
      c. Growth plate injuries are common and may lead to permanent disability.
      d. Compartment syndrome is an emergency in children.
      e. Any sites of active bleeding must be controlled.
      f. Splinting should be performed to prevent further injury and blood loss.
      g. PASG may be useful in unstable pelvic fractures with hypotension.
   5. Burns
      a. Second leading cause of death in children
      b. Leading cause of accidental death in the home in children under age 14
      c. Thermal, electrical, and chemical mechanisms
      d. Scalding is the most common cause.

POINT TO EMPHASIZE
Children tend to develop pulmonary contusions, sometimes massive, following blunt trauma to the chest.

POINT TO EMPHASIZE
Burns are the second leading cause of death in children.

e. Rule of nines must be modified to account for child's larger head size. (**Fig. 2-45**)
   f. Rule of palm can be used to estimate size of smaller burns.
   g. Management priorities
      i. Prompt management of the airway is required, because swelling can develop rapidly.
      ii. If intubation is required, an endotracheal tube up to two sizes smaller than what would normally be used may be required.
      iii. Thermally burned children are very susceptible to hypothermia; maintain normal body temperature.
      iv. Suspect musculoskeletal injuries in electrical burn patients and perform spine immobilization techniques.

X. Sudden infant death syndrome (SIDS). (pp. 130–131)

A. Epidemiology (pp. 130–131)
   1. Sudden death of infant during first year of life from an illness of unknown etiology
   2. Leading cause of death from 2 weeks to 1 year old
   3. Prevention strategies
      a. Infants should sleep in supine position.
      b. Avoid overwrapping infants.
      c. Avoid smoking before and after pregnancy.
      d. Avoid filling cribs with soft bedding.
B. Assessment (p. 131)
   1. No external signs of injury
   2. Lividity
   3. Frothy blood-tinged drainage from nose/mouth
   4. Rigor mortis
   5. Evidence that the baby was very active just before death (rumpled bed clothes, unusual position or location in the bed)
C. Management (p. 131)
   1. Initiate CPR unless the infant is obviously dead (unquestionably dead to a layperson).
   2. Perform ALS as indicated.
   3. Be prepared for the range of possible family emotional reactions.
   4. Parents/caregiver should be allowed to accompany baby in ambulance.
   5. Explain that certain information about infant's health is necessary to determine care to be given.
   6. Use the baby's name.
   7. Phrase questions so that blame is not implied.
   8. Critical incident stress debriefing of responders may be needed.

XI. Child abuse and neglect. (pp. 131–134)

A. Epidemiology (p. 131)
   1. Leading cause of death in infants <6 months old
   2. Between 2,000 and 5,000 children die each year as a result of abuse and neglect.
B. Perpetrators of abuse or neglect (pp. 131–132)
   1. Parent, legal guardian, foster parent; person, institution, agency, or program having custody of the child; person serving as a caretaker (e.g., babysitter)
   2. Perpetrators can come from any geographic, religious, ethnic, racial, occupational, educational, or social background.
C. Types (pp. 132–133) (**Fig. 2-46; Fig. 2-47**)
   1. Psychological
   2. Physical

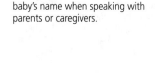

POINT TO EMPHASIZE

At all points in a SIDS case, use the baby's name when speaking with parents or caregivers.

POINT TO EMPHASIZE

In SIDS, active and aggressive care should continue until delivery to the ER unless the infant is obviously dead.

POWERPOINT PRESENTATION

Volume 5, Chapter 2, PowerPoint slides 221–227

3. Sexual
   4. Neglect (either physical or emotional)
D. Assessment of potentially abused or neglected child (pp. 133–134)
   1. Physical indicators of abuse
      a. Obvious or suspected fractures in child <2 years old
      b. Multiple injuries in various stages of healing, especially burns and bruises (**Fig. 2-48**)
      c. More injuries than usually seen in children of same age and size
      d. Injuries scattered on many areas of body
      e. Bruises or burns in patterns that suggest intentional infliction
      f. Increased ICP in infants
      g. Suspected intraabdominal trauma in a young child
      h. Any injury that does not fit the description given of the cause
   2. Indicators of abuse in the history
      a. History does not match nature or severity of injury.
      b. History is vague or changes during the interview.
      c. Accusations that child injured himself intentionally
      d. Delay in seeking help
      e. Child dressed inappropriately for situation
      f. Revealing comments by bystanders, especially siblings
   3. Indicators of neglect
      a. Extreme malnutrition
      b. Multiple insect bites
      c. Long-standing skin infections
      d. Extreme lack of cleanliness
      e. Verbal or social skills far below those expected of a child of similar age and background
      f. Lack of appropriate medical care (**Fig. 2-49**)
E. Management of the potentially abused or neglected child (p. 134)
   1. Assess the injuries/neglect and render appropriate care.
   2. Look at the environment for condition and cleanliness.
   3. Look for evidence of anything out of the ordinary.
   4. Look and listen to caregiver/family members.
   5. Assess whether the explanation fits the injury.
   6. Do not "cross-examine" the parents.
   7. Try to be supportive of parents if this will help you to transport the child.
   8. Never leave transport to the alleged abuser.
   9. Document all findings thoroughly.
   10. Report suspicions to appropriate personnel.
F. Resources for abuse and neglect (p. 134)
   1. State, regional, and local child protection agencies
   2. Hospital social service department

XII. Infants and children with special needs. (pp. 134–138)

A. Types (pp. 134–135)
   1. Premature babies
   2. Lung diseases
   3. Heart diseases
   4. Neurologic diseases
   5. Chronic diseases
      a. Cystic fibrosis
      b. Asthma
      c. Childhood cancers
      d. Cerebral palsy

POINT TO EMPHASIZE
Never leave transport of an abused child to an alleged abuser.

POINT TO EMPHASIZE
In many states, paramedics are mandatory reporters of child (and other) abuse and neglect. Check your state laws.

6. Altered functions from birth

    a. Cerebral palsy

    b. Spina bifida

B. Common home care devices (pp. 135–138)

    1. Tracheostomy tube (**Fig. 2-51**)

        a. Complications may include

            i. Obstruction

            ii. Bleeding

            iii. Air leak

            iv. Dislodgement

            v. Infection

        b. Management

            i. Maintain an open airway.

            ii. Suction the tube, as needed.

            iii. Maintain position of comfort.

            iv. Give oxygen if respiratory distress is present.

            v. Intubation orally in absence of upper airway obstruction.

            vi. Intubate via stoma if upper airway obstruction is present.

            vii. Transport.

    2. Apnea monitors (**Fig. 2-51**)

        a. Used to alert parents and caregivers to cessation of breathing in an infant

    3. Home artificial ventilators

        a. Complications include

            i. Mechanical failure

            ii. Power outages

         b. Management

            i. Ensure airway.

            ii. Artificially ventilate with BVM and oxygen.

            iii. Transport.

    4. Central venous lines

        a. Intravenous lines that are placed in superior vena cava for long-term use

        b. Uses

            i. Antibiotics

            ii. Chemotherapy

            iii. IV nutrition

         c. Complications

            i. Cracked line

            ii. Infection

            iii. Clots

            iv. Bleeding

            v. Air embolism

         d. Management

            i. If cracked line

               • Clamp between crack and patient.

            ii. If altered mental status following cracked line

               • Position on left side with head down.

            iii. If bleeding

               • Apply pressure.

            iv. Transport.

    5. Gastric feedings and gastrostomy tubes (**Fig. 2-52**)

        a. Tubes placed directly into stomach for feeding

        b. Complications

            i. Bleeding at site

            ii. Dislodged tube

POINT TO EMPHASIZE

Most parents who have infants on apnea monitors have received training in pediatric CPR.

   iii. Respiratory distress secondary to aspiration
   iv. Altered mental status in diabetics due to missed feedings.
  c. Management
   i. Ensure adequate airway.
   ii. Administer 100 percent oxygen.
   iii. Suction if needed.
   iv. Consider hypoglycemia in diabetic patient who cannot be fed.
   v. Transport sitting or lying on right side, head elevated.
 6. Shunts
  a. Device running from the brain to abdomen to drain excess cerebrospinal fluid
  b. Complications
   i. Shunt connections may separate due to child's growth.
   ii. Increase in intracranial pressure occurs, producing altered mental status, respiratory distress, and posturing.
  c. Management
   i. Manage airway.
   ii. Ensure adequate artificial ventilation.
   iii. Transport with head elevated if possible.
C. General assessment and management procedures (p. 138)
 1. Patients with special needs require the same assessment as other patients.
 2. The child's special need is often an ongoing process.
 3. Concentrate on the acute problem.
 4. Ask the parent or caregiver, "What unusual situation caused you to call an ambulance?"
 5. Most parents or caregivers will be very knowledgeable about the patient's condition.
 6. Avoid using the term "disability."
 7. Never assume the patient cannot understand what you are saying.
 8. Involve the parents or caregivers and the patient.
 9. Treat the patient with a special need with the same respect as any other patient.

XIII. Mass/multiple-casualty incidents (MCIs) involving children. (pp. 138–141)

A. JumpSTART Pediatric MCI Triage Tool
 1. Objective tool developed specifically for the triage of children in the multicasualty/disaster setting
 2. Developed in 1995 to parallel the structure of the START system
 3. Designed for use in disaster/multicasualty settings and not for daily EMS or hospital triage
 4. Intended for the triage of children with acute injuries and may not be appropriate for the primary triage of children with medical illnesses in a disaster setting
B. JumpSTART's objectives
 1. Optimize the primary triage of injured children in the MCI setting
 2. Enhance the effectiveness of resource allocation for all MCI victims
 3. Reduce the emotional burden on triage personnel who may have to make rapid life-or-death decisions about the injured
C. Using the JumpSTART System (**Fig. 2-53**)
 1. Identify and direct all ambulatory patients to the designated minor (GREEN) area for secondary triage and treatment.
 2. Assess breathing.
  a. If the child is breathing spontaneously, go on to the next step (assessing respiratory rate).

POINT TO EMPHASIZE

In most cases, concentrate on the acute problem rather than the ongoing special need.

POWERPOINT PRESENTATION

Volume 5, Chapter 2, PowerPoint slides 228–230

b. If the child is apneic or with very irregular breathing, open the airway using standard positioning techniques.

    i. If positioning results in resumption of spontaneous respirations, tag the patient immediate (RED) and move on to the next patient.

    ii. If the child is not breathing after airway opening, check for peripheral pulse.

        • If there is no pulse, tag the patient deceased/nonsalvageable (BLACK) and move on to the next patient.

        • If there is a peripheral pulse, give 5 mouth-to-barrier ventilations.

            ○ If apnea persists, tag the patient deceased/nonsalvageable (BLACK) and move on to the next patient.

            ○ If breathing resumes after the "jumpstart" (ventilatory trial), tag the patient immediate (RED) and move on to the next patient.

3. Assess respiratory rate.

    a. If the child's respiratory rate is 15–45 per minute, proceed to the next step (assess perfusion).

    b. If the respiratory rate is <15 or >45 per minute or irregular, tag the patient as immediate (RED) and move on to the next patient.

4. Assess perfusion.

    a. If a peripheral pulse is palpable, proceed to the next step (assess mental status).

    b. If no peripheral pulse is present (in the least injured limb), tag the patient immediate (RED) and move on to the next patient.

5. Assess mental status.

    a. Use the AVPU scale to assess mental status.

    b. If Alert, responsive to Verbal, or appropriately responsive to Pain, tag the patient as delayed (YELLOW) and move on to the next patient.

    c. If inappropriately responsive to Pain or Unresponsive, tag the patient as immediate (RED) and move on to the next patient.

D. Modifications for nonambulatory children

    1. If any meet immediate (RED) criteria, tag as RED. If the child meets the delayed (YELLOW) criteria, classify further:

        a. Delayed (YELLOW) if significant external signs of injury are found

        b. Minor (GREEN) if no significant external injury is found

E. Reassessing victims tagged as dead/nonsalvageable

    1. Unless clearly suffering from injuries incompatible with life, victims tagged in the dead/nonsalvageable (BLACK) category should be reassessed once critical interventions have been completed for immediate (RED) and delayed (YELLOW) patients.

    2. Care should be taken to preserve the dignity of the dead, at the same time being careful not to disturb any forensic evidence present.

F. Families who can't or won't be separated

    1. If the family can't or won't be separated, send them all to the triage/treatment area corresponding to the category of the most injured family member.

XIV. Summary. Pediatric emergencies are among the most stressful a paramedic will face. Most pediatric emergencies result from trauma, respiratory distress, ingestion of poisons, or febrile seizure activity. Child abuse and neglect are also significant problems. Remember that it will be necessary to modify the approaches to assessment and management when dealing with pediatric patients. (pp. 141–142)

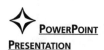

PowerPoint

PRESENTATION
Volume 5, Chapter 2, PowerPoint slide 231

 ©2009 Pearson Education, Inc.
Paramedic Care: Principles & Practice, Vol. 5, 3rd. Ed.

SKILLS DEMONSTRATION AND PRACTICE

Students can practice the skills discussed in this chapter in the following settings.

Skills Lab One: Divide the class into as many groups as appropriate. Have the groups circulate through the stations. Monitor the groups to be sure that all groups have a chance to practice each of the skills.

Station	Equipment and Personnel Needed	Activities
Station 1–1	Stethoscopes	After demonstrating how to perform a pediatric assessment, have students perform an initial assessment, taking vital signs and identifying IV and IO sites on an infant, toddler, preschooler, grade-school-aged child, and adolescent.
Pediatric	Blood pressure cuffs	Children of instructors, students, or community members may be recruited to serve as models. They should be accompanied by a parent, and a consent form should be signed by the parent, agreeing to the physical exam and accepting responsibility for the child's supervision during the workshop.
Assessment	Chairs for parents and children "Exam" table Blankets Pen lights Rewards for children (crayons, books, Legos) Toys/snacks for children to play with/eat during station time 1 instructor 1 infant 1 preschooler 1 grade-school-aged child 1 adolescent	
Station 1–2	Child manikins	After demonstrating basic life support techniques, have each student practice and demonstrate one-rescuer infant and child CPR, two-rescuer child CPR, infant FBAO management, and child FBAO management. Demonstration should be kept simple to reinforce the priorities and techniques of CPR.

Station	Equipment and Personnel Needed	Activities
Basic life support	Infant manikins Alcohol wipes Extra lungs CPR skills sheets	
Station 1–3	Infant manikins	After demonstrating pediatric airway adjuncts, have each student give return demonstrations of the use of oxygen delivery systems, oral airways, bag-valve-mask devices, and suctioning devices.
Pediatric airway adjuncts	Child manikins Infant, child, and adult bag-valve-mask devices Oropharyngeal airways: 00, 0, 1, 2, 3, 4 Suction devices: Bulb syringe, DeLee suction, tonsil-tip suction device, meconium aspiration adaptor, and standard suction catheters (5, 6, 8, 10, 14 French) Pediatric and adult oxygen masks Pediatric and adult nasal cannulas Pocket masks	
Station 1–4	Infant intubation manikins	After demonstrating endotracheal intubation, have each student give a return demonstration of proper intubation technique for an infant and child.
Endotracheal intubation	Child intubation manikins BVM device for each manikin Stethoscopes Tape Laryngoscope handles Laryngoscope blades: Curved 2, 3; straight 0, 1, 2, 3 Endotracheal tubes: 2.5, 3.0, 3.5, 4.0, 4.5, 5.0, 6.0, 6.5, 7.0 Stylets of appropriate sizes Pediatric and adult Magill forceps	

Station	Equipment and Personnel Needed	Activities
Station 1–5	Equipment for peripheral IV	After demonstrating peripheral vascular access, have each student give a return demonstration of pediatric vascular access techniques, including:
Peripheral vascular access	Over-the-needle catheters: 18-, 20-, 22-, 24-gauge Butterfly needles: 19-, 21-, 23-, 25-gauge Pediatric IV arms Model head for scalp vein IV insertion IV solutions 3-mL syringes Solution administration sets Alcohol prep pads Tourniquets Materials for securing IVs: arm boards, tape Sharps container IV poles Equipment for intraosseous infusion Raw chicken legs Bone marrow needles 5-mL syringes Exam gloves Flush solution (250-mL bag of NS)	1. Cannulation of an arm vein 2. Cannulation of a scalp vein 3. Placement of an intraosseous line
Station 1–6	Long backboard with attached straps	After demonstrating pediatric immobilization, have students demonstrate effective techniques for adapting adult equipment to immobilizing children.
Pediatric immobilization	Short spinal immobilization device (preferably a KED) 2-inch tape Blankets Pediatric cervical collars: small, medium, and large Towels Pillows Scissors Infant car seat Infant manikin 1 child, age 4 to 8	

Hospital: Begin patient assessments in emergency department.

Field Internship: Begin patient assessments on simple emergency calls.

YOU MAKE THE CALL

Review student responses to the You Make the Call scenario on text page 142. Suggested responses to the questions that follow the scenario are given below. Point out to students that these are acceptable answers but not necessarily the only ones. Discuss with students pros and cons of points where their responses differ from these.

1. What are your assessment priorities for this patient?

   (You should immediately pick up on the fact that the family dynamics in this case are stressed and that this is a potentially dangerous situation. The story is a little odd in that the neighbors called 911 because they heard "loud cries" coming from the house. Your assessment priorities are to ensure your own safety and that of your partner. Identify an exit and be ready to leave if violence erupts. Leave your equipment until law enforcement personnel arrive. Your assessment should follow the standard approach taught in this book. Assess the airway, breathing, and circulation as well as other components of the initial assessment. Regardless of your suspicions, your primary responsibility is to care for the child. However, carefully monitor the environment and note any clues that might point to child abuse. The rule "eyes open, mouth shut" really applies here. Document your findings and prepare for transport.)

2. What interventions would you perform on-scene and en route to the receiving hospital?

   (The child should be transported if at all possible. Provide any indicated care including airway management, spinal immobilization, bandaging and splinting, IV therapy, emotional support, and any other steps. Report your suspicions to hospital and law enforcement personnel. Do not spend a great deal of time quizzing the parents about the event as it may make them suspicious. The parents may refuse transport, arguing that they will take the child to the doctor later. If this occurs, you should gently remind them that emergency care can't wait. The child may need tests that are only available in the ED. Try to gain the trust of the parents. If the family steadfastly refuses, inform the parents of the risks of refusing transport and have a refusal document signed by both parents and witnessed by a police officer. Remind the parents that they can call you back at any time and you will immediately respond. If the child is "at risk" in your mind, and the parent(s) refuse transport, notify the appropriate agencies. Withdraw from the scene and arrange to meet the supportive personnel at a location a safe distance from the house. Remember, a good law enforcement officer can be very effective in convincing the parents to take the child to the ED. Employ this strategy early.)

3. Describe possible transport considerations, including a potential refusal of transport by the angry parents.

   (As discussed in question 2, the ideal situation is for the child to be transported to an appropriate ED accompanied by the parents. If the situation turns ugly, the police may arrest one of the parents if the person becomes problematic. Following this, the mother or father can grant consent to treat and transport. If both refuse, document all actions. Have the informed refusal witnessed by a law enforcement officer. Again, as noted in question 2, assure the family that they can call EMS at any time if they change their minds.)

4. What are the important factors for reporting this incident and documenting the call?
(You are so busy that many important details may escape your memory. It is best to immediately document the call in detail before taking the next assignment. Be sure to identify all personnel at the scene and the reason they were there. Remember, this information will be your primary reminder of what happened if and when you are called to court.)

ASSIGNMENTS

Assign the students to complete Chapter 2, "Pediatrics," of the Workbook. Also assign them to read Chapter 3, "Geriatric Emergencies," before the next class.

EVALUATION

Chapter Quiz and Scenario Distribute copies of the Chapter Quiz and scenario provided in Handouts 2-2 and 2-3 to evaluate student understanding of this chapter. Make sure each student reads the scenario to reinforce critical thinking on the scene. Remind students not to use their notes or textbooks while taking the quiz.

Student CD Quizzes for every chapter are contained on the dynamic and highly visual in-text student CD.

Companion Website Additional quizzes for every chapter are contained on this exciting website.

TestGen You may wish to create a custom-tailored test using *Prentice Hall TestGen for Paramedic Care: Principles & Practice,* 3rd edition, to evaluate student understanding of this chapter.

Online Test Preparation (for students and instructors) Additional test preparation is available through Brady's new online product, EMT Achieve: Paramedic Test Preparation, at *http://www.prenhall.com/emtachieve.* Instructors can also monitor student mastery online.

Success! for the Paramedic Keyed to *Paramedic Care: Principles & Practice* and *Essentials of Paramedic Care,* this comprehensive exam review contains hundreds of test questions and rationales.

REINFORCEMENT

Handouts If classroom discussion or performance on the quiz indicates that some students have not fully mastered the chapter content, you may wish to assign some or all of the Reinforcement Handouts for this chapter.

Student CD (for students) A wide variety of material on this CD-ROM will reinforce and also expand student knowledge and skills.

PowerPoint Presentation (for instructors) The PowerPoint material developed for this chapter offers useful reinforcement of chapter content.

WORKBOOK
Chapter 2 Activities

READING/REFERENCE
Textbook Chapter 3, pp. 146–217

HANDOUT 2-2
Chapter 2 Quiz

HANDOUT 2-3
Chapter 2 Scenario

PARAMEDIC STUDENT CD
Student Activities

COMPANION WEBSITE
http://www.prenhall.com/bledsoe

TESTGEN
Volume 5, Chapter 2

EMT ACHIEVE:
PARAMEDIC TEST PREPARATION
Mistovich & Beasley. *EMT Achieve: Paramedic Test Preparation*
http://www.prenhall.com/emtachieve.

SUCCESS! FOR THE PARAMEDIC
Cherry. *SUCCESS! for the Paramedic,* 4th edition.

HANDOUTS 2-4 TO 2-8
Reinforcement Activities

PARAMEDIC STUDENT CD
Student Activities

POWERPOINT PRESENTATION
Volume 5

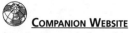

COMPANION WEBSITE
http://www.prenhall.com/bledsoe

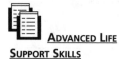
OneKey
Volume 5, Chapter 2

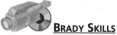
ADVANCED LIFE SUPPORT SKILLS
Larmon & Davis. *Advanced Life Support Skills.*

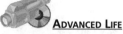
ADVANCED LIFE SKILLS REVIEW
Larmon & Davis. *Advanced Life Skills Review.*

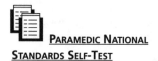
BRADY SKILLS SERIES: ALS
Larmon & Davis. *Brady Skills Series: ALS.*

PARAMEDIC NATIONAL STANDARDS SELF-TEST
Miller. *Paramedic National Standards Self-Test,* 5th edition.

Companion Website (for students)   Additional review quizzes and links to EMS resources will contribute to further reinforcement of the chapter.

OneKey   Online support is offered for this course on one of three platforms: CourseCompass, Blackboard, or WebCT. Includes the IRM, PowerPoints, Test Manager, and Companion Website for instruction. Ask your local sales representative for more information.

Brady Skills Series: Advanced Life Skills (Video or CD).   Have your students watch the skills come to life on VHS or CD-ROM, or they can purchase the highly visual, full-color text with step-by-step procedures with rationales.

Paramedic National Standards Self-Test   Another comprehensive review manual containing hundreds of review questions with page references keyed to several Brady texts.

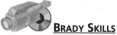

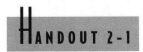

Student's Name _____

CHAPTER 2 OBJECTIVES CHECKLIST

Knowledge Objective	Date Mastered
1. Discuss the paramedic's role in the reduction of infant and childhood morbidity and mortality from acute illness and injury.	
2. Identify methods/mechanisms that prevent injuries to infants and children.	
3. Describe Emergency Medical Services for Children (EMSC) and how it can affect patient outcome.	
4. Identify the common family responses to acute illness and injury of an infant or child.	
5. Describe techniques for successful interaction with families of acutely ill or injured infants and children.	
6. Identify key anatomical, physiological, growth, and developmental characteristics of infants and children and their implications.	
7. Outline differences in adult and childhood anatomy, physiology, and "normal" age-group-related vital signs.	
8. Describe techniques for successful assessment and treatment of infants and children.	
9. Discuss the appropriate equipment utilized to obtain pediatric vital signs.	
10. Determine appropriate airway adjuncts, ventilation devices, and endotracheal intubation equipment; their proper use; and complications of use for infants and children.	
11. List the indications and methods of gastric decompression for infants and children.	
12. Define pediatric respiratory distress, failure, and arrest.	
13. Differentiate between upper airway obstruction and lower airway disease.	
14. Describe the general approach to the treatment of children with respiratory distress, failure, or arrest from upper airway obstruction or lower airway disease.	
15. Discuss the common causes and relative severity of hypoperfusion in infants and children.	

OBJECTIVES

Knowledge Objective	Date Mastered
16. Identify the major classifications of pediatric cardiac rhythms.	
17. Discuss the primary etiologies of cardiopulmonary arrest in infants and children.	
18. Discuss age-appropriate sites, equipment, techniques, and complications of vascular access sites for infants and children.	
19. Describe the primary etiologies of altered level of consciousness in infants and children.	
20. Identify common lethal mechanisms of injury in infants and children.	
21. Discuss anatomical features of children that predispose or protect them from certain injuries.	
22. Describe aspects of infant and child airway management that are affected by potential cervical spine injury.	
23. Identify infant and child trauma patients who require spinal immobilization.	
24. Discuss fluid management and shock treatment for infant and child trauma patients.	
25. Determine when pain management and sedation are appropriate for infants and children.	
26. Define sudden infant death syndrome (SIDS), child abuse, and child neglect.	
27. Discuss the parent/caregiver responses to the death of an infant or child.	
28. Define children with special health care needs and technology-assisted children.	
29. Discuss basic cardiac life support (CPR) guidelines for infants and children.	
30. Integrate advanced life support skills with basic cardiac life support for infants and children.	
31. Discuss the indications, dosage, route of administration, and special considerations for medication administration in infants and children.	
32. Discuss appropriate transport guidelines for low- and high-risk infants and children.	

©2009 Pearson Education, Inc.
Paramedic Care: Principles & Practice, Vol. 5, 3rd. Ed.

Knowledge Objective	Date Mastered
33. Describe the epidemiology, including the incidence, morbidity/mortality, risk factors, prevention strategies, pathophysiology, assessment, and treatment of infants and children with:	
a. Respiratory distress/failure	
b. Hypoperfusion	
c. Cardiac dysrhythmias	
d. Neurologic emergencies	
e. Trauma	
f. Abuse and neglect	
g. Special health care needs, including technology-assisted children	
h. SIDS	

Skill Objective	Date Mastered
34. Given several preprogrammed simulated pediatric patients, provide the appropriate assessment, treatment, and transport.	

OBJECTIVES

CHAPTER 2 QUIZ

Write the letter of the best answer in the space provided.

_____ 1. You respond to a private residence to find a 4-month-old infant with a fractured humerus. Your examination also reveals numerous bruises and abrasions in various stages of healing on the child's back and buttocks and what appear to be cigarette burns on the child's palms and soles. The child's mother says the fracture was a result of the infant's rolling off the bed onto the floor. You should:
   A. call the police and have the mother arrested for child abuse.
   B. lecture the mother sternly about her treatment of the child.
   C. transport the child and report your suspicions to the physician at the emergency department.
   D. keep what you suspect to yourself, because you may be liable if you falsely report child abuse.

_____ 2. Headache, seizures, a stiff neck, bulging fontanelles, and a rash consisting of tiny pinpoint hemorrhages under the skin indicate:
   A. meningitis.   C. pneumonia.
   B. epiglottitis.   D. laryngotracheobronchitis.

_____ 3. The patient is a 5-year-old female who developed severe respiratory distress with inspiratory stridor about 30 minutes ago. Her mother tells you that the patient "seemed to be perfectly healthy" until about 3 hours earlier when she began to complain of a severe sore throat. The patient is sitting on the side of her bed, leaning forward with her neck slightly extended. Respiratory distress with accessory muscle use and intercostal retractions is present. The child is drooling profusely, and when she tries to talk, her voice sounds "muffled." She is suffering from a life-threatening emergency due to potential:
   A. seizures.   C. airway obstruction.
   B. cardiac dysrhythmias.   D. respiratory arrest.

_____ 4. The patient is a 3-year-old male who awakened about 10 minutes ago with respiratory distress and stridor. He is sitting bolt upright in bed. Accessory muscle use and intercostal retractions are present, but drooling is absent. Cyanosis of the lips and nail beds is present. The patient coughs frequently, producing a sound similar to a seal's bark. When he attempts to talk, he sounds very hoarse. His mother tells you that the patient has had a cold with a low-grade fever for "2 or 3 days." The treatment for this patient would include:
   A. systemic drug therapy with 1:1000 epinephrine.
   B. intubation and high-concentration oxygen.
   C. humidified oxygen and nebulized bronchodilators.
   D. systemic drug therapy with aminophylline.

_____ 5. The patient is a 7-year-old female who experienced a sudden onset of coughing and expiratory wheezing about 20 minutes ago. She has no history of pulmonary or cardiovascular disease. She states that she was eating peanuts immediately before the onset of the symptoms and that she "almost choked on one." Auscultation of her chest reveals localized wheezing in the right lung field. She is most likely suffering from:
   A. an acute asthma attack.
   B. anaphylaxis.
   C. aspiration of a foreign body into the lower airways.
   D. pneumonia.

©2009 Pearson Education, Inc.
Paramedic Care: Principles & Practice, Vol. 5, 3rd. Ed.

_____ **6.** To select the proper-size pediatric endotracheal tube, choose one that is:
   A. the same size as the patient's age in months.
   B. the same size as the patient's little finger.
   C. as long as the distance from nose to ear.
   D. the same size as the base of the child's thumb.

_____ **7.** The patient is a 3-month-old infant who suddenly developed cyanosis and audible expiratory wheezing. Retractions and nasal flaring with a respiratory rate of 80/min are present. The patient's mother reports that he has had a mild cold with a cough for 2 or 3 days. The patient has had a low-grade fever. There is no family history of asthma or allergies. The initial treatment of choice for this patient would be:
   A. epinephrine 1:1000 subcutaneous.
   B. humidified oxygen.
   C. nebulized racemic epinephrine.
   D. immediate endotracheal intubation.

_____ **8.** Before administering epinephrine to a patient who is having an asthma attack, you should always obtain a medication history from the patient because:
   A. the patient already may have severe cardiac irritability from an overdose of bronchodilators from a home inhaler.
   B. medication in inhalers tends to antagonize the effects of epinephrine.
   C. the combination of epinephrine with drugs the patient has already taken may worsen bronchospasm.
   D. the combination of epinephrine with drugs the patient has already taken may slow the patient's heart.

_____ **9.** To defibrillate a child, you should use pediatric paddles. If for some reason these special paddles are not available, you would use adult paddles. Which of the following positions best explains how you modify paddle placement in this situation?
   A. below right clavicle; at apex   **C.** anterior thorax; posterior thorax
   B. below right nipple; below left nipple **D.** below left clavicle; at apex

_____ **10.** Status epilepticus refers to:
   A. a severe seizure that cannot be stopped with diazepam.
   B. two or more seizures without a period of consciousness between them.
   C. a very mild type of seizure that is caused by fever.
   D. a type of grand mal seizure produced by hypoglycemia.

_____ **11.** A prolonged asthma attack that cannot be broken with epinephrine is:
   A. status asthmaticus.
   B. beta-resistant primary bronchospasm.
   C. status epilepticus.
   D. sympathorefractory asthma.

_____ **12.** The purpose of administering humidified oxygen in the treatment of asthma is to:
   A. dilate the bronchi.
   B. avoid drying of mucus secretions in the airway.
   C. increase the respiratory rate.
   D. correct alveolar dehydration.

_____ **13.** Bronchiolitis is best described as a:
   A. viral infection causing inflammation of the larynx, trachea, and bronchi.
   B. bacterial infection causing inflammation of the bronchioles.
   C. bacterial infection causing inflammation of the larynx, trachea, and bronchi.
   D. viral infection causing inflammation of the bronchioles.

_____ 14. Asthma is best described as an:
  A. obstructive pulmonary disease characterized by distention of the pulmonary air spaces with destructive changes in their walls.
  B. obstructive pulmonary disease characterized by episodes of severe bronchospasm, bronchial edema, and hypersecretion of mucus in the lower airways.
  C. obstructive pulmonary disease characterized by excessive mucus production in the bronchial tree with a chronic productive cough.
  D. inflammation of the bronchioles caused by a viral infection.

_____ 15. Croup is best described as a:
  A. bacterial infection causing inflammation of the larynx.
  B. viral infection causing inflammation of the larynx.
  C. bacterial infection causing inflammation of the oropharynx and epiglottis.
  D. viral infection causing inflammation of the oropharynx and epiglottis.

_____ 16. The initial endotracheal dose of epinephrine for cardiac arrest in children is:
  A. 0.01 mg/kg of 1:10,000 solution.   C. 0.01 mg/kg of 1:1000 solution.
  B. 0.1 mg/kg of 1:10,000 solution.   D. 0.1 mg/kg of 1:1000 solution.

_____ 17. The initial intravenous dose of epinephrine for cardiac arrest in children is:
  A. 0.01 mg/kg of 1:10,000 solution.   C. 0.01mg/kg of 1:1000 solution.
  B. 0.1 mg/kg of 1:10,000 solution.   D. 0.1 mg/kg of 1:1000 solution.

_____ 18. The usual dose of lidocaine for ventricular fibrillation in children is:
  A. 0.01 mg/kg.   C. 0.3 mg/kg.
  B. 0.5 mg/kg.   D. 1 mg/kg.

_____ 19. The most common cause of death following seizures is:
  A. hyperthermia.   C. dehydration.
  B. anoxia.   D. head injury.

_____ 20. Which of the following groups of activities best describes the prehospital management of a patient with epiglottitis?
  A. Restrain the patient in a supine position and intubate immediately.
  B. Administer humidified oxygen, allow the patient to assume the most comfortable position, and transport.
  C. Administer humidified oxygen for 5 minutes, and start a TKO IV if doing this does not increase the patient's distress, and attempt to intubate.
  D. Administer humidified oxygen, establish an IV with LR wide open, allow the patient to assume the most comfortable position, and transport.

_____ 21. The least desirable vein to use during CPR is a(n):
  A. scalp vein.   C. femoral vein.
  B. antecubital vein.   D. saphenous vein.

_____ 22. Which of the following combinations of laryngoscope blades and endotracheal tubes should be used when intubating a 2-year-old?
  A. straight blade; uncuffed tube
  B. curved blade; uncuffed tube
  C. straight blade; cuffed tube
  D. curved blade; cuffed tube

_____ 23. The patient is a 6-month-old infant found unconscious by his mother. The infant has no pulse, no blood pressure, and no respirations. You should begin two-rescuer CPR using a rate of at least:
  A. 100/minute; ratio 15:2; depth 1/3 to 1/2 the depth of the chest.
  B. 100/minute; ratio 15:2; depth 1/2 to 1 inch.
  C. 100/minute; ratio 30:2; depth 1/3 to 1/2 the depth of the chest.
  D. 80/minute; ratio 5:1; depth 1 to 11/2 inches.

 ©2009 Pearson Education, Inc.
Paramedic Care: Principles & Practice, Vol. 5, 3rd. Ed.

_____ **24.** Cardiac arrest in infants and children usually results from:
  A. heart attack.
  B. respiratory failure or arrest.
  C. electric shock.
  D. drowning.

_____ **25.** How many watt-seconds should be used initially to defibrillate a 12-kg infant?
  A. 25 watt-seconds
  B. 50 watt-seconds
  C. 100 watt-seconds
  D. 200 watt-seconds

_____ **26.** The initial attempt to defibrillate a 30-kg child is unsuccessful. How many watt-seconds should be used to repeat the defibrillation of the child?
  A. 60 watt-seconds
  B. 120 watt-seconds
  C. 300 watt-seconds
  D. 360 watt-seconds

_____ **27.** Which of the following actions is associated with diazepam?
  A. anticonvulsant
  B. antiarrhythmic
  C. bronchodilator
  D. antihistamine

_____ **28.** The patient is a 4-year-old female who received an electrical shock. The child has no pulse and no respirations. You should begin two-rescuer CPR using a rate of:
  A. at least 100/minute; ratio 30:2; depth 1/3 to 1/2 chest diameter.
  B. 100/minute; ratio 15:2; depth 1/2 to 1 inch.
  C. 100/minute; ratio 15:2; depth 1/3 to 1/2 chest diameter.
  D. 100/minute; ratio 5:1; depth 1 to 11/2 inches.

_____ **29.** If an infant has a complete airway obstruction not relieved by back blows, the rescuer should:
  A. administer five abdominal thrusts.
  B. administer five additional back blows.
  C. administer five chest thrusts.
  D. perform a finger sweep.

_____ **30.** Before beginning chest compressions on an infant, you should check for the presence of a pulse at which artery?
  A. temporal
  B. carotid
  C. brachial
  D. femoral

_____ **31.** Before beginning chest compressions on a child, you should check for the presence of a pulse at which artery?
  A. temporal
  B. carotid
  C. brachial
  D. femoral

_____ **32.** When compressing the chest of a child, you most typically use the:
  A. tips of the index and middle fingers of one hand.
  B. heel of one hand.
  C. heels of both hands.
  D. thumbs of both hands.

_____ **33.** Which of the following statements best defines sudden infant death syndrome (SIDS)?
  A. the sudden, unexplained, and unexpected death of an infant before an autopsy to determine cause of death
  B. the sudden, unexplained, and unexpected death of an infant where a thorough autopsy fails to reveal the cause of death
  C. the sudden, unexpected death of an infant where the autopsy reveals the cause of death to be cardiovascular disease
  D. the sudden, unexpected death of an infant in its sleep caused by suffocation in the bed clothing

_____ **34.** Which of the following statements about asthma and bronchiolitis is correct?
  A. Asthma usually is associated with a family history of the disease, whereas bronchiolitis is not.
  B. Bronchiolitis is common in infants less than 1 year of age, but asthma is uncommon in that age group.
  C. Asthma produces generalized wheezes, but bronchiolitis produces localized wheezes.
  D. Both A and B.

_____ **35.** Assessment of a patient who is having an asthma attack would include examination for:
   A. state of consciousness, general appearance, vital signs, respiratory movement, skin turgor, dryness of mucous membranes.
   B. state of consciousness, vital signs, general appearance, respiratory movement, pedal edema.
   C. state of consciousness, general appearance, vital signs, respiratory movement, abdominal rebound tenderness.
   D. general appearance, state of consciousness, vital signs, respiratory movement, jugular vein distention.

_____ **36.** Differences in the anatomy of the airway that warrant differences in intubation techniques for infants and adults include:
   A. the infant's tongue being larger in relation to other structures in the airway.
   B. the glottis being higher in the infant than in the adult.
   C. the epiglottis being narrower in the infant and its vocal cords slanting upward and backward.
   D. all of the above.

_____ **37.** In which of the following age groups does sudden infant death syndrome (SIDS) most commonly occur?
   A. birth to 2 weeks
   B. 2 months to 4 months
   C. 6 months to 12 months
   D. 12 months to 18 months

_____ **38.** What question(s) would be appropriate to ask about a child who has had a seizure?
   A. Does the child have a history of previous seizures, head trauma, diabetes, recent headache, or stiff neck?
   B. Is the child taking any medications?
   C. How many seizures has the child had, and what did they look like?
   D. All of the above.

_____ **39.** Which of the following statements about specific age groups of pediatric patients is correct?
   A. 2- to 3-year-olds are usually cooperative and like to be touched by strangers.
   B. 4- to 5-year-olds are usually cooperative and like to "help out" the paramedic.
   C. School-age children usually do not like to be told what is being done to them.
   D. Adolescents usually are not concerned about lasting effects of injury or illness.

_____ **40.** The endotracheal tube used in infant intubation is often not cuffed because of anatomical differences in the infant's:
   A. pharynx.   **C.** glottis.
   B. trachea.   **D.** mandible.

_____ **41.** What procedure would be appropriate when examining a toddler?
   A. Decide which parts of the physical exam are essential and get through them as quickly as possible.
   B. Establish ground rules, for example, "It's all right to cry, but not to bite or kick."
   C. Obtain as much information as possible before touching the child.
   D. All of the above.

_____ **42.** The patient is a 5-year-old child who is in respiratory arrest. The child should be ventilated once every:
   A. 3–5 seconds.   **C.** 5–6 seconds.
   B. 2–4 seconds.   **D.** 6–8 seconds.

_____ **43.** How many times a minute should an infant who is not breathing be ventilated?
   A. 10–12   **C.** 12–20
   B. 15–20   **D.** 25–30

©2009 Pearson Education, Inc.
Paramedic Care: Principles & Practice, Vol. 5, 3rd. Ed.

_____ 44. A patient with epiglottitis would typically exhibit:
   A. inspiratory stridor, pain on swallowing, high fever, and drooling.
   B. expiratory wheezing, coughing, rales, and cyanosis.
   C. inspiratory stridor, "seal-bark" cough, low-grade fever, and orthopnea.
   D. expiratory wheezing, rales, coughing, high fever.

_____ 45. A patient with laryngotracheobronchitis would typically exhibit:
   A. inspiratory stridor, pain on swallowing, high fever, drooling.
   B. expiratory wheezing, coughing, rales, cyanosis.
   C. inspiratory stridor, "seal-bark" cough, low-grade fever, orthopnea.
   D. expiratory wheezing, rales, coughing, high fever.

_____ 46. Which of the following age groups is usually associated with croup?
   A. 0 to 6 months   C. 4 years to 12 years
   B. 6 months to 4 years   D. over 12 years

_____ 47. The physical exam of a child who has had a seizure should include a check for:
   A. level of consciousness.
   B. evidence of fever or dehydration.
   C. signs of an injury that caused or was caused by the seizures.
   D. all of the above.

_____ 48. Which group of pediatric patients would generally be expected to be uncooperative?
   A. 2 to 3 years old   C. 6 to 10 years old
   B. 4 to 5 years old   D. 10 to 14 years old

_____ 49. A pediatric patient is seen by paramedics for a seizure. The child has a fever of 101°F, was lethargic and irritable before the seizure, and has had no previous seizure activity. The child complained of a headache earlier in the day. What is the most likely problem?
   A. febrile seizure   C. hypoglycemia
   B. meningitis   D. hypoxia

_____ 50. You are called to see a 6-month-old infant. The mother's chief complaint is that the child has been irritable for the last few days, is not feeding well, is sweaty, and is "just not acting right." On exam, you find a fussy infant who wants the bottle. Respirations are 40/min. The skin is pink but is cool distally. Capillary refill is 2 seconds. Pulses are very rapid at about 300/min. The ECG shows a narrow complex tachycardia with no P waves visible. You should:
   A. administer oxygen and transport.
   B. cardiovert immediately at 0.5 to 1 J/kg.
   C. administer verapamil.
   D. administer 20 mL/kg lactated Ringer's solution.

_____ 51. You respond to a mottled, cyanotic 3-month-old, 5-kg infant who responds only to painful stimuli. Proximal pulses are too rapid to count and thready proximally. Distal pulses are absent. The skin is pale and cold distally. Capillary refill is 5 seconds. Respirations are 65/min, and the patient is working hard to breathe. ECG shows a narrow complex tachycardia with no P waves visible. You should:
   A. administer oxygen and transport.
   B. cardiovert at 0.5 to 1 J/kg.
   C. administer verapamil.
   D. administer 20 mL/kg lactated Ringer's solution.

_____ 52. You are called to evaluate an 8-month-old infant with a 5-day history of vomiting and diarrhea. Mom states that the infant is "not acting right." On initial observation, you note a lethargic infant with mottled skin and no spontaneous movement. Respirations are 60, unlabored. Pulse is 170, weak. Capillary refill is 4 seconds. Extremities are cool. The ECG shows a narrow complex tachycardia P waves are visible and the rhythm is slightly irregular. You should:
   A. administer oxygen and transport.
   B. cardiovert at 0.5 to 1 J/kg.
   C. administer verapamil.
   D. administer 20 mL/kg lactated Ringer's solution.

_____ 53. A 2-year-old male fell into a swimming pool and was submersed for about 2 minutes. The child is unresponsive, cyanotic, apneic, and pulseless. A firefighter who first responded on an engine is performing CPR. You are not able to quickly obtain vascular access, but you are able to place an endotracheal tube. EKG shows a sinus bradycardia with a rate of 32. You should:
   A. start an intraosseous line immediately.
   B. administer 0.01 mg/kg epinephrine 1:10,000 down the endotracheal tube.
   C. administer 0.1 mg/kg epinephrine 1:1000 down the endotracheal tube.
   D. administer 0.02 mg/kg atropine down the endotracheal tube.

_____ 54. A 5-year-old boy was struck by an automobile when he ran into the street from between two parked cars. He is pale, confused, and sweating heavily. Capillary refill time is 5 seconds. Breath sounds are present bilaterally. The upper left quadrant of the abdomen is bruised and tender. Fluid resuscitation should consist of:
   A. two large-bore IVs with lactated Ringer's infused as rapidly as possible.
   B. a single IV with lactated Ringer's to avoid overhydrating the child.
   C. 20 mL/kg of lactated Ringer's while monitoring him for signs of improved perfusion.
   D. two large-bore IVs of D$_5$W infused as rapidly as possible, because lactated Ringer's should not be given to small children.

_____ 55. Children and infants who are burned are more likely to suffer more significant fluid loss than adults because:
   A. a larger portion of a pediatric patient's body mass consists of water.
   B. IVs cannot be established as easily.
   C. their body surface area is larger in proportion to their body volume.
   D. crying associated with pain and anxiety will add to volume loss.

_____ 56. A 3-year-old and his brother were walking along a frozen irrigation ditch. The 3-year-old tried to retrieve a dropped toy and fell through the ice. He is apneic and pulseless with fixed, dilated pupils. No one knows how long he was underwater. ECG shows asystole. You should:
   A. start CPR immediately and transport.
   B. call for the police and the coroner.
   C. attempt to rewarm the patient as rapidly as possible.
   D. transport without doing CPR.

_____ 57. A 4-month-old male infant has been vomiting and having watery diarrhea for 2 days. His mother says the infant has not urinated at all today. The baby's lips and oral mucosa are dry, and his fontanelles are sunken. The infant's extremities are cold to the elbows and knees. Capillary refill is 5 seconds. Heart rate is 170. ECG shows a narrow complex tachycardia with P waves visible. Management should include:
   A. infusion of 20 mL/kg lactated Ringer's.
   B. cardioversion at 0.5 to 1 J/kg.
   C. checking a "dex" stick with possible administration of D$_{25}$W for hypoglycemia.
   D. both A and C.

©2009 Pearson Education, Inc.
Paramedic Care: Principles & Practice, Vol. 5, 3rd. Ed.

_____ **58.** A 3-year-old female ingested six 0.25-mg digoxin tablets about 2 hours ago. She is awake, alert, and taking the bottle. Pulse is 50, strong, regular. Respirations are 30, regular, unlabored. Capillary refill is less than 2 seconds. Skin is pink and warm. BP is 90 by palpation. ECG shows a sinus bradycardia with a first-degree AV block. You should administer:

    A. 0.2 mg/kg atropine IV push.   **C.** 5 mg/kg calcium chloride IV push.

    B. 0.01 mg/kg epinephrine IV push.   **D.** oxygen by blow-by, monitor, and transport.

_____ **59.** Indications that an intraosseous line has been successfully placed include which of the following?

    A. A change in resistance is felt as the marrow cavity is entered.

    B. The needle stands on its own without support.

    C. Bone marrow can be aspirated from the needle.

    D. All of the above.

_____ **60.** You are called to see a 9-month-old baby who has stopped breathing. The mother's boyfriend is babysitting and states that the infant fell off the couch. The baby is lying in the crib. There are no obvious signs of trauma. The child is lethargic and breathing slowly at a rate of 8/min. Skin is warm, and capillary refill is normal. Heart rate is 140. The left pupil is dilated and fixed. The right pupil is mid-position and reactive. Linear bruises are present on both upper arms. Management of the infant should include all of the following, EXCEPT:

    A. stabilization of the cervical spine.

    B. intubation and hyperventilation with high-concentration oxygen.

    C. infusion of 20 mL/kg of lactated Ringer's solution.

    D. reporting of possible child abuse to the ER physician.

_____ **61.** A 15-year-old male has been involved in a swimming accident at a spot that is popular with local teenagers. The boy was reported to have jumped or dove from a rock outcropping into the river. He did not surface immediately and was pulled from the water a few minutes later about 25 yards downstream. The patient is unresponsive. His respiratory rate is 8/min. His heart rate is 120/min. His extremities are cold. Management should include all of the following, EXCEPT:

    A. opening of the airway with a jaw thrust and stabilization of the cervical spine.

    B. drying and wrapping in warm blankets.

    C. assisted ventilations with a bag-valve mask and oxygen, followed by possible endotracheal intubation.

    D. administration of sodium bicarbonate to correct acidosis.

_____ **62.** All of the following statements about the physical assessment of a patient with an acute asthma attack are true, EXCEPT:

    A. sleepiness or stupor indicates severe hypercarbia, hypoxia, and acidosis.

    B. the disappearance of wheezing during a severe asthma attack is a good sign, because it indicates that bronchospasm has stopped.

    C. tenting of the skin and dryness of the mucous membranes can indicate dehydration due to the asthma attack.

    D. young children may not show the positional preferences of older children.

_____ **63.** You are called to see a 6-year-old child because he has a very high fever. His mother tells you that he became ill about 4 hours ago and has been complaining of a severe sore throat. He will not eat or drink because he says it hurts to swallow. You find the child sitting upright in bed, crying and drooling noticeably. He appears very frightened. His axillary temperature is 104°F. His respirations are 30 and shallow, and there is flaring of his nostrils on inhalation. His chest is clear to auscultation. All of the following are part of the management of this child, EXCEPT:

    A. administering high-concentration, humidified oxygen.

    B. deferring starting an IV, because this may worsen the patient's distress.

    C. carefully examining the throat to determine whether inflammation is present.

    D. transporting the child in the sitting position.

_____ **64.** A call comes in late at night for a sick child. When you arrive, a very distraught mother tells you that her 6-year-old son has been "having fits." He has been ill today with an upper respiratory infection and about half an hour ago began having seizures. He has had three seizures so far. The mother did not notice how the seizures started. You find the child apparently asleep on his bed. He is difficult to arouse. As you examine him, his eyes suddenly open and deviate sharply to the right, and he rapidly develops another grand mal seizure. All of the following should be considered, EXCEPT:

    A. administration of high-concentration, humidified oxygen.

    B. placing a bite-block between his teeth to protect his tongue.

    C. checking blood glucose level and giving glucose if he is hypoglycemic.

    D. administering diazepam to terminate the seizures.

_____ **65.** You are called to see a 3-year-old child who is in moderate respiratory distress. His mother says he has appeared well during the day, but for the past two nights he has been waking up around midnight with a high-pitched cough that sounds like a dog barking. You find the child lying in bed, looking very tired and miserable. Axillary temperature is 99.7°F. Respirations are stridorous at 30/min, with suprasternal retractions and accessory muscle use. On auscultation of the chest, no wheezing or crackles are heard. All of the following would be included in the management of this patient, EXCEPT:

    A. administration of high-concentration, humidified oxygen.

    B. performing direct laryngoscopy to be sure the airway is not obstructed.

    C. administering racemic epinephrine by nebulizer.

    D. transporting to the hospital in the position of comfort.

©2009 Pearson Education, Inc.
Paramedic Care: Principles & Practice, Vol. 5, 3rd. Ed.

CHAPTER 2 SCENARIO

Review the following real-life scenario. Then answer the questions that follow.

At 2330 hours you are called to evaluate a 2-year-old male with a 5-Day history of vomiting and diarrhea. The patient's mother says that she called because the child "is not acting right." On initial observation, you note that the child has mottled skin and no spontaneous movement. He is unresponsive to painful stimuli. Respirations are 60/min, shallow, and regular. Radial pulses are absent. Carotid pulse is 170, weak, and regular. Capillary refill is 5 seconds. The patient's extremities are cool. The ECG shows a narrow complex tachycardia at rate of 170. P waves are visible.

1. What problem does the patient appear to have?

2. What is the significance of the patient's cool, mottled skin?

3. Why is the patient tachypneic?

4. When you attempt to start an IV on this patient, you cannot find any veins. What alternative route is available for vascular access?

5. How do you know you have achieved vascular access via this route?

6. Once you have achieved vascular access, what method would you use to infuse fluid? Why?

7. You decide to endotracheally intubate the patient. How would you select the proper endotracheal tube size?

HANDOUT 2-4

CHAPTER 2 REVIEW

Write the word or words that best complete each sentence in the space(s) provided.

1. In assessing and treating pediatric patients, it is important to keep in mind that they are not simply _____ _____.

2. The federally funded program aimed at improving the health of pediatric patients who suffer from life-threatening illnesses and injuries is _____ _____ _____ for _____.

3. Foremost in approaching any pediatric emergency is consideration of the patient's _____ and _____ development.

4. When assessing or treating a pediatric patient, always use _____ that is appropriate for the age of the child.

5. An infant up to 1 month of age is known as a(n) _____.

6. Infants should have _____ their birth weight by 5 or 6 months of age.

7. _____ are the leading cause of injury deaths in patients aged 1 to 15 years.

8. When examining school-age children, give _____ the responsibility of providing the history.

9. If you must perform a detailed physical exam on an adolescent patient, respect the patient's sense of _____.

10. The pediatric patient's head is proportionally _____ than the adult's, and the occipital region is significantly _____.

11. A child's larynx is _____ than an adult's and extends into the _____.

12. Pediatric patients are prone to _____ because of their greater BSA-to-weight ratio.

13. The three components of the _____ _____ _____ are appearance, breathing, and circulation.

14. _____ and _____ problems are the most common cause of cardiac arrest in infants and children.

15. The normal respiration rate for a preschooler is _____ to _____ breaths per minute.

16. For a patient under 5 years, one of the signs of a risk of cardiopulmonary arrest is a heart rate greater than _____ or less than _____ per minute.

17. A severe patient would be one with a Glasgow coma scale score of less than or equal to _____.

18. _____ is a late and often sudden sign of cardiovascular decompensation in pediatric patients.

19. For conscious infants less than 1 year old with foreign body airway obstruction, deliver 5 _____ _____, followed by 5 _____ _____.

20. Never do _____ _____ _____ in infant or child FBAO patients.

21. Never use a(n) _____ _____ on a child with midface or head trauma.

22. The length of an endotracheal tube for a patient 4 to 6 years old should be _____ cm measured from the teeth to the midtrachea.

23. When intubating a pediatric patient, you should use a laryngoscope with a(n) _____ blade.

24. If gastric distention is present in a pediatric patient, consider placement of a(n) _____ _____.

25. One indication for intraosseous infusion is a child patient less than _____ _____ old.

26. The initial dosage of fluid in a pediatric patient suffering from hypovolemia should be _____ of an isotonic fluid.

27. The last stage of respiratory compromise, to which the patient will progress if not treated, is respiratory _____.

28. The viral infection common in children from 6 months to 4 years of age that usually occurs in fall and winter months is _____.

29. If the pediatric patient with epiglottitis is maintaining the airway, do not put anything _____ _____ _____.

30. In severe asthma attacks, an ominous sign is a lack of _____.

31. Common causes of lower airway distress include FBAO, asthma, bronchiolitis, and _____.

32. A slight increase in _____ _____ is one of the earliest signs of shock in the pediatric patient.

33. The child in septic shock may require _____ therapy.

34. _____ _____ _____ is an abnormality or defect in the heart that is present at birth.

35. Most of the pediatric seizures that paramedics encounter are _____.

36. Bacteria and viruses can cause the infection of the GI system known as _____.

37. In the prehospital setting, hypoglycemia in pediatric patients usually results from _____ _____ diabetes.

38. Most poisonings treated by EMS result from accidental _____.

39. _____ are the single most common cause of injury in children.

40. The second leading cause of death in infants less than 6 months of age is _____ _____.

Student's Name _____

CHAPTER 2 SHORT ANSWER A

Answer each of the following questions.

1. Why do infants and small children require special precautions to prevent them from becoming cold?

2. Match the age group with the typical characteristics of that group.

   Adolescents _____   **a.** Dislike strange people; strong assertiveness; high mobility, low common sense

   Toddlers _____   **b.** Totally subjective worldview; think magically; do not separate fantasy and reality; intense fear of injury, pain, blood loss

   School-age children _____   **c.** Master environment through information; can make compromises, think objectively

   Preschoolers _____   **d.** Seeking self-determination; fragile self-esteem; very acute body image; high need for modesty

3. What is the most common form of shock in pediatric patients?

4. What are the fontanelles? What change occurs in the fontanelles of a dehydrated infant?

5. What is status asthmaticus?

6. Why should skin turgor be checked in patients who are having an asthma attack?

7. Why is it important to determine the medications taken by an asthmatic before beginning any therapy?

8. Why should oxygen be humidified when it is administered to an asthma patient?

9. What is the prehospital treatment for croup?

10. What is the principal danger facing a patient with epiglottitis?

REINFORCEMENT

Student's Name _____

CHAPTER 2 SHORT ANSWER B

Answer each of the following questions.

1. What is the proper finger position for performing chest compressions on an infant?

2. What are the proper depth and rate for chest compressions on an infant? On a child?

3. How is hypovolemic shock corrected in pediatric patients? Why is this technique used?

4. Should flow-restricted, oxygen-powered breathing devices (demand valves) be used to ventilate children? Why?

5. How is the proper size of endotracheal tube selected for pediatric patients?

6. Why are uncuffed endotracheal tubes sometimes used on infants and children less than 8 years old?

7. What is the suggested initial setting for defibrillation of pediatric patients? What energy is used on subsequent shocks?

8. What three routes are available for drug administration to children during cardiopulmonary arrest?

9. What drug is always used FIRST in the management of symptomatic bradycardia in pediatric patients?

10. What is the initial IV dose of epinephrine in pediatric cardiac arrest?

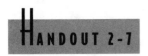 ANDOUT 2-7

Student's Name _____

CHAPTER 2 PEDIATRIC CARE SCENARIOS

Answer each of the following questions.

1. A 6-month-old infant was found unconscious and unresponsive. The baby's skin is cool and pale. Capillary refill is greater than 5 seconds. Radial pulses are absent. Carotid and femoral pulses are thready. The ECG shows a narrow complex tachycardia with a rate of 300 and no visible P waves. How would you manage this patient?

2. A 9-month-old infant's mother called you because she says the baby "turns a funny color and sweats" when he feeds and won't take the entire bottle. The infant is awake and alert. His skin is warm and pink. Capillary refill is less than 2 seconds. Radial and pedal pulses are palpable but very fast. How would you manage this patient?

3. A 2-year-old was found floating facedown in a neighbor's swimming pool. He is unconscious and unresponsive. Pulses and respirations are absent. The ECG shows a sinus bradycardia. How would you manage this patient?

4. A 7-month-old infant responds only to painful stimuli. The skin is pale and mottled. Peripheral pulses are weak, and capillary refill is greater than 4 seconds. The infant's respirations are 52/min but are unlabored. Rectal temperature is 105°F. What problem do you suspect? How would you manage this patient?

5. An 18-month-old male with a history of nausea, vomiting, and diarrhea for 3 days presents with listlessness and a decreased level of consciousness. Skin and mucous membranes are dry. Skin turgor is decreased. Respirations are rapid and shallow. Peripheral pulses are rapid and weak. Capillary refill is slow. Describe your management of this patient.

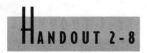

Student's Name _____

CHAPTER 2: PEDIATRIC JUMPSTART MATCHING

Match the following pediatric patients using the JumpSTART system with the appropriate triage tag color.

A. Green
B. Yellow
C. Red
D. Black

_____ **1.** Patient with a minor laceration to the left leg. Bleeding is controlled. Patient is to walk and follow directions.

_____ **2.** Patient is found unresponsive and is not breathing. After opening the airway, spontaneous respirations return.

_____ **3.** Infant who is crying. There are no apparent injuries.

_____ **4.** Unresponsive patient who is not breathing. Spontaneous respirations do not return after opening the airway and there are peripheral pulses noted. After five ventilations, apnea persists.

_____ **5.** Nonambulatory patient who is spontaneously breathing at a rate of 11 breaths per minute.

_____ **6.** Unresponsive patient found not breathing. Spontaneous respirations do not return after opening the airway and there are peripheral pulses noted. After five ventilations, spontaneous respirations return but the patient remains unresponsive.

_____ **7.** Patient with spontaneous respirations of 28 who complains of right ankle pain. Upon exam, you notice swelling and discoloration to the right ankle.

_____ **8.** Nonambulatory patient with spontaneous respirations at a rate of 48 breaths per minute.

_____ **9.** Patient with spontaneous respirations of 32, obvious left leg deformity and absent peripheral pulses in the left leg.

_____ **10.** Unresponsive patient who is not breathing. Spontaneous respirations do not return after opening the airway and there are no peripheral pulses.

©2009 Pearson Education, Inc.
Paramedic Care: Principles & Practice, Vol. 5, 3rd. Ed.

REINFORCEMENT

Chapter 2 Answer Key

Handout 2-2: Chapter 2 Quiz

1. C	18. D	35. A	52. D
2. A	19. B	36. D	53. C
3. C	20. B	37. B	54. C
4. C	21. A	38. D	55. C
5. C	22. A	39. B	56. A
6. B	23. A	40. B	57. D
7. B	24. B	41. D	58. D
8. A	25. A	42. A	59. D
9. C	26. B	43. C	60. C
10. B	27. A	44. A	61. D
11. A	28. D	45. C	62. B
12. B	29. C	46. B	63. C
13. D	30. C	47. D	64. B
14. B	31. B	48. A	65. B
15. B	32. B	49. B	
16. D	33. B	50. A	
17. A	34. D	51. B	

Handout 2-3: Chapter 2 Scenario

1. The patient is suffering from volume depletion (dehydration) and hypovolemic shock.
2. Early in hypovolemic shock, patients vasoconstrict to shunt blood to the body core. As shock persists, compensatory mechanisms begin to fail and dilation begins to occur in localized parts of the periphery. This produces the patchy appearance called mottling. Mottling suggests decompensated shock.
3. Hypoperfusion causes cells to convert to anaerobic metabolism. A by-product of anaerobic metabolism is lactic acid. This lactic acid is buffered by the carbonate buffer system to produce carbon dioxide. Removal of this carbon dioxide by increased respirations helps compensate for the metabolic acidosis produced by shock.
4. The intraosseous route.
5. Resistance is lost as the needle passes through the cortex of the bone; the needle stands by itself; marrow can be aspirated through the needle; IV fluid will flow freely through the needle.
6. 20 mL/kg boluses of lactated Ringer's or normal saline would be infused. After each bolus, perfusion would be reassessed. This technique restores adequate volume while minimizing the risk of volume overload.
7. Use a device like the Broselow tape; use the formula (age + 16)/4; select a tube the same size as the child's little finger.

Handout 2-4: Chapter 2 Review

1. small adults
2. Emergency Medical Services, Children
3. emotional, psychological
4. language
5. neonate
6. doubled
7. Accidents
8. them (the patients)
9. privacy
10. larger, larger

11. higher, pharynx
12. hypothermia
13. pediatric assessment triangle
14. Airway, respiratory
15. 22, 34
16. 180, 80
17. 8
18. Hypotension
19. back blows, chest thrusts
20. blind finger sweeps
21. nasopharyngeal airway
22. 16
23. straight
24. nasogastric tube
25. 6 years
26. 20 mL/kg
27. arrest
28. croup
29. in the mouth
30. wheezing
31. pneumonia
32. heart rate
33. pressor
34. Congenital heart disease
35. febrile
36. gastroenteritis
37. type I
38. ingestion
39. Falls
40. child abuse

Handout 2-5: Chapter 2 Short Answer A

1. Infants and small children have a high surface-to-volume ratio; therefore, they tend to lose heat more rapidly than adults.
2. B, D, C, A
3. hypovolemic
4. The fontanelles are areas in the infant's skull that have not yet fused. The fontanelles of a dehydrated infant become sunken.
5. Status asthmaticus is a severe, prolonged asthma attack that cannot be broken by aggressive use of beta-adrenergic agonists.
6. Increased respiratory water losses and decreased fluid intake during an asthma attack can lead to dehydration.
7. Asthmatics in distress frequently overuse their inhalers; therefore, an asthmatic may be suffering from increased cardiac irritability from the effects of beta agonists.
8. If oxygen is not humidified, it will tend to dry the mucus in the asthmatic's airways, worsening the plugging that already is present.
9. Humidified high-concentration oxygen, nebulized racemic epinephrine or albuterol, continuous monitoring of oxygen saturation and ECG, transport. An IV should not be established, because it will increase the patient's anxiety.
10. Loss of airway.

Handout 2-6: Chapter 2 Short Answer B

1. One finger-width below the nipple line.
2. Compression depth is 1/3 to 1/2 the diameter of the chest at a rate of 100 compressions/min for both infants and children.
3. With 20 mL/kg fluid boluses, reassessing perfusion between boluses. Because children have smaller cardiovascular systems, they are at increased risk for volume overload.
4. No. Flow-restricted, oxygen-powered breathing devices deliver high pressures and do not allow the operator to feel pulmonary compliance. Therefore, they are more likely to cause pneumothorax in children.
5. Use a length-based resuscitation system such as the Broselow tape; compare the tube to the child's little finger; use the formula (age +16)/4.
6. The narrowest part of the child's airway is below the glottis at the cricoid ring. This structure can form a functional cuff on the endotracheal tube.
7. 2 J/kg, 4 J/kg
8. endotracheal, intravenous, intraosseous
9. oxygen
10. 0.01 mg/kg of 1:10,000 solution

Handout 2-7: Pediatric Care Scenarios

1. Give high-concentration oxygen. Perform synchronized cardioversion at 0.5 to 1 J/kg.
2. Give high-concentration oxygen and transport.
3. Begin chest compressions and ventilations with high-concentration oxygen. If child does not respond, place an endotracheal tube. If child still does not respond, establish vascular access and administer epinephrine. Remember that epinephrine also can be given via the endotracheal tube.
4. Septic shock. Give high-concentration oxygen. Establish vascular access. Give 20 mL/kg isotonic crystalloid. Reassess perfusion, respirations, and lung sounds. Repeat fluid boluses until adequate perfusion is restored.
5. Give high-concentration oxygen. Consider assisting ventilations. Establish vascular access. Give 20 mL/kg isotonic crystalloid. Reassess perfusion, respirations, and lung sounds. Repeat fluid boluses until adequate perfusion is restored. Also check blood glucose level. If patient is hypoglycemic secondary to decreased intake, give $D_{25}W$.

Handout 2-8: Pediatric JumpSTART Matching

1. A
2. C
3. A
4. D
5. C
6. C
7. B
8. C
9. C
10. D

©2009 Pearson Education, Inc.
Paramedic Care: Principles & Practice, Vol. 5, 3rd. Ed.

Chapter 3

Geriatrics

INTRODUCTION

Today, approximately one in every eight persons in the United States is over age 65. By the year 2030, one in every four persons will be a member of this age group. The elderly are four times more likely than the nonelderly to use ambulance services. For example, in 1987, 36 percent of ambulance transports to hospital emergency departments were for patients over age 65, and more than 50 percent of all ambulance transports of any kind were for elderly patients. It has been projected that by the year 2030, patients who are 65 or older will represent 70 percent of all ambulance transports. Paramedic students must master the assessment and management of geriatric patients because the practice of paramedics in the 21st century will focus heavily on the special problems and needs of the elderly.

CHAPTER OBJECTIVES

Knowledge Objectives

1. Discuss the demographics demonstrating the increasing size of the elderly population in the United States. (pp. 150–152)
2. Assess the various living environments of elderly patients. (pp. 153–155)
3. Discuss society's view of aging and the social, financial, and ethical issues facing the elderly. (pp. 150–155)
4. Describe the resources available to assist the elderly and create strategies to refer at-risk patients to appropriate community services. (pp. 155–159)
5. Discuss common emotional and psychological reactions to aging, including causes and manifestations. (pp. 152–155, 204–205, 208–210)
6. Apply the pathophysiology of multiple system failure to the assessment and management of medical conditions in the elderly patient. (p. 160)
7. Compare the pharmacokinetics of an elderly patient to that of a young patient, including drug distribution, metabolism, and excretion. (pp. 160–162)
8. Discuss the impact of polypharmacy, dosing errors, increased drug sensitivity, and medication noncompliance on assessment and management of the elderly patient. (pp. 160–162)
9. Discuss the use and effects of commonly prescribed drugs for the elderly patient. (pp. 160–162, 201–206)
10. Discuss the problem of mobility in the elderly and develop strategies to prevent falls. (p. 162)

TOTAL TEACHING TIME: 9.66 HOURS

The total teaching time is only a guideline based on the didactic and practical lab averages in the National Standard Curriculum. Instructors should take into consideration such factors as: the pace at which students learn, the size of the class, and breaks. The actual time devoted to teaching objectives is the responsibility of the instructor.

11. Discuss age-related changes in sensations in the elderly and describe the implications of these changes for communication and patient assessment. (pp. 162, 163, 166–169)

12. Discuss the problems with continence and elimination in the elderly patient and develop communication strategies to provide psychological support. (pp. 162–164)

13. Discuss factors that may complicate the assessment of the elderly patient. (pp. 160, 164–169)

14. Describe the principles that should be employed when assessing and communicating with the elderly. (pp. 155, 162, 164–169)

15. Compare the assessment of a young patient with that of an elderly patient. (pp. 164–169)

16. Discuss common complaints of elderly patients. (pp. 160–164)

17. Discuss the normal and abnormal changes with age in relation to the:

   a. Pulmonary system (pp. 170–172)
   b. Cardiovascular system (p. 172)
   c. Nervous system (p. 173)
   d. Endocrine system (pp. 173–174)
   e. Gastrointestinal system (p. 174)
   f. Thermoregulatory system (p. 174)
   g. Integumentary system (p. 174)
   h. Musculoskeletal system (p. 175)

18. Describe the incidence, morbidity/mortality, risk factors, prevention strategies, pathophysiology, assessment, need for intervention and transport, and management for elderly medical patients with:

   a. Pneumonia, chronic obstructive pulmonary disease, pulmonary edema, lung cancer, and pulmonary embolism (pp. 178–182)
   b. Angina pectoris, myocardial infarction, heart failure, dysrhythmias, aneurysm, hypertension, and syncope (pp. 182–186)
   c. Cerebral vascular disease, seizures, dizziness, delirium, dementia, Alzheimer's disease, and Parkinson's disease (pp. 186–191)
   d. Diabetes and thyroid diseases (pp. 192–193)
   e. Gastrointestinal problems, GI hemorrhage, bowel obstruction, and mesenteric infarct (pp. 193–194)
   f. Skin diseases and pressure ulcers (pp. 194–196)
   g. Osteoarthritis and osteoporosis (pp. 196–199)
   h. Hypothermia and hyperthermia (pp. 200–201)
   i. Toxicological problems, including drug toxicity, substance abuse, alcohol abuse, and drug abuse (pp. 201–207)
   j. Psychological disorders, including depression and suicide (pp. 208–210)

19. Describe the incidence, morbidity/mortality, risk factors, prevention strategies, pathophysiology, assessment, need for intervention and transport, and management of the elderly trauma patient with:

   a. Orthopedic injuries (pp. 212–214)
   b. Burns (p. 214)
   c. Head injuries (pp. 214–215)

Skill Objective

20. Given several preprogrammed simulated geriatric patients with various complaints, provide the appropriate assessment, management, and transport. (pp. 150–215)

©2009 Pearson Education, Inc.
Paramedic Care: Principles & Practice, Vol. 5, 3rd. Ed.

FRAMING THE LESSON

Begin by reviewing the important points from Chapter 2, "Pediatrics." Discuss any points that the class does not completely understand. Then move on to Chapter 3. Ask students to describe images that come to mind when they hear the phrases "senior citizen" or "older person." Frequently, EMS students have a very limited range of experience with older people and assume that almost everyone over the age of 65 is confined to a nursing home. Ask students to continue to provide images and impressions until they are describing the entire range of situations in which they are likely to encounter older persons—from the frail, chronically ill patient in the nursing home to the vigorous older adult who has injured himself engaging in a sport normally associated with younger persons. Emphasize to students that providing for the health care needs of the elderly is going to be a critical element of paramedic practice in the 21st century.

CONSIDERING THE CASE STUDY

Ask a volunteer to read aloud the Case Study that begins on text page 148. Suggest that students close their eyes as the scenario is read to help them mentally visualize the events described in it. You can use the following questions about the Case Study as a starting point for teaching the chapter—a chapter preview in a functional setting.

When the chapter is completed, you may wish to return to the Case Study and encourage further discussion aimed at answering the questions or solving the problems.

CASE STUDY DISCUSSION QUESTIONS (AND ANSWERS)

1. Why is the paramedic intern's quip about "too many beers and a taco" a source of concern for his preceptor?
   (Younger people frequently have a number of misconceptions about the aging process and older persons. Stereotypes about how the elderly "do and don't" act can lead to incomplete histories and missed diagnoses, which in turn can result in poor patient outcomes.)
2. What is the immediate significance of the patient's obviously being in severe pain?
   (As people age, natural deterioration in the nervous system frequently results in a decrease in the ability to feel pain. Therefore, when an older person complains of severe pain, it probably is associated with a very severe problem.)
3. Why did the paramedic ask if the patient had fallen recently?
   (Older persons who live alone are at particular risk for falls. Pain in these patients should always raise the possibility of trauma.)
4. What is the significance of this patient's atrial fibrillation?
   (Atrial fibrillation is a risk factor for developing emboli. Although the most common presentations of this problem are stroke and pulmonary embolism, it is possible for patients to embolize blood vessels supplying other organs, including the bowel.)
5. What is the key symptom that suggests bowel infarction?
   (Pain out of proportion to physical findings during the abdominal exam.)

TEACHING STRATEGIES

People learn in a variety of ways. Some do better with the spoken word, while others prefer the written. Some prefer to work alone, whereas others profit from working in groups. Recognizing these different ways of acquiring knowledge, the authors of this *Instructor's Resource Manual* have provided a variety of teaching strategies for the different types of learners. These strategies are intended to foster higher-level cognitive skills and encourage creative learning and problem solving.

For greatest effectiveness, incorporate these strategies into your class lecture. Marginal notes in the Teaching Outline indicate the points at which various exercises might be most appropriate. Other strategies can be used to preview the lesson or to summarize it.

The following strategies are keyed to specific sections of the lesson:

1. Interview an Elderly Person. In cooperation with your local senior center or nursing home, have students interview an elderly person. Arm them with a questionnaire that covers such things as the subject's demographic information, occupations, and education. Be sure to ask additional questions about the person's perspective on issues today such as technology and health care. Discuss the findings of the interviews in class. This activity will lay a foundation of empathy for this unit, broadening each student's perspective on aging.

2. Defining "Old." Ask students to define "when a person becomes old." Many will associate "old" with a number, such as 55 or retirement age. Others will define "old" by the state of mind, such as when a person ceases to socialize or care for himself. Discuss the findings in class. You will likely find that those who have elders close in their lives, such as aging parents or grandparents, respect an elder's knowledge and abilities. In contrast, those with little exposure to the elderly define old by one's illnesses and disabilities.

3. Film Clip: **On Golden Pond.** This movie provides some nice illustrations of changes that take place during the aging process. Show the first 20 minutes, and then ask the students to contrast Henry Fonda's experiences with Katherine Hepburn's.

4. Threats to the Elderly. Make a list of threats or concerns that plague the elderly. Include topics such as hopelessness, loneliness, loss of independence, lack of choices, and institutionalization. Have students create solutions to these concerns in the context of an ambulance call. For example, to combat fear and loneliness, a paramedic could summon a family member to the scene or hospital to sit with the patient during tests and procedures. Or, to empower the patient, allow him to walk to the stretcher if possible, choose which hospital to go to, or gather important belongings before leaving the scene. These practices will improve the relationship between patient and provider.

5. Investigating Housing for the Elderly. Have students visit a variety of homes for aging adults. Create a list of questions for them to ask residents and staff. Information gathered might include: average age of resident, number of rooms or full apartments or houses, level of nursing care (if any), meals provided, social activities planned, most interesting resident, pets allowed, and so on. Have them bring brochures and information to share with the class. This activity requires students to get acquainted with the facilities in their neighborhood or response district, exercise interviewing skills, and practice oral communication skills in the classroom report.

6. Ethical Decisions about Caring for the Elderly. Create a set of case studies involving ethical decisions about caring for the elderly. Consider

©2009 Pearson Education, Inc.
Paramedic Care: Principles & Practice, Vol. 5, 3rd. Ed.

including issues such as caring for an incompetent person in the home, gaining access to health care for a poor elderly person, dealing with an Alzheimer's patient, getting care for a severely ill but competent elder refusing care, and DNR orders and living wills. Give the same set of case studies to each of several groups and compare the care plans arrived at by each group. This critical thinking activity improves cooperative learning and oral communication skills.

7. *Health Care Financing and the Elderly.* Paramedics are easily frustrated by patients who do not comply with their medication regimen or who fail to seek health care promptly. Help students understand the financial limitations of health care financing and fixed incomes by having each seek health insurance. Give students a set of demographics and have them use the Internet or an insurance broker to seek health care coverage for their fictitious person. Be sure to compare the cost of coverage and elements covered by the policies. Offer a prize for the most economical and most comprehensive coverage sought. Most likely, everyone will be amazed at the cost and limitations of coverage for older adults.

8. *Designing a Safety or Prevention Program.* Divide the class into work teams and ask them to design a safety or prevention program that focuses on needs of the elderly. Be sure they address issues of researching the need, identifying the population to be served, financing the project, implementation, data collection and sharing, measuring the impact on the target population, and benefits to EMS providers. These projects should be documented and presented to the class. This activity encourages critical thinking and creative problem solving. Communication skills also are exercised.

9. *Explaining the Inconvenience of Aging.* Allow students to experience the inconveniences of aging by giving each a disability of aging for the day. Create arthritics by placing Popsicle sticks in the fingers of exam gloves. Imitate cataracts and glaucoma patients by placing clear tape on goggles. The hearing impaired should use disposable earplugs. Emphysema patients can be simulated by wearing a nasal cannula and portable oxygen tank. Be sure to have students do daily activities such as dressing, toileting, eating, and socializing.

The following strategy relates to Special Features in the student textbook and can be used to enhance the student's understanding:

Cultural Considerations: How Well Are They Living? Take a field trip to a local senior citizen or adult day care center to interact with the seniors to develop a better understanding of situations affecting this patient group. Alternatively, your community may have a senior citizen outreach program that will provide a speaker or allow a field trip to interact with senior patients.

The following strategies can be used at various points throughout the lesson or to help summarize and demonstrate what students have learned:

What Might Explain? Encourage students to exercise cause-and-effect thinking by asking them to consider what might explain an event.

Guest Speaker. Several options are available for using guest speakers. A gerontologist might discuss the biologic and social aspects of the aging process. An internist or family physician with a special interest in geriatrics might be asked to present a program on disease processes affecting a particular organ system. Recognizing elder abuse might be an appropriate topic for a police investigator or adult protective services officer to discuss. Representatives from local or state agencies that provide services to the elderly might be asked to briefly discuss their programs and the resources they have available.

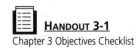

HANDOUT 3-1
Chapter 3 Objectives Checklist

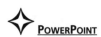
READING/REFERENCE
Criss, E., and L. Honeycutt. "20 Challenges of Geriatric Care," *JEMS*, Apr. 2000.

Kauder, D. "The Geriatric Puzzle," *JEMS*, July 2000.

POWERPOINT PRESENTATION
Volume 5, Chapter 3, PowerPoint slides 1–2

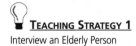
POWERPOINT PRESENTATION
Volume 5, Chapter 3, PowerPoint slides 3–14

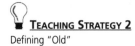
TEACHING STRATEGY 1
Interview an Elderly Person

TEACHING STRATEGY 2
Defining "Old"

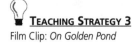
SLIDES/VIDEOS
"What It's Like to Get Old," *Pulse: Emergency Medical Update*, Aug. 1996.

TEACHING STRATEGY 3
Film Clip: *On Golden Pond*

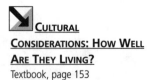
CULTURAL CONSIDERATIONS: HOW WELL ARE THEY LIVING?
Textbook, page 153

Clinical Rotations. Clinical rotations in nursing homes can provide students with an opportunity to interact with older persons and observe the interplay between normal effects of aging, acute illness, and chronic illness. Rotations with home health services offer students a chance to see older persons living in the community who require varying levels of ongoing health services. A rotation at a community center that serves seniors could give students the chance to interact with older persons who are healthy and living independently and to learn about issues and life changes to which older persons may adapt.

TEACHING OUTLINE

Chapter 3 is the third lesson in Volume 5, *Special Considerations/Operations*. Distribute Handout 3-1 so that the students can familiarize themselves with the learning goals for this chapter. If the students have any questions about the objectives, answer them at this time.

Then present the chapter. One possible lecture outline follows. In the outline, the parenthetical references in regular type are references to text pages; those in bold type are to figures, tables, or procedures.

I. Introduction. Aging is a complex process that has many implications for EMS, for which it represents a fast-growing number of users. (p. 150)

II. Epidemiology and demographics. (pp. 150–159)

A. Population characteristics (pp. 150–152)
    1. Great impact of aging on society (**Fig. 3-1**)
    2. Gerontology
        a. Scientific study of effects of aging and age-related disease on humans
    3. Geriatrics
        a. Study and treatment of diseases of the aged
B. Societal issues (pp. 152–155) (**Fig. 3-2**)
    1. Living environments
        a. Poverty and loneliness
            i. Factors that heavily affect the aged
        b. Social support (**Fig. 3-3**)
            i. Friends and family
                • Decreasing numbers of each
            ii. Life-care communities
            iii. Congregate care
            iv. Personal-care homes
            v. Independent vs. dependent living
    2. Ethics (**Fig. 3-4**)
        a. Advance directives
            i. Applicability to the elderly
        b. Paramedics should follow state laws and local EMS protocols when dealing with the elderly.
        c. Financing and resources for health care (pp. 155–159)
    3. Government programs
        a. Medicare
        b. Medicaid
        c. Veterans Administration (**Fig. 3-5**)
    4. Health care alternatives
        a. The growing costs of health care need to be contained.
        b. Home care offers the possibility of cost cutting.

5. Prevention and self-help (**Table 3-1**)
   a. Senior centers (**Fig. 3-6**)
      i. Social atmosphere
      ii. Health care endeavors
      iii. Nutrition programs
   b. Religious organizations
   c. National and state organizations
      i. AARP
      ii. Alzheimer's Association
      iii. Association for Senior Citizens
   d. Government agencies
      i. Local Departments of Health, and so on (**Fig. 3-7**)

III. General pathophysiology, assessment, and management. (pp. 160–170)

A. Pathophysiology of the elderly patient (pp. 160–164)
  1. Multiple-system failure produces common complaints.
    a. Fatigue/weakness
    b. Dizziness/vertigo/syncope
    c. Falls
    d. Headaches
    e. Insomnia
    f. Dysphagia
    g. Loss of appetite
    h. Inability to void
    i. Constipation/diarrhea
  2. Pharmacology in the elderly
    a. Often use multiple medications for multiple problems
    b. Be alert for problems that may cause lack of compliance with drug programs. (**Fig. 3-8**)
    c. Limited income
    d. Memory loss
    e. Limited mobility
    f. Sensory impairment
    g. Multiple or complicated drug therapies
    h. Fear of toxicity
    i. Childproof containers
    j. Duration of drug therapy
  3. Problems with mobility and falls (contributing factors) (**Table 3-2**)
    a. Poor nutrition
    b. Difficulty with elimination
    c. Poor skin integrity
    d. Greater predisposition for falls
    e. Loss of independence and/or confidence
    f. Depression from feeling old
    g. Isolation and lack of social network
  4. Communication difficulties (**Table 3-3**)
  5. Problems with continence and elimination
    a. Incontinence causes
       i. Medical disorders
       ii. Medications
       iii. Age-related physical changes
    b. Elimination (**Table 3-4**)

B. Assessment considerations (pp. 164–170)
  1. General health assessment
    a. Living situation
    b. Level of activity

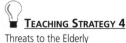

TEACHING STRATEGY 4
Threats to the Elderly

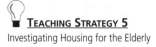

TEACHING STRATEGY 5
Investigating Housing for the Elderly

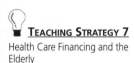

TEACHING STRATEGY 6
Ethical Decisions about Caring for the Elderly

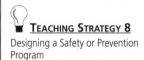

TEACHING STRATEGY 7
Health Care Financing and the Elderly

POWERPOINT PRESENTATION
Volume 5, Chapter 3, PowerPoint slides 15–112

TEACHING STRATEGY 8
Designing a Safety or Prevention Program

TEACHING STRATEGY 9
Explaining the Inconvenience of Aging

POINT TO EMPHASIZE
The elderly often suffer from more than one illness or disease at a time.

POINT TO EMPHASIZE
In taking a medical history of an elderly patient, remember to ask if the patient is taking a prescribed medication as directed.

READING/REFERENCE
"Drug Therapy in the Elderly," in Beers, M. H., et al., eds. *The Merck Manual of Diagnosis and Therapy,* 17th ed. Whitehouse Station, NJ: Merck Research Laboratories, 1999.

POINT TO EMPHASIZE
In treating incontinence, remember to respect the patient's modesty and dignity.

POINT TO EMPHASIZE
Because of the increased risk of tuberculosis in patients who are in nursing homes, consider using a HEPA or N95 respirator.

READING/REFERENCE

Emmett, K. R. "Non-specific and Atypical Presentations of Diseases in the Older Patient," *Geriatrics* 53(2), Feb. 1998.

POINT TO EMPHASIZE

Try to distinguish the patient's chief complaint from the primary problems.

POINT TO EMPHASIZE

Be prepared to spend more time obtaining a history from an elderly patient.

POINT OF INTEREST

Patients who have experienced gradual hearing loss may have compensated by unconsciously learning to read lips.

POINT OF INTEREST

Because initial hearing loss frequently involves high-frequency sounds, some elderly patients may have difficulty hearing higher-pitched voices. This may present a problem for female paramedics when they try to take a history from a geriatric patient.

POINT TO EMPHASIZE

In treating respiratory disorders in the elderly patient, DO NOT FLUID OVERLOAD.

POINT TO EMPHASIZE

DO NOT assume that a confused, disoriented patient is "just senile." This constitutes failing to assess for a serious underlying problem.

---

      c. Network of social support
      d. Level of independence
      e. Medication history
      f. Sleep patterns
  2. Pathophysiology and assessment
      a. Take extra time in gathering a history, which may be difficult but is extremely vital.
  3. History
      a. Communication challenges (**Fig. 3-9; Fig. 3-10; Fig. 3-11; Fig. 3-12**)
        i. Vision difficulties
        ii. Hearing loss
        iii. Trouble speaking
      b. Altered mental status and confusion (**Fig. 3-13**)
        i. On-scene confusion
        ii. Medical conditions
        iii. Drugs
        iv. Depression
      c. Conclude the history by verifying with a credible source if one is available and the confirmation can be done discreetly.
  4. Physical examination
      a. Always respect the needs of the elderly patient when performing a physical exam.
C. Management considerations (p. 170)
  1. ABCs
  2. Remain alert for changes in patient's condition.
  3. Provide emotional support.
  4. Treatment based on assessment and history

IV. System pathophysiology in the elderly. (pp. 170–173)

A. Respiratory system (pp. 170–177)
  1. Age-related changes (**Fig. 3-14**) (**Table 3-5**)
  2. Complications
  3. Management
      a. Positioning
      b. Teach breathing patterns.
      c. Use bronchodilators as needed.
      d. Provide supplemental oxygen as needed.
      e. Monitor patient closely.
B. Cardiovascular system (p. 173)
  1. Age-related changes
  2. Complications
  3. Management
      a. Provide high-concentration supplemental oxygen.
      b. Start IV for medication administration.
      c. Inquire about age-related dosages.
      d. Monitor vital signs and rhythm.
      e. Acquire a 12-lead ECG.
      f. Remain calm, professional, and empathetic.
C. Nervous system (p. 174)
  1. Age-related changes
  2. Complications
  3. Management
      a. Monitor patient closely.
      b. Assign priority if possible stroke victim.
      c. Provide supplemental oxygen as needed.
      d. Administer medications per protocols and medical direction.

D. Endocrine system (pp. 174–175)
   1. Age-related changes
   2. Complications
      a. Hormonal Replacement Therapy (HRT)
         i. Can increase risk of breast cancer and stroke in menopausal woman
      b. Thyroid disorders
      c. Marfan's syndrome
         i. Abnormal growth of distal tissues
   3. Management
      a. Monitor patient carefully.
E. Gastrointestinal system (p. 175)
   1. Age-related changes
   2. Complications
   3. Management
F. Thermoregulatory system (p. 175)
   1. Age-related changes
   2. Complications
   3. Management
G. Integumentary system (pp. 175–176)
   1. Age-related changes
   2. Complications
   3. Management
H. Musculoskeletal system (p. 176)
   1. Age-related changes
   2. Complications
   3. Management
I. Renal system (p. 176)
   1. Age-related changes
   2. Complications
   3. Management
      a. Oxygenation
      b. Fluid status
      c. Monitoring
J. Genitourinary system (pp. 176–177)
   1. Age-related changes
   2. Complications
   3. Management
K. Immune system (p. 177)
   1. Age-related changes
   2. Complications
   3. Management
L. Hematology system (p. 177)
   1. Age-related changes
   2. Complications
   3. Management

V. Common medical problems in the elderly. (pp. 177–210)

A. Pulmonary/respiratory disorders (pp. 177–182) (**Fig. 3-15**)
   1. Pneumonia (**Fig. 3-16**)
      a. Fourth leading cause of death in elderly
      b. Signs and symptoms
         i. Increasing dyspnea
         ii. Congestion
         iii. Fever/chills
         iv. Tachypnea

POINT TO EMPHASIZE
Many endocrine emergencies encountered in the field present as altered mental status, especially with insulin-related disorders.

POINT TO EMPHASIZE
DO NOT transmit an illness—even a mild cold—to an elderly patient

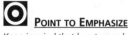

       v. Sputum production

      vi. Altered mental status

    c. Treatment

       i. Manage all life threats.

      ii. Maintain adequate oxygenation.

     iii. Transport and monitor.

2. Chronic obstructive pulmonary disease (**Fig. 3-17**)

    a. Signs and symptoms

       i. Cough

      ii. Increased sputum production

     iii. Dyspnea

     iv. Accessory muscle use

      v. Pursed lip breathing

     vi. Tripod positioning

    vii. Exercise intolerance

   viii. Wheezing

     ix. Pleuritic chest pain

      x. Tachypnea

    b. Treatment

       i. Oxygen

      ii. Drug therapy

3. Pulmonary embolism (**Fig. 3-18**)

    a. Signs and symptoms

       i. Dyspnea

      ii. Pleuritic chest pain

     iii. Right heart failure

     iv. Cardiac dysrhythmias

    b. Treatment

       i. Morphine sulfate for anxiety

      ii. Anticoagulants

     iii. Rapid transport

4. Pulmonary edema

    a. Signs and symptoms

       i. Severe dyspnea

      ii. Congestion

     iii. Rapid labored breathing

     iv. Cough with blood-stained sputum

      v. Cyanosis

     vi. Cold extremities

    b. Treatment is directed toward altering the cause of the condition.

5. Lung cancer

    a. Signs and symptoms

       i. Progressive dyspnea

      ii. Hemotypsis

     iii. Chronic cough

     iv. Weight loss

    b. Treatment is in hospital.

B. Cardiovascular disorders (pp. 182–186)

   1. Angina pectoris

   2. Myocardial infarction

    a. Presentations in elderly

       i. Absence of pain

      ii. Exercise intolerance

     iii. Confusion/dizziness

     iv. Syncope

      v. Dyspnea

      vi. Neck, dental, and/or epigastric pain
      vii. Fatigue/weakness
   3. Heart failure
     a. Signs and symptoms
       i. Fatigue
      ii. Two-pillow orthopnea
      iii. Dyspnea on exertion
      iv. Dry, hacking cough progressing to productive cough
      v. Dependent edema
      vi. Nocturia
      vii. Anoxeria, hepatomegaly, ascites
   4. Dysrhythmias
   5. Aortic dissection/aneurysms
     a. Due largely to atherosclerosis combined with hypertension
     b. IV medication and rapid transport
   6. Hypertension
     a. Often no clinically obvious signs or symptoms
     b. Management often with beta-blockers
   7. Syncope
     a. Common presentations
       i. Vasopressor
         • Common faint
      ii. Orthostatic
         • On rising from a supine or seated position
      iii. Vasovagal
         • Result of a Valsalva maneuver
      iv. Cardiac
         • Sudden decrease in cardiac output
      v. Seizures
         • Syncope may result from a seizure disorder.
         • Syncope may cause seizures.
      vi. Transient ischemic attack
         • May cause syncope
C. Neurologic disorders (pp. 186–191)
   1. Cerebrovascular disease (stroke/brain attack) (**Fig. 3-19**)
     a. Two major categories
       i. Brain ischemia (80 percent of strokes)
      ii. Brain hemorrhage
     b. Be highly suspicious of this condition in the elderly patient with a sudden change in mental status.
     c. Complete Glasgow coma scale for later comparison in ER.
   2. Seizures
     a. Easily mistaken for stroke; cause often cannot be determined in field.
   3. Dizziness/vertigo
   4. Delirium (**Table 3-6**)
     a. Signs and symptoms
       i. Acute anxiety
      ii. Inability to focus
      iii. Disordered thinking
      iv. Irritability
      v. Inappropriate behavior
      vi. Fearfulness
      vii. Excessive energy
      viii. Psychotic behavior
      ix. Aphasia/speaking disorders

POINT TO EMPHASIZE

The elderly patient with myocardial infarction is less likely to present with classic symptoms than a younger counterpart.

TEACHING TIP

Ask students why the elderly are more likely to present with "silent" myocardial infarctions.

TEACHING TIP

Some older persons who have CHF present with recurring episodes of nocturnal confusion. Why?

TEACHING TIP

Ask students to explain the relationship between major types of antihypertensives and orthostatic syncope.

TEACHING TIP

Ask students to explain why a syncopal episode could trigger a seizure.

TEACHING TIP

Strokes caused by thrombus formation frequently occur when older patients are sleeping. Why?

POINT TO EMPHASIZE

Whenever you suspect stroke, it is essential that you complete the Glasgow coma scale for later comparison in the emergency department.

READING/REFERENCE

Schneider, S. M. "Altered Mental Status in the Elderly: Current Assessment and Management Strategies for a Complex Clinical Syndrome," *Emergency Medicine Reports, 17*(5), Mar. 4, 1996.

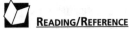
5. Dementia
   a. Signs and symptoms
      i. More prevalent in elderly than delirium
      ii. Progressive disorientation
      iii. Shortened attention span
      iv. Aphasia/nonsense talking
      v. Hallucinations
6. Alzheimer's disease (**Fig. 3-20**)
   a. Signs and symptoms
      i. Particular type of dementia
      ii. Early stage
         • Memory loss
         • Inability to learn new material
         • Mood swings
         • Personality changes
         • Aggression/hostility common
      iii. Intermediate stage
         • Complete inability to learn new material
         • Wandering
         • Increased falls
         • Loss of ability for self-care
         • Inability to walk
         • Regression to infant stage
7. Parkinson's disease (**Fig. 3-21**)
   a. Degenerative disorder characterized by changes in muscle response
   b. Common signs and symptoms
      i. Impossible to distinguish primary and secondary in field setting
      ii. Resting tremor with pill-rolling motion
      iii. Slowed, jerky movements
      iv. Shuffling gait
      v. Kyphotic deformity
      vi. Mask-like face devoid of expression

D. Metabolic and endocrine disorders (pp. 192–193)
   1. Diabetes mellitus
      a. Affects 20 percent of older adults
      b. Do not manage the diabetic and hypoglycemic emergencies differently for older patients than for others.
   2. Thyroid disorders
      a. Condition experienced by 2 to 3 percent of older patients
      b. Must be cared for in hospital.

E. Gastrointestinal disorders (pp. 193–194)
   1. Common among elderly and require prompt management
   2. Treatment
      a. Airway management
      b. Support of breathing and circulation
      c. High-flow oxygen therapy
      d. IV fluid replacement with crystalloid
      e. PASG if indicated
      f. Rapid transport
   3. Causes of upper GI bleed
      a. Peptic ulcer disease
      b. Gastritis
      c. Esophageal varices
      d. Mallory-Weiss tear

4. Lower GI bleed
   a. Diverticulosis
   b. Tumors
   c. Ischemic colitis
   d. Arterio-venous malformations
5. Bowel obstruction signs and symptoms
   a. Diffuse abdominal pain
   b. Bloating
   c. Nausea
   d. Vomiting
   e. Distended abdomen
   f. Hypoactive/absent bowel sounds
6. Mesenteric infarct signs and symptoms
   a. Pain out of proportion to physical exam
   b. Bloody diarrhea
   c. Some tachycardia
   d. Abdominal distention
F. Skin disorders (pp. 194–196)
   1. Skin diseases
      a. Itching may camouflage other conditions.
      b. Slower healing and compromised tissue perfusion make the elderly more susceptible to bacterial infection and fungal infections.
      c. Disorders may be drug-induced.
         i. For example, beta-blockers and psoriasis
   2. Pressure ulcers (decubitus ulcers) (**Fig. 3-22**)
      a. Most common in people over 70
      b. Care
         i. Change patient's position frequently.
         ii. Use a pull sheet to move patient.
         iii. Pad skin before movement.
         iv. Clean and dry areas of excessive moisture.
         v. Clean ulcers with normal saline and cover with hydrocolloid or hydrogel dressings.
G. Musculoskeletal disorders (pp. 196–199)
   1. Osteoarthritis
      a. Leading cause of disability of those 65 and older
      b. Initially presents as joint pain, worsened by exercise, improved by rest. (**Fig. 3-23**)
      c. Treatment involves stretching, drug therapy and, as a last resort, surgery.
   2. Osteoporosis (**Fig. 3-24**)
      a. Softening of bone tissue due to loss of essential minerals
      b. Affects 20 million Americans
      c. Usually asymptomatic until fracture occurs
      d. Management involves prevention through exercise and drug therapy.
   3. Ankylosing spondylitis (**Fig. 3-25**)
      a. Inflammation of the joints between the vertebrae of the spine and the sacroiliac joints in the pelvis
      b. Bamboo spine
      c. Progresses to spinal fusion
         i. No flexion, extension, or lateral movement
      d. Management considerations
H. Renal disorders (p. 199)
   1. Common problems
      a. Renal failure
      b. Glomerulonephritis
      c. Renal blood clots

2. Precipitating conditions
   a. Hypotension
   b. Heart failure
   c. Major surgery
   d. Sepsis
   e. Angiographic procedures
   f. Use of nephrotoxic antibiotics
I. Urinary disorders (pp. 199–200)
   1. Affects 10 percent of the elderly
   2. Signs and symptoms
      a. Cloudy, foul-smelling urine
      b. Bladder pain
      c. Frequent urination
      d. Signs of septic shock with urosepsis
   3. Treatment
      a. Placement of large-bore IVs for administration of fluids and antibiotics
      b. Prompt transport
J. Environmental emergencies (pp. 200–201)
   1. Hypothermia
      a. Elderly may fail to note or report signs/symptoms of hypothermia; may not shiver.
      b. Rewarm as with other patients and provide rapid transport.
   2. Hyperthermia (heatstroke)
      a. Nearly half of all heatstroke deaths are to people over age 50.
      b. Signs and symptoms may be masked.
      c. Treat as with other patients and provide rapid transport.
K. Toxicological emergencies (pp. 201–206)
   1. Aging alters pharmacokinetics and pharmacodynamics in the elderly, while medical conditions lead them to take more medications.
   2. Common drugs that cause problems for elderly patients
      a. Lidocaine
      b. Beta-blockers
      c. Antihypertensives/diurectics
         i. Hydrochlorothiazide
         ii. Furosemide
         iii. Ethacrynic acid
         iv. Bumetanide
         v. Torsemide
      d. Angiotensin-Converting Enzyme (ACE) inhibitors
      e. Digitalis (Digoxin, Lanoxin)
      f. Antipsychotropics/antidepressants
         i. SSRIs:
            • Prozac
            • Wellbutrin
         ii. Tricyclic antidepressants
            • Elavil
            • Tofranil
         iii. Monamine oxidase inhibitors
            • Marplan
            • Nardil
            • Lithium
         iv. Antipsychotics
            • Thorazine
            • Mellaril
            • Taractan

POINT TO EMPHASIZE

Remember that the elderly hypothermic patient often does not shiver.

READING/REFERENCE

Criss, E. "The Elderly & Drug Interactions." *JEMS*, Mar. 2002

- • Navane
- • Haldol
- **v.** Benzodiazepines
  - • Flurazepam
  - • Temazepam
  - • Triazolam
- **vi.** Antianxiety
  - • Diazepam
  - • Lorazepam
  - • Chlordiazepoxide
- **g.** Medications for Parkinson's disease
  - **i.** Carbidopa/levadopa
  - **ii.** Bromocriptine
  - **iii.** Benzotropine mesylate
  - **iv.** Amantadine
  - **v.** Tsmar
  - **vi.** Sinemet
- **h.** Antiseizure medications
  - **i.** Analgesics and anti-inflammatory agents
  - **ii.** Narcotic analgesics
    - • Codeine
    - • Meperidine
    - • Morphine
    - • Oxycodone
    - • Propoxyphene
  - **iii.** NSAIDs
  - **iv.** Acetaminophen
- **j.** Corticosteroids
  - **i.** Cortisone
  - **ii.** Hydrocortisone
  - **iii.** Prednisone
- **L.** Substance abuse (pp. 206–207)
  - **1.** Up to 17 percent of the elderly are addicted to substances.
  - **2.** Drug abuse
    - **a.** Polypharmacy
    - **b.** Signs and symptoms
      - **i.** Memory changes
      - **ii.** Drowsiness
      - **iii.** Decreased vision/hearing
      - **iv.** Orthostatic hypotension
      - **v.** Poor dexterity
      - **vi.** Mood changes
      - **vii.** Falling
      - **viii.** Restlessness
      - **ix.** Weight loss
  - **3.** Alcohol abuse
    - **a.** 15 percent of men and 12 percent of women exceed guidelines for use of alcohol.
    - **b.** High risk of toxicity in elderly with abuse of alcohol
    - **c.** Signs and symptoms
      - **i.** Mood swings, denial, hostility
      - **ii.** Confusion
      - **iii.** History of falls
      - **iv.** Anorexia
      - **v.** Insomnia
      - **vi.** Visible anxiety
      - **vii.** Nausea

 POINT TO EMPHASIZE

Unless an elderly person is openly intoxicated, discovery of alcohol abuse often depends upon a thorough history.

M. Behavioral/psychological disorders (pp. 207–210)
    1. Common classifications of disorders related to aging include
        a. Organic brain syndrome
        b. Affective disorders
            i. Depression
        c. Personality disorders
            i. Dependent personality
        d. Dissociative disorders
            i. Paranoid
            ii. Schizophrenia
    2. Depression
        a. Up to 15 percent of the elderly experience depression.
        b. Rising to 30 percent among the institutionalized
    3. Suicide
        a. Highest suicide rates in United States are in those over 65, especially men.
        b. Third leading cause of death among the elderly
        c. Warning signs
            i. Loss of interest in once-pleasurable activities
            ii. Curtailing of social interaction, grooming, self-care
            iii. Breaking from medical or exercise regimens
            iv. Grieving a personal loss
            v. Feeling useless
            vi. Putting affairs in order, finalizing things
            vii. Stockpiling medications or other means of self-destruction

VI. Trauma in the elderly patient. (pp. 210–215)

A. Contributing factors for severe injury and complications (p. 210)
    1. Osteoporosis
    2. Reduced cardiac reserve
    3. Decreased respiratory function, ARDS
    4. Impaired renal function
    5. Decreased elasticity in blood vessels
B. General assessment (pp. 210–211)
    1. Proceed as with other patients, but remember that signs and symptoms in the elderly can be deceptive
    2. Observe for abuse/neglect; report suspected cases. (**Fig. 3-26**)
    3. Average abused patient
        a. Over 80
        b. Has multiple medical problems
        c. Senile dementia is common
C. General management (pp. 211–212)
    1. Cardiovascular considerations
        a. Elderly trauma patients may require higher-than-usual arterial pressures for perfusion of vital organs.
        b. Take care in IV fluid administration because of decreased myocardial reserves.
    2. Respiratory considerations
        a. Remember age-related changes in the respiratory system.
        b. Make necessary adjustments in treatment to provide adequate oxygenation and CO_2 removal.
        c. Use positive-pressure ventilations cautiously.
    3. Renal considerations
        a. Remember age-related changes in the renal system.
        b. Injured elderly patients are at greater risk for fluid overload and pulmonary edema.
        c. Toxins and medications accumulate more readily in the elderly.

POINT TO EMPHASIZE

All suicidal elderly patients should be transported to the hospital.

READING/REFERENCE

Criss, E. "Trauma in the Elderly," *JEMS*, Jul. 2002.

POINT TO EMPHASIZE

In assessing elderly trauma patients, remember that blood pressure and pulse readings can be deceptive indicators of hypoperfusion.

POINT TO EMPHASIZE

Many states have laws that require prehospital personnel to report suspected cases of geriatric abuse and/or neglect.

READING/REFERENCE

"Geriatric Trauma" and "Abuse in the Elderly and Impaired," in Tintinalli, J. E., et al., eds., *Emergency Medicine: A Comprehensive Study Guide,* 5th ed., New York: McGraw-Hill, 1999.

4. Transport considerations
- **a.** Remember frailty of the elderly.
- **b.** Move gently.
- **c.** Keep the patient warm.
- **d.** Package appropriately. (**Fig. 3-27**)

D. Specific injuries (pp. 212–215)
- **1.** Orthopedic injuries (**Fig. 3-28**)
  - **a.** The elderly suffer the greatest mortality and disability from falls.
    - **i.** Most commonly a fracture of hip or pelvis
  - **b.** When treating orthopedic injuries, remain alert for cardiac emergencies.
- **2.** Burns
  - **a.** The elderly more likely to suffer deaths from burns than any other age group except neonates and infants.
  - **b.** Factors affecting burns in elderly
    - **i.** Slowed reaction time among elderly
    - **ii.** Preexisting diseases
    - **iii.** Age-related skin changes
    - **iv.** Immunological and metabolic changes
    - **v.** Reductions in physiological function and reduced reserve of organ systems
  - **c.** Management is the same as for other patients but remember:
    - **i.** Elderly are at increased risk for shock.
    - **ii.** Fluids are important to prevent renal tubular damage.
- **3.** Head and spinal injuries
  - **a.** Remember that the elderly are at increased risk of brain injury because of decrease in brain size.
  - **b.** The spine is also more subject to injury because of osteoporosis and spondylosis.

VII. Summary. The elderly are a growing part of EMS, and paramedics must be prepared for special concerns in their assessment and care. (p. 215)

POINT TO EMPHASIZE

Keep in mind that trauma places an elderly person at increased risk of hypothermia. Ensure that the patient is kept warm at all times.

POWERPOINT PRESENTATION

Volume 5, Chapter 3, PowerPoint slide 113

SKILLS DEMONSTRATION AND PRACTICE

Give the students a chance to experience some of the effects of aging by rotating them through the following stations in a skills lab.

Station 1: Vision Obtain a set of swimmer's goggles or safety goggles and:

- Paste yellow transparent cellophane or lubricating jelly on the lenses to represent yellowing of the lens of the eye and to simulate cataracts.
- Paste strips of black paper on the sides for left and/or right obstruction of peripheral vision.
- Paste black paper in a circle around each eye to depict tunnel vision.
- Paste spots of black paper on the goggles to represent spotted vision commonly experienced by patients with certain forms of retinal disorders.
- Totally blacken the lens to represent blindness.
- Have students wearing the totally blackened goggles take a "blind walk" to illustrate dependence on a companion, the importance of cues and barriers, and the use of handrails.
- Shake a slide in a projector as the slide is shown on a screen to simulate an inability to control ocular motion.

- Have students read or perform other detailed work in a dimly lit room to illustrate effects of reduction in light to the eyes.

Station 2: Hearing

- Obtain a set of swimmer's earplugs, a pair of earmuffs, or a stocking hat to dull the sound of people talking. After the student inserts the earplugs, verbally give him directions for accomplishing a task. Time the students to illustrate how hearing loss may even affect how fast a person can accomplish an assignment or process directions.
- Do not forget the interrelation of vision and hearing. Have a blindfolded person listen to instructions given at a fast pace. This will illustrate how often we depend on nonverbal as well as verbal communication cues.

Station 3: Touch

- Have students don plastic or rubber gloves to work in different water temperatures and to pick up small objects, so that they may experience the difficulties the elderly may experience in distinguishing water temperatures and in grasping small objects.
- Ask a person wearing a pair of gloves to tie shoelaces or to perform any other similar task such as buttoning a shirt or buckling a belt.
- Place masking tape around several fingers and/or joints to simulate a missing finger or stiffened joint. Use elastic bandages to limit the functioning of the hand or wrist.
- Set up some one-handed tasks to demonstrate the difficulty encountered by a person who is missing an arm or who has lost the use of an arm through a stroke.

Station 4: Taste
After blocking out the student's visual and olfactory capacities by use of a blindfold and cotton in the nose:

- Have the student eat and identify raw pieces of apple and potato (foods that have similar textures); a potato chip and a corn chip.
- Ask the student to distinguish between a variety of foods that have been put through a blender so they cannot be recognized by their texture.

Station 5: Smell
The close relationship between smell, taste, and vision makes designing simulation exercises for smell alone difficult.

- As a variation of the exercise suggested for taste, ask students to identify substances by smell. Substances used can range from apples and oranges to peanut butter, mustard, and chocolate as long as they have distinctive odors. Cotton or swimmer's nose clips can be used to simulate loss of smell.
- Blindfold students and present them with a variety of odors to identify. Be certain to use a range of distinctive odors.
- Use one strong odor, such as musk oil, to mask other odors. Have the blindfolded student try to identify the other odors.

Station 6: Mobility and Gait

- Using a wheelchair and a door, ask the student to maneuver the wheelchair through the door using only one arm or leg, as would a person who had experienced a stroke. While the student is sitting in the wheelchair, have another person come from behind and move the chair without telling the student where they are going.
- Have students attempt to carry packages in their hands while using a walker or cane.

- Have a student sit in a desk chair. After spinning the chair around rapidly a few times, ask the student to walk a straight line. The dizziness experienced is similar to that of a person who has a mobility or balance problem.
- Paste thick sponge rubber on the bottom of a pair of shoes and have the person walk in them. This simulates dizziness or a lack of stability.
- Use elastic bandages on the knees and other joints to simulate stiffness. Then have the student attempt to walk across the room or rise from a low chair.
- Use a combination of these activities and those recommended for vision and touch training to demonstrate the effect of the interrelationship among the senses on mobility and balance.

YOU MAKE THE CALL

Review student responses to the You Make the Call scenario on text page 215. Suggested responses to the questions that follow the scenario are given below. Point out to students that these are acceptable answers but not necessarily the only ones. Discuss the pros and cons of points where their responses differ from these.

1. What general impression do you have of this patient?
   (The patient has fallen, leaving him at risk for head injury or fracture of the hip or pelvis. He may also have sustained blunt trauma to the chest or abdomen. A question exists as to how this patient fell. Alcohol use is prevalent among the elderly population, but the man could have experienced a syncopal episode or stroke.)

2. Do you suspect that this is an acute or chronic problem? Explain.
   (Probably acute. The house is clean and well cared for, and the wife implied that he does the cleaning.)

3. Aside from the patient's presentation and response to your interventions, what other information must be included in your hospital report?
   (The hospital staff needs to know that Mr. Jones is the primary caregiver for his disabled wife. Arrangements for her care must be made.)

4. What support do you provide for Mrs. Jones?
   (Keep in mind the devastating effect of an ill spouse on an elderly patient. You could soon have two patients instead of one. Provide Mrs. Jones with psychological support and tell her that everything possible will be done for her husband. Ask if she can call anybody to help her. Assure her that you will make the hospital aware of her need for home care.)

ASSIGNMENTS

Assign students to complete Chapter 3, "Geriatric Emergencies," of the Workbook. Also assign them to read Chapter 4, "Abuse and Assault," before the next class.

EVALUATION

Chapter Quiz and Scenario Distribute copies of the Chapter Quiz and Scenario provided in Handouts 3-2 to 3-4 to evaluate student understanding of this chapter. Make sure each student reads the scenario to reinforce critical thinking on the scene. Remind students not to use their notes or textbooks while taking the quiz.

WORKBOOK
Chapter 3 Activities

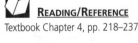
READING/REFERENCE
Textbook Chapter 4, pp. 218–237

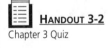
HANDOUT 3-2
Chapter 3 Quiz

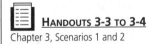
HANDOUTS 3-3 TO 3-4
Chapter 3, Scenarios 1 and 2

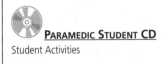
PARAMEDIC STUDENT CD
Student Activities

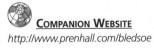
COMPANION WEBSITE
http://www.prenhall.com/bledsoe

TestGen
Volume 5, Chapter 3

EMT Achieve:
Paramedic Test Preparation
Mistovich & Beasley. *EMT Achieve:*
Paramedic Test Preparation,
http://www.prenhall.com/
emtachieve.

Success! for the
Paramedic
Cherry. *SUCCESS! for the Paramedic,*
4th edition

Handouts 3-5 to 3-6
Reinforcement Activities

Paramedic Student CD
Student Activities

PowerPoint
Presentation
Volume 5

Companion Website
http://www.prenhall.com/bledsoe

OneKey
Volume 5, Chapter 3

Advanced Life
Support Skills
Larmon & Davis. *Advanced Life*
Support Skills

Advanced Life
Skills Review
Larmon & Davis. *Advanced Life Skills*
Review

Brady Skills
Series: ALS
Larmon & Davis. *Brady Skills Series:*
ALS

Paramedic National
Standards Self-Test
Miller. *Paramedic National Standards*
Self-Test, 5th edition

Student CD   Quizzes for every chapter are contained on the dynamic and highly visual in-text student CD.

Companion Website   Additional quizzes for every chapter are contained on this exciting website.

TestGen   You may wish to create a custom-tailored test using *Prentice Hall TestGen for Paramedic Care: Principles & Practice,* 3rd edition, to evaluate student understanding of this chapter.

Online Test Preparation (for students and instructors)   Additional test preparation is available through Brady's new online product, EMT Achieve: Paramedic Test Preparation, at *http://www.prenhall.com/emtachieve.* Instructors can also monitor student mastery online.

Success! for the Paramedic   Keyed to *Paramedic Care: Principles & Practice* and *Essentials of Paramedic Care,* this comprehensive exam review contains hundreds of test questions and rationales.

REINFORCEMENT

Handouts   If classroom discussion or performance on the quiz indicates that some students have not fully mastered the chapter content, you may wish to assign some or all of the Reinforcement Handouts for this chapter.

Student CD (for students)   A wide variety of material on this CD-ROM will reinforce and also expand student knowledge and skills.

PowerPoint Presentation (for instructors)   The PowerPoint material developed for this chapter offers useful reinforcement of chapter content.

Companion Website (for students)   Additional review quizzes and links to EMS resources will contribute to further reinforcement of the chapter.

OneKey   Online support is offered for this course on one of three platforms: CourseCompass, Blackboard, or WebCT. Includes the IRM, PowerPoints, Test Manager, and Companion Website for instruction. Ask your local sales representative for more information.

Brady Skills Series: Advanced Life Skills (Video or CD)   Have your students watch the skills come to life on VHS or CD-ROM, or they can purchase the highly visual, full-color text with step-by-step procedures with rationales.

Paramedic National Standards Self-Test   Another comprehensive review manual containing hundreds of review questions with page references keyed to several Brady texts.

©2009 Pearson Education, Inc.
Paramedic Care: Principles & Practice, Vol. 5, 3rd. Ed.

CHAPTER 3 OBJECTIVES CHECKLIST

Knowledge Objective	Date Mastered
1. Discuss the demographics demonstrating the increasing size of the elderly population in the United States.	
2. Assess the various living environments of elderly patients.	
3. Discuss society's view of aging and the social, financial, and ethical issues facing the elderly.	
4. Describe the resources available to assist the elderly and create strategies to refer at-risk patients to appropriate community services.	
5. Discuss common emotional and psychological reactions to aging, including causes and manifestations.	
6. Apply the pathophysiology of multisystem failure to the assessment and management of medical conditions in the elderly patient.	
7. Compare the pharmacokinetics of an elderly patient to that of a young patient, including drug distribution, metabolism, and excretion.	
8. Discuss the impact of polypharmacy, dosing errors, increased drug sensitivity, and medication noncompliance on assessment and management of the elderly patient.	
9. Discuss the use and effects of commonly prescribed drugs for the elderly patient.	
10. Discuss the problem of mobility in the elderly, and develop strategies to prevent falls.	
11. Discuss age-related changes in sensations in the elderly, and describe the implications of these changes for communication and patient assessment.	
12. Discuss the problems with continence and elimination in the elderly patient, and develop communication strategies to provide psychological support.	
13. Discuss factors that may complicate the assessment of the elderly patient.	
14. Describe principles that should be employed when assessing and communicating with the elderly.	
15. Compare the assessment of a young patient with that of an elderly patient.	
16. Discuss common complaints of elderly patients.	

OBJECTIVES

Knowledge Objective	Date Mastered
17. Discuss the normal and abnormal changes of age in relation to the:	
a. Pulmonary system	
b. Cardiovascular system	
c. Nervous system	
d. Endocrine system	
e. Gastrointestinal system	
f. Thermoregulatory system	
g. Integumentary system	
h. Musculoskeletal system	
18. Describe the incidence, morbidity/mortality, risk factors, prevention strategies, pathophysiology, assessment, need for intervention and transport, and management for elderly medical patients with:	
a. Pneumonia, chronic obstructive pulmonary disease, pulmonary edema, lung cancer, and pulmonary embolism	
b. Angine pectoris, myocardial infarction, heart failure, dysrhythmias, aneurysm, hypertension, and syncope	
c. Cerebral vascular disease, seizures, dizziness, delirium, dementia, Alzheimer's disease, and Parkinson's disease	
d. Diabetes and thyroid diseases	
e. Gastrointestinal problems, GI hemorrhage, bowel obstruction, and mesenteric infarct	
f. Skin diseases and pressure ulcers	
g. Osteoarthritis and osteoporosis	
h. Hypothermia and hyperthermia	
i. Toxicological problems, including drug toxicity, substance abuse, alcohol abuse, and drug abuse	
j. Psychological disorders, including depression and suicide	

Knowledge Objective	Date Mastered
19. Describe the incidence, morbidity/mortality, risk factors, prevention strategies, pathophysiology, assessment, need for intervention and transport, and management of the elderly trauma patient with:	
a. Orthopedic injuries	
b. Burns	
c. Head injuries	

Skill Objective	Date Mastered
20. Given several preprogrammed simulated geriatric patients with various complaints, provide the appropriate assessment, management, and transport.	

OBJECTIVES

CHAPTER 3 QUIZ

Write the letter of the best answer in the space provided.

_____ 1. A 78-year-old nursing home patient is found to have severe pedal edema. His neck veins are flat. No adventitious sounds are present in the lung fields. There is no abdominal distention. The patient reportedly spends 12 to 14 hours a day sitting in front of the TV with his feet in a dependent position. The edema of his ankles and feet probably results from:
  A. right-sided heart failure.
  B. immobility and the dependent position of his feet.
  C. liver disease.
  D. left-sided heart failure.

_____ 2. Kyphosis in a geriatric patient will most likely result in the paramedic having to modify:
  A. interviewing techniques because kyphosis causes hearing loss.
  B. methods for spinal stabilization because kyphosis results in excessive curvature of the upper back and neck.
  C. drug dosages because kyphosis is a result of liver damage.
  D. sedation because kyphosis is associated with manic-depressive disorder.

_____ 3. In the United States, the most common cause of dementia among older persons is:
  A. psychosis.   **C.** drug and alcohol abuse.
  B. Alzheimer's disease.   **D.** depression.

_____ 4. Which of the following medications poses the greatest risk of adverse effects in the geriatric patient if given at normal adult doses?
  A. Lidocaine   **C.** Midazolam
  B. Adenosine   **D.** Narcan

_____ 5. The most common psychiatric disorder among geriatric patients is:
  A. schizophrenia.
  B. paranoia.
  C. depression.
  D. posttraumatic stress disorder.

_____ 6. A 90-year-old female has been experiencing episodes of nocturnal confusion for several weeks. Her lower extremities are swollen, with large, translucent fluid-filled areas resembling blisters on the skin. These areas probably are caused by:
  A. an allergic reaction to medication.
  B. toxicity from an antidepressant medication the patient is taking.
  C. increased hydrostatic pressure caused by right-sided CHF and sleeping sitting up.
  D. degenerative effects of old age on the skin of the lower extremities.

_____ 7. A 77-year-old male has been experiencing dizziness and weakness when he attempts to stand quickly. Causes that should be considered include:
  A. beta-blocker use.
  B. use of vasodilators for treatment of hypertension.
  C. hypovolemia secondary to diuretic use or depressed thirst mechanisms.
  D. all of the above.

_____ 8. An 89-year-old female presents with multiple bruises on her face and upper extremities. She lives with her son, who tells you that the patient is always falling down and is just generally clumsy. The patient appears malnourished and frightened. She cowers when you approach and is reluctant to allow you to examine her. Her son seems to be hostile toward you and your

©2009 Pearson Education, Inc.
Paramedic Care: Principles & Practice, Vol. 5, 3rd. Ed.

partner and nervously attempts to explain each bruise. In this case you should do all of the following, EXCEPT:
- A. obtain a complete patient and family history.
- B. report suspicions of elder abuse to the emergency department staff.
- C. be honest and open with the patient's son about your concerns.
- D. listen carefully for inconsistencies in stories.

_____ 9. When you are assessing or managing an older patient, you should:
- A. use physical contact to compensate for loss of sight or hearing.
- B. talk louder than normal because most of the elderly have hearing loss.
- C. separate the patient from friends or family as quickly as possible to reduce anxiety.
- D. call the patient "dear" or "honey" to make the patient feel cared for.

_____ 10. Patients taking diuretics such as furosemide are at special risk for developing which of the following electrolyte imbalances?
- A. hypocalcemia
- B. hypokalemia
- C. hypercalcemia
- D. hyperkalemia

_____ 11. Which of the following combinations of signs and symptoms would be most suggestive of acute myocardial infarction in a geriatric patient?
- A. extreme weakness, malaise, syncope, jaundice
- B. extreme weakness, syncope, loss of bowel and bladder control, malaise
- C. syncope, loss of bowel and bladder control, confusion, stiff neck and headache
- D. extreme weakness, confusion, syncope, stiff neck and headache

_____ 12. Which of the following statements about medical emergencies in geriatric patients is NOT true?
- A. Dyspnea may be the only symptom with which acute myocardial infarction presents.
- B. Syncope in the elderly is rarely significant.
- C. Congestive heart failure may present with episodes of nocturnal restlessness and confusion.
- D. Occlusive strokes (thrombus formation) tend to be more common in the elderly.

_____ 13. What effect will hypokalemia have if a patient is taking digitalis?
- A. It will enhance the effects of digitalis, possibly resulting in digitalis toxicity.
- B. It will antagonize the action of digitalis, making the digitalis ineffective.
- C. It will not produce any significant effects.
- D. It will antagonize the effects of digitalis if the patient is digitalis toxic, but will enhance the effects if the patient is not digitalis toxic.

_____ 14. Which of the following statements about the care of geriatric trauma patients is NOT true?
- A. The heart's ability to increase its rate and stroke volume to compensate for hypovolemia may be decreased.
- B. The patient may require a greater amount of IV fluid to support the higher arterial pressures needed to perfuse the vital organs.
- C. In the geriatric patient, tissues and organs have less tolerance of hypoxia and hypoperfusion.
- D. Physical deformities may require modification of packaging procedures.

_____ 15. A 73-year-old female has been experiencing episodes of weakness and dizziness. You have placed her on oxygen by nonrebreather mask and attached an ECG monitor. As you continue to take her history, she suddenly complains of feeling light-headed and weak. You look at the monitor and notice that the patient has gone into complete AV block with no escape rhythm. After about 15 seconds of generating only P waves, the patient returns to a sinus rhythm, and her symptoms quickly resolve. The patient has experienced a problem called:
- A. Stokes-Adams syndrome.
- B. transient ischemic attack.
- C. sick sinus syndrome.
- D. autonomic dysreflexia.

_____ 16. Which of the following statements about elder abuse is NOT true?
  A. Elder abuse generally is limited to low socioeconomic situations.
  B. Injuries that cannot be explained are the primary finding.
  C. The victim frequently is no longer able to be independent, and the family has difficulty upholding commitments to provide care.
  D. It may be important to note inconsistencies between the histories obtained from the patient and from family members.

_____ 17. A 67-year-old male fell while trying to get up from a chair. He had begun to experience pain in his lower back about 15 minutes before. When he tried to get up, he discovered that his legs were weak and numb. The patient has a history of hypertension for about 15 years. He smokes two packs of cigarettes a day. Vital signs are BP 102/60; pulse 120 weak, regular; respirations 18 shallow, regular. He is awake, alert, and responds appropriately to questions. Breath sounds are present and equal bilaterally with no adventitious sounds. Abdomen is very obese and nontender. The lower abdomen is mottled. The lower extremities are mottled and have no spontaneous movement and no response to pain. There are no pedal pulses. The back is nontender to palpation. Upper extremities move spontaneously with equal grip strengths and normal sensation. What problem do you suspect?
  A. cerebrovascular accident
  B. lumbar spine fracture
  C. abdominal aortic aneurysm
  D. silent acute myocardial infarction

_____ 18. A 76-year-old male called 911 because he could not breathe. He pants as he speaks and must take several breaths between each word. He is diaphoretic, and his lips and nailbeds are cyanotic. The problem has been worsening for about 4 days. When he breathes, he has a sharp pain in his left lower chest that is not constant and lasts only a few seconds at a time. He has a chronic cough and smokes three packs of cigarettes a day. He says he has no history of cardiovascular disease. Vital signs are BP 130/88; pulse 130 strong, regular; respirations 42 labored. The patient's temperature is 102°F. Crackles (rales) and wheezes are present in the left lower chest. The most appropriate medications to use in managing this patient would be:
  A. oxygen, nitroglycerin, morphine.
  B. oxygen, nitroglycerin, morphine, furosemide.
  C. oxygen, morphine.
  D. oxygen, albuterol.

_____ 19. In distinguishing between delirium and dementia, you should recall that delirium:
  A. is a chronic, slowly progressive process; dementia is rapid in onset and has a fluctuating course.
  B. tends not to affect memory; dementia tends to impair memory.
  C. may be reversed if treated early; dementia is an irreversible disorder.
  D. causes global cognitive deficits; dementia causes focal cognitive deficits.

_____ 20. Special problems that may be encountered in geriatric patients may include:
  A. increased susceptibility to general deterioration as a result of illness.
  B. depressed pain and temperature-regulating mechanisms.
  C. increased susceptibility to confusion and depression.
  D. all of the above.

_____ 21. The key symptom in patients with bowel infarction is:
  A. vomiting of fecal material.
  B. pain out of proportion to physical findings.
  C. uncontrollable diarrhea.
  D. melena.

_____ 22. Which of the following findings is NOT typical of a patient with Parkinson's disease?
  A. tremor combined with pill-rolling motion of the hands
  B. shuffling gait with short steps
  C. mask-like face with no expression
  D. tendency to speak rapidly and loudly

©2009 Pearson Education, Inc.
Paramedic Care: Principles & Practice, Vol. 5, 3rd. Ed.

Student's Name _____

THE START TRIAGE SYSTEM

The following diagram represents the operation of the START triage system. Fill in each missing label to complete the flow chart.

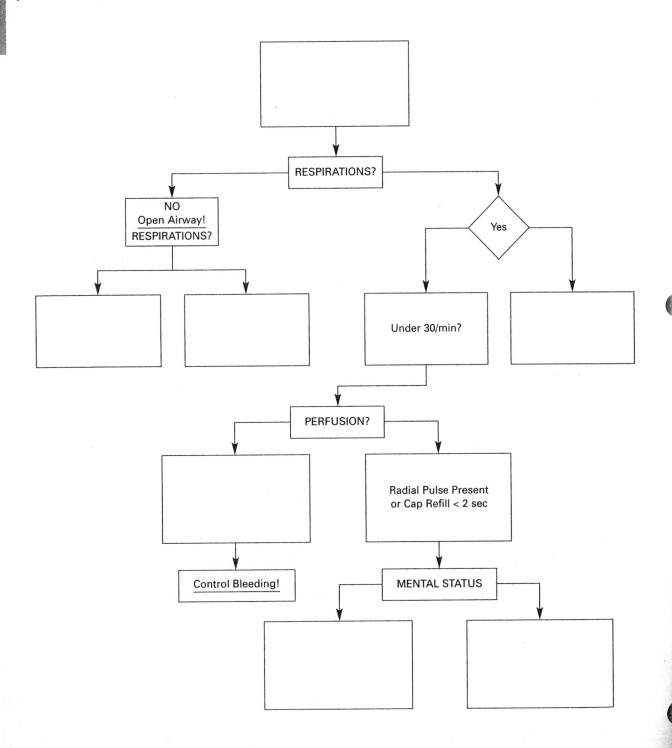

Student's Name _____

THE START TRIAGE SYSTEM

The following diagram represents the operation of the START triage system. Fill in each missing label to complete the flow chart.

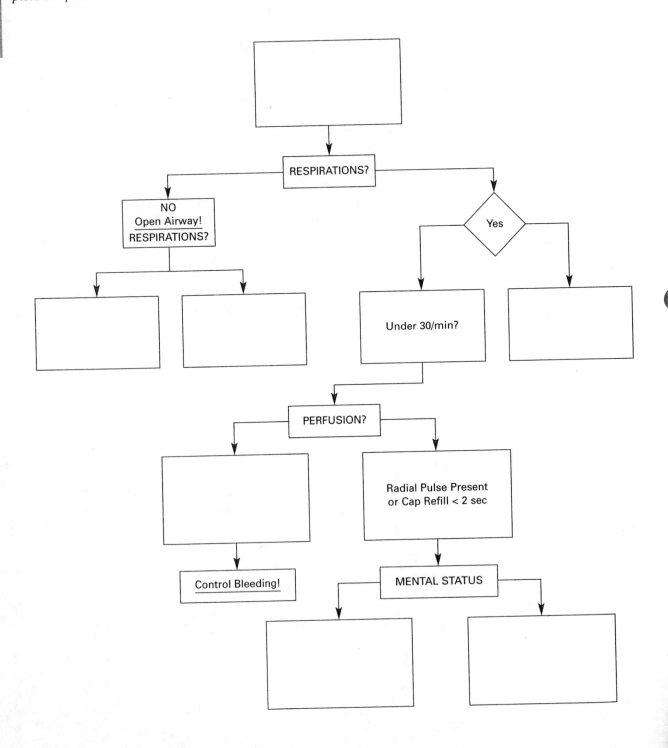

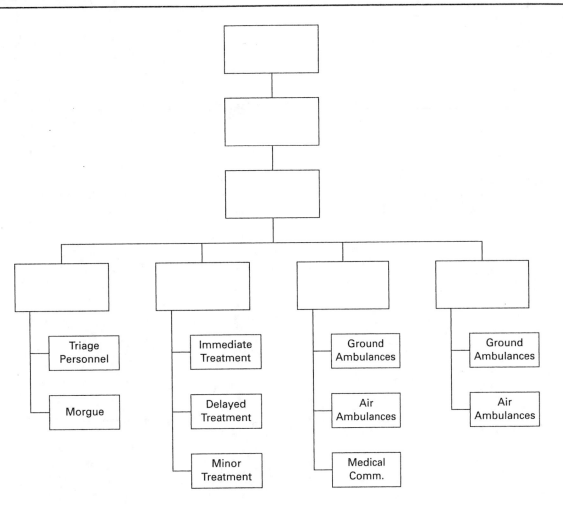

IMS EMS Branch

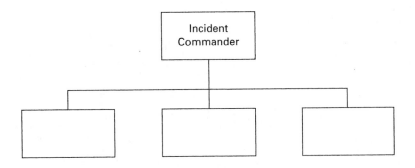

**Basic IMS Organization
EMS Operations**

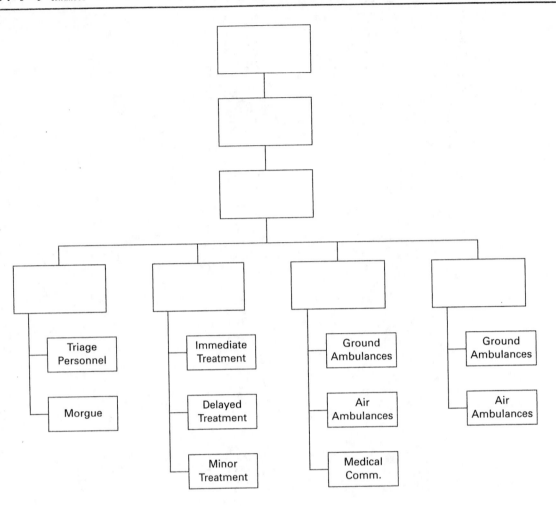

IMS EMS Branch

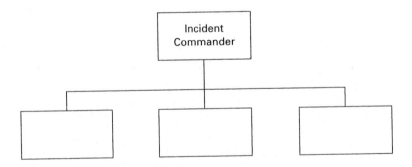

**Basic IMS Organization
EMS Operations**

STRUCTURES OF THE INCIDENT MANAGEMENT SYSTEM

Each of the following diagrams represents a figure from the text that highlights key information about IMS. Fill in each box with the missing labels.

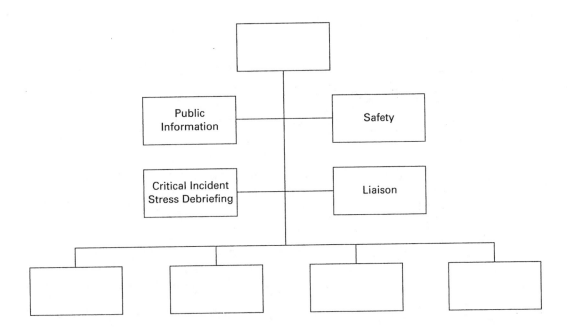

Basic Elements of the Incident Management System

©2009 Pearson Education, Inc.
Paramedic Care: Principles & Practice, Vol. 5, 3rd. Ed.

HANDOUT 9-6

Student's Name _____

STRUCTURES OF THE INCIDENT MANAGEMENT SYSTEM

Each of the following diagrams represents a figure from the text that highlights key information about IMS. Fill in each box with the missing labels.

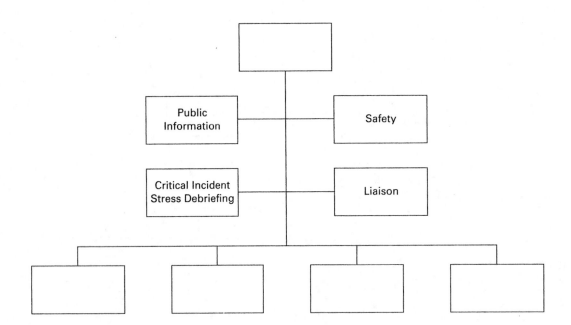

Basic Elements of the Incident Management System

©2009 Pearson Education, Inc.
Paramedic Care: Principles & Practice, Vol. 5, 3rd. Ed.

- Know how long it takes for your ambulance to cross an intersection. This will help you judge whether you have enough time to pass through safely.

- Watch pedestrians at an intersection carefully. If they all seem to be staring in another direction, rather than at your ambulance, they may well be looking at the fire truck headed your way.

- Remember that there is no such thing as a rolling stop in an ambulance weighing over 10,000 pounds or a medium-duty vehicle weighing some 24,000 pounds. Even at speeds as slow as 30 miles per hour, these vehicles will not stop on a dime. When negotiating an intersection, consider "covering the brake" to shorten the stopping distance.

- Know how long it takes for your ambulance to cross an intersection. This will help you judge whether you have enough time to pass through safely.

- Watch pedestrians at an intersection carefully. If they all seem to be staring in another direction, rather than at your ambulance, they may well be looking at the fire truck headed your way.

- Remember that there is no such thing as a rolling stop in an ambulance weighing over 10,000 pounds or a medium-duty vehicle weighing some 24,000 pounds. Even at speeds as slow as 30 miles per hour, these vehicles will not stop on a dime. When negotiating an intersection, consider "covering the brake" to shorten the stopping distance.

REINFORCEMENT

Student's Name _____

LIGHTS, SIRENS, AND INTERSECTIONS

GUIDELINES ON USE OF LIGHTS AND SIREN

Consider the following before turning on the siren:

- Motorists are less inclined to yield to an ambulance when the siren is continually sounded.
- Many motorists feel that the right-of-way privileges given to ambulances are abused when sirens are sounded.
- Inexperienced motorists tend to increase their driving speeds by 10 to 15 miles per hour when a siren is sounded.
- The continuous sound of a siren can possibly worsen sick or injured patients by increasing their anxiety.
- Ambulance operators may also develop anxiety from sirens used on long runs, not to mention the possibility of hearing problems.

Some useful guidelines on use of sirens include the following:

- Use the siren sparingly and only when you must.
- Never assume all motorists hear your siren.
- Assume that some motorists will hear your siren, but choose to ignore it.
- Be prepared for panic and erratic maneuvers when drivers do hear your siren.
- Never use the siren to scare someone.

INTERSECTIONS

Helpful tips for negotiating an intersection include the following:

- Stop at all red lights and stop signs and then proceed with caution.
- Always proceed through an intersection slowly.
- Make eye contact with other motorists to ensure they understand your intentions.
- If you are using any of the exemptions offered to you as an emergency vehicle, such as passing through a red light or a stop sign, make sure you warn motorists by appropriately flashing your lights and sounding the siren.
- Remember that lights and siren only "ask" the public to yield the right of way. If the public does not yield, it may be because they misunderstand your intentions, cannot hear the siren because of noise in their own vehicles, or cannot see your lights. Never assume that other motorists have a clue as to what you plan on doing at the intersection.
- Always go around cars stopped at the intersection on their left (driver's) side. In some instances, this may involve passing into the oncoming lane, which should be done slowly and very cautiously. You invite trouble when you use a clear right lane to sneak past a group of cars at an intersection. If motorists are doing what they should do under motor vehicle laws, they may pull into the right lane just as you attempt to pass.

©2009 Pearson Education, Inc.

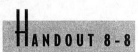

Student's Name _____

LIGHTS, SIRENS, AND INTERSECTIONS

GUIDELINES ON USE OF LIGHTS AND SIREN

Consider the following before turning on the siren:

- Motorists are less inclined to yield to an ambulance when the siren is continually sounded.
- Many motorists feel that the right-of-way privileges given to ambulances are abused when sirens are sounded.
- Inexperienced motorists tend to increase their driving speeds by 10 to 15 miles per hour when a siren is sounded.
- The continuous sound of a siren can possibly worsen sick or injured patients by increasing their anxiety.
- Ambulance operators may also develop anxiety from sirens used on long runs, not to mention the possibility of hearing problems.

Some useful guidelines on use of sirens include the following:

- Use the siren sparingly and only when you must.
- Never assume all motorists hear your siren.
- Assume that some motorists will hear your siren, but choose to ignore it.
- Be prepared for panic and erratic maneuvers when drivers do hear your siren.
- Never use the siren to scare someone.

INTERSECTIONS

Helpful tips for negotiating an intersection include the following:

- Stop at all red lights and stop signs and then proceed with caution.
- Always proceed through an intersection slowly.
- Make eye contact with other motorists to ensure they understand your intentions.
- If you are using any of the exemptions offered to you as an emergency vehicle, such as passing through a red light or a stop sign, make sure you warn motorists by appropriately flashing your lights and sounding the siren.
- Remember that lights and siren only "ask" the public to yield the right of way. If the public does not yield, it may be because they misunderstand your intentions, cannot hear the siren because of noise in their own vehicles, or cannot see your lights. Never assume that other motorists have a clue as to what you plan on doing at the intersection.
- Always go around cars stopped at the intersection on their left (driver's) side. In some instances, this may involve passing into the oncoming lane, which should be done slowly and very cautiously. You invite trouble when you use a clear right lane to sneak past a group of cars at an intersection. If motorists are doing what they should do under motor vehicle laws, they may pull into the right lane just as you attempt to pass.

_____ **23.** You respond to a report of a "person seizing." The patient is a 74-year-old female who is experiencing uncontrollable movements of the skeletal muscles in her extremities and face. She is awake, alert, and extremely agitated and restless. The patient has no history of cerebrovascular accident, seizures, or other neurologic disease. You discover that the patient's physician recently placed her on a new medication, but neither she nor her family can remember what the name of the drug is. Which of the following drugs would be most likely to produce these effects?
   A. Elavil
   B. Thorazine
   C. Librium
   D. Lithium carbonate

_____ **24.** Which of the following statements about suicide and suicide risk in the elderly is TRUE?
   A. The elderly have the lowest suicide rate of any age group in the United States.
   B. The elderly are less likely to seek help for depression and suicidal ideation than younger people.
   C. Elderly women are more likely to commit suicide than elderly men.
   D. The elderly are less likely to turn anger and sorrow inward rather than expressing these emotions outward.

_____ **25.** An 82-year-old female presents with vague complaints about feeling weak and fatigued. She denies chest pain, dizziness, nausea, or shortness of breath. She has a long history of cardiovascular and respiratory problems. She takes numerous medications but cannot recall their names or which ones she has taken today. During the physical exam, you note pedal edema, weak pedal pulses, and fine bibasilar crackles (rales). Which of the following statements about this patient is true?
   A. Absence of chest pain excludes myocardial infarction as a possible problem.
   B. Her crackles and peripheral edema may be normal findings for her.
   C. Her risk of death is highest during the first few hours following the onset of symptoms.
   D. All of the above.

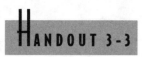
Student's Name _____

CHAPTER 3 SCENARIO 1

Review the following real-life situation. Then answer the questions that follow.

On a Saturday morning at 0930, you respond to a report of "difficulty breathing" in a residential neighborhood. The patient is a 68-year-old female who complains of weakness and shortness of breath that have increased gradually over the previous 3 days. She denies any history of heart or lung disease. Her only past history has been severe osteoarthritis for which she has been taking "a lot of aspirin." The patient is awake and alert, and she responds to questions appropriately. Vital signs are pulse 114 strong, regular; respirations 22 regular, unlabored; BP 116/86. Her skin is pale, warm, and dry. Pupils are equal and react briskly to light. Breath sounds are present and equal bilaterally with no adventitious sounds. The abdomen is soft and nontender.

1. What problem should you suspect?

2. What questions might you ask?

3. What other problem should you consider as a possible cause for her weakness and dizziness?

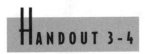

Student's Name _____

CHAPTER 3 SCENARIO 2

Review the following real-life situation. Then answer the questions that follow.

At 1030 on a Tuesday morning, you respond to a report of a motor vehicle collision. The patient is an 82-year-old male who appears to have lost control of his vehicle, which struck a utility pole. The patient is awake, alert, restless, and anxious. Respirations are rapid and shallow at 24 breaths/min. Radial pulses are weak at 80 beats/min. The patient's blood pressure is 128/86. The left lower chest is bruised and is tender to palpation. The left upper abdominal quadrant is tender. Breath sounds are present and equal bilaterally. The patient also complains of pain in his left shoulder. However, there is no bruising, tenderness, or deformity of this area. The patient takes a "blood pressure pill," but he cannot remember its name and does not have the bottle with him.

1. Based on the mechanism of injury and your physical findings, what problem do you suspect?

2. Is the patient's heart rate consistent with this problem? Why or why not?

3. If the patient's heart rate is not consistent with the problem you suspect, how do you explain your findings?

4. Is the patient's blood pressure consistent with the suspected problem? If not, how do you explain your findings?

CHAPTER 3 REVIEW

Write the word or words that best complete the following sentences in the space(s) provided.

1. The elderly who are 80 or older are referred to as the _____ - _____.

2. The scientific study of the effects of aging and age-related diseases on humans is known as _____.

3. Discrimination against old people is termed _____.

4. A living arrangement in which the elderly live in, but do not own, individual apartments or rooms and receive select services is _____ _____.

5. A legal document prepared when a person is alive, competent, and able to make informed decisions about health care is a(n) _____ _____.

6. When a paramedic is presented with a DNR, he should follow state laws and local EMS system _____.

7. The program under which federal and state governments share responsibility for providing health care to the aged poor, the blind, the disabled, and low-income families with dependent children is _____.

8. In treating the elderly, the best intervention is _____.

9. A person with a decreased ability to meet daily needs on an independent basis suffers from a(n) _____ _____.

10. A complicating factor in the assessment of the elderly is having more than one disease at a time, a condition known as _____.

11. Another complicating factor in the assessment and care of the elderly is _____, in which there is concurrent use of a number of drugs.

12. _____ - _____ injuries represent the leading cause of accidental death among the elderly.

13. The inability to retain urine or feces because of loss of sphincter control or cerebral or spinal lesions is _____.

14. In the elderly, efforts to force a bowel movement can lead to _____ _____ _____ or _____.

15. Elderly patients are more likely to suffer from _____, a ringing in the ears, or from _____ _____, a condition characterized by vertigo, nerve deafness, and a roar or buzzing in the ears.

16. The condition that can mimic senility and organic brain syndrome and can inhibit patient cooperation with the paramedic is _____.

17. By the time people reach age 65, vital capacity may be reduced by as much as _____ percent.

18. Overall there is an average _____ percent reduction in brain weight from age 20 to age 90.

19. _____ _____, in which a portion of the stomach protrudes upward into the mediastinal cavity, while not age-related per se, can have severe consequences for the elderly.

20. _____ _____ primarily causes inflammation of the joints between the vertebrae of the spine and the sacroiliac joints in the pelvis.

©2009 Pearson Education, Inc.
Paramedic Care: Principles & Practice, Vol. 5, 3rd. Ed.

21. The diminished vigor of the immune response to the challenge and rechallenge by pathogens is referred to as _____ _____.

22. The fourth leading cause of death among those 65 and older is _____.

23. The leading cause of death in the elderly is _____ _____.

24. Unlike younger cardiac patients, the elderly are more apt to suffer a(n) _____ _____ _____.

25. The best-known form of dementia is _____ _____.

26. The most common initial sign of _____ _____ is a resting tremor combined with a pill-rolling motion.

27. The paramedic should not rule out _____ as a complicating factor in cases of hypoglycemia.

28. Gastritis and esophageal varices are likely causes of _____ GI bleeding.

29. Elderly patients are more likely to develop the ischemic damage and subsequent necrosis affecting the skin that is known as a(n) _____ - _____.

30. The leading cause of disability among those 65 and older is _____.

31. The drugs that are widely used to treat hypertension, angina pectoris, and dysrhythmias and that are commonly associated with toxicity in the elderly are _____-_____.

32. An exaggerated feeling of depression or unrest, characterized by a mood of general dissatisfaction, restlessness, discomfort, and unhappiness, is _____.

33. The syndrome in which an elderly person is physically or psychologically injured by another is _____ _____.

34. The most common fall-related fracture is of the _____ or _____.

35. _____, a degeneration of the vertebral body, is common in the elderly.

Student's Name _____

THE PHYSIOLOGY OF AGING

Answer each of the following questions in the space provided.

1. What effect does aging have on dermal blood supply and thickness? How does this affect wound healing? How does this affect severity of burn injuries in the elderly?

2. What effect does aging have on bone resorption? Which gender is particularly affected? What effect does this have in victims of sudden deceleration trauma?

3. What effect does aging have on respiratory reserve capacity? What effect does this have on the ability of older patients to compensate for chest trauma or acute respiratory disease such as pulmonary embolism, spontaneous pneumothorax, or pneumonia?

4. What effect does aging have on myocardial reserve capacity? What effect does this have on volume resuscitation of the older trauma patient?

5. What effect does aging have on the peripheral blood vessels? What effect does this have on the older patient's ability to compensate for volume loss? What effect does this have on the older patient's ability to tolerate hot or cold environments?

6. What effect does aging have on the kidneys? What effect does this have on the response of the patient to drugs? What effect does this have on the response of the patient to fluid therapy for hypovolemia?

7. What effect does aging have on the conduction velocity of the nerves? What effect does this have on the ability of the older patient to feel pain?

8. What effect does aging have on the thirst mechanisms? What effect does this have on patients?

9. What effect does aging have on the size of the brain relative to the size of the cranial cavity? What effect does this produce regarding the onset of signs and symptoms from a subdural hematoma?

10. If a patient is on beta-blocker therapy, what effect does this have on your ability to detect the early signs of shock? Why?

11. What effect does aging have on the cervical spine and spinal canal? What effect do these changes have on the risk of an older person sustaining a cervical spinal cord injury?

12. What effect does aging have on hepatic blood flow and on the ability of the liver to metabolize drugs? What change does this effect dictate for the dosing of most drugs?

Chapter 3 Answer Key

Handout 3-2: Chapter 3 Quiz

1. B	8. C	14. B	20. D
2. B	9. A	15. A	21. B
3. B	10. B	16. A	22. D
4. A	11. B	17. C	23. B
5. C	12. B	18. D	24. B
6. C	13. A	19. C	25. D
7. D			

Handout 3-3: Chapter 3 Scenario 1

1. Anemia caused by gastrointestinal hemorrhage caused by excessive aspirin use.
2. Ask the patient about changes in her stool. A dark, tarry consistency helps confirm your suspicions.
3. Silent myocardial infarction.

Handout 3-4: Chapter 3 Scenario 2

1. Intra-abdominal hemorrhage and hypovolemic shock, probably from an injury to the spleen.
2. No. If the patient is compensating for volume loss secondary to hemorrhage, the heart rate should be increased.
3. If the "blood pressure pill" is a beta-blocker, the patient may be unable to accelerate his heart rate adequately in response to hypovolemia.
4. It does not appear to be, until the history of hypertension is considered. Even with treatment, a hypertensive patient may have a blood pressure significantly above "normal." Therefore, this patient may be hypotensive relative to his "normal" blood pressure.

Handout 3-5: Chapter 3 Review

1. old-old
2. gerontology
3. ageism
4. congregate care
5. advance directive
6. protocols
7. Medicaid
8. prevention
9. functional impairment
10. comorbidity
11. polypharmacy
12. Fall-related
13. incontinence
14. transient ischemic attack, syncope
15. tinnitus, Meniere's disease
16. depression
17. 50
18. 10
19. Hiatal hernia
20. Ankylosing spondylitis
21. immune senescence
22. pneumonia
23. cardiovascular disease
24. silent myocardial infarction
25. Alzheimer's disease
26. Parkinson's disease
27. alcohol
28. upper
29. pressure ulcer
30. osteoarthritis
31. beta-blockers
32. dysphoria
33. geriatric abuse
34. hip, pelvis
35. Spondylosis

Handout 3-6: The Physiology of Aging

1. The dermal blood supply decreases, and the dermis thins. Wound healing takes longer. The elderly burn more quickly and more severely at lower temperatures.
2. The rate of bone resorption increases, resulting in a decrease in bone mass and density. Females tend to be affected more frequently. Fractures can occur with less force and at lower velocities than in younger patients.
3. Respiratory reserve capacity in the elderly decreases. This diminishes the ability to compensate for chest trauma or acute respiratory disease.
4. Myocardial reserve capacity decreases. The elderly develop volume overload more easily than younger patients. Volume resuscitation must be carried out cautiously, with careful monitoring for signs of overload, particularly pulmonary edema.
5. Peripheral vessel walls become sclerotic and less able to vary the diameter of the vessel. Older patients cannot vasoconstrict as efficiently in response to volume loss. Because the elderly cannot vary the diameter of their peripheral blood vessels effectively, they cannot thermoregulate as well as younger patients.
6. Reductions in the number of nephrons and in renal blood flow occur. Drugs are excreted less effectively via the renal route, so drug action is prolonged. Excess fluid is excreted less effectively, so patients are prone to volume overload.
7. Nerve conduction velocity decreases. Pain sensation in the elderly is diminished.
8. Thirst diminishes with age. The elderly frequently do not have adequate fluid intake and often are chronically dehydrated.
9. The brain decreases in size relative to the cranial cavity. Onset of signs and symptoms of subdural hematoma may be delayed.
10. Detection of shock may be more difficult. By blocking the beta effects of sympathetic stimulation, beta-blockers mask early signs and symptoms of shock.
11. The spinal canal tends to narrow, and degeneration tends to occur in the vertebral bodies. The risk of cervical spine fracture and of spinal cord injury increases.
12. Hepatic blood flow and ability to metabolize drugs decrease. Doses of most drugs must be decreased to compensate.

©2009 Pearson Education, Inc.
Paramedic Care: Principles & Practice, Vol. 5, 3rd. Ed.

Abuse and Assault

INTRODUCTION

Abuse (which can be physical, psychological, or both) and assault (physical violence toward another person) are overwhelmingly serious and common problems. These are complex situations for paramedics to handle because the provider must address physical and psychological issues of medical care and provide appropriate management from the perspective of law enforcement. It can be very difficult to support a distraught patient, perform an adequate assessment and medical intervention, and obtain evidence for possible legal action. In some cases, providers must also remain aware that the patient's safety, and perhaps their own, is not secure. This chapter discusses incidence rates and categories of abuse, as well as profiles of perpetrators and persons at risk for abuse. It details medical aspects of care and a provider's legal responsibilities, as well as lists the resources that a provider may be able to access to assist patients who are victims of abuse and assault.

CHAPTER OBJECTIVES

Knowledge Objectives

1. Discuss the incidence of abuse and assault. (p. 220)
2. Describe the categories of abuse. (pp. 220–231)
3. Discuss examples of spouse, elder, child, and sexual abuse. (pp. 220–233)
4. Describe the characteristics associated with the profile of a typical spouse, elder, or child abuser and the typical assailant of sexual abuse. (pp. 221–222, 226, 232)
5. Identify the profile of the at-risk spouse, elder, and child. (pp. 222–223, 225, 226–227, 231–232)
6. Discuss the assessment and management of the abused patient. (pp. 223, 224, 227–230, 233)
7. Discuss the legal aspects associated with abuse situations. (pp. 220, 223, 230–231, 234)
8. Identify community resources that are available to assist victims of abuse and assault. (pp. 220, 223, 230–231, 234–235)
9. Discuss the documentation necessary when caring for abused and assaulted patients. (pp. 217, 220, 234–235)

FRAMING THE LESSON

Begin teaching of the lesson by asking students to name types of abuse and the typical victims associated with abuse and assault. Encourage all students to

TOTAL TEACHING TIME: 4.25 HOURS
The total teaching time is only a guideline based on the didactic and practical lab averages in the National Standard Curriculum. Instructors should take into consideration such factors as: the pace at which students learn, the size of the class, and breaks. The actual time devoted to teaching objectives is the responsibility of the instructor.

participate and stretch themselves on points of age, gender, or type of partner relationship. Persons of any age may be victims of abuse, as can males or females. Partner relationships can include heterosexual ones (with either the male or female as victim) or homosexual ones (again, including male or female victims). If you have time, encourage students who wish to mention a case with which they are personally familiar to discuss these instances; doing so will make personal the complex and sad situations that they will encounter as paramedics in the field. (Be prepared that one or more students may confide in you that they have been abused or are in an abusive relationship.) After this exercise is complete, students will have a better understanding of the scope of the problems of abuse and assault as well as its seriousness as a medical and legal emergency.

CONSIDERING THE CASE STUDY

Ask a volunteer to read aloud the Case Study that begins on text page 219. Suggest that students close their eyes as the scenario is read to help them visualize the events described in it. You can use the following questions as a starting point for teaching the chapter—a sort of chapter preview in a functional setting.

In the case of this particular chapter, you may wish, either before or after the discussion of questions and answers, to get students to discuss their emotional reactions to hearing the Case Study read aloud. It is not only nearly impossible for paramedics to remain completely emotionally distant when involved in abuse situations, but it may also impair their handling of such incidents. (For example, what if the female provider hadn't thought of the patient's wish for privacy and dignity and used a blanket to protect her from the gaze of others at the scene?)

When the chapter is completed, you may wish to return to the Case Study and encourage further discussion aimed at answering the questions.

CASE STUDY DISCUSSION QUESTIONS (AND ANSWERS)

1. What medical and legal aspects of this case should be apparent to the team as they make their initial scene size-up while walking toward the patient and the officer?
   (The initial impression of the patient is that she is a possible abuse victim [she is partially clothed] and a possible trauma patient [if bruises, lacerations, or other evidence of being thrown from a vehicle are present], as well as that she is definitely in need of emotional and psychological support [on the basis of the previous impressions and her apparent emotional state, crying and incoherent].)

2. What steps are taken by the team that are appropriate and specific to an incidence of abuse or assault?
   (The provider performing the physical is of the same gender, she responds to the patient's particular emotional needs [use of blanket to provide a sense of privacy and security], and she is proficient in performing tasks associated with the legal aspects of the case [handling removed clothing as possible evidence]. In addition, the team notifies an appropriate receiving facility of the patient's condition, so proper personnel will be present when the patient arrives, and takes the time to complete detailed documentation of the case as soon as possible so details are fresh in their minds.)

3. Are there any medical possibilities that might have been overlooked if the team were not prepared to handle their medical and legal roles in this emotionally trying situation?
(They might have overlooked or downplayed the trauma elements of the case because the woman didn't have severe, obvious trauma injury. If that had happened, they might not have remembered to perform spinal immobilization, a vital precaution for a patient ejected from a moving vehicle.)

TEACHING STRATEGIES

People learn in a variety of ways. Some do better with the spoken word, while others prefer the written. Some prefer to work alone, whereas others profit from working in groups. Recognizing these different ways of acquiring knowledge, the authors of this *Instructor's Resource Manual* have provided a variety of teaching strategies for the different types of learners. These strategies are intended to foster higher-level cognitive skills and encourage creative learning and problem solving.

For greatest effectiveness, incorporate these strategies into your class lecture. Marginal notes in the Teaching Outline indicate the points at which various exercises might be most appropriate. Other strategies can be used to preview the lesson or to summarize it.

The following strategies are keyed to specific sections of the lesson:

1. Understanding Victims of Abuse. It is important for students to learn that the victims of abuse are often regular people, not so different from themselves. To do this, they must spend time with people who have suffered abuse and assaults. Have the class create a volunteer project, fundraiser, or social event for a local shelter or survivor program. The gift of their time will be much appreciated, but the cooperation shared between your students and these people in need will go a long way the next time one cares for a victim of abuse or assault.

2. Creating a Reporting System for Identifying Abuse. Suggest to students that they create a reporting structure for victims that begins in the field and transfers to the hospital. For example, Rural/Metro of Syracuse, New York, has a simple half sheet of colored paper that can be removed from the run report that includes the facts surrounding suspicion of abuse or assault. Whenever the ED staff sees the report on this special colored paper, the patient gets a consult with social services, a division of the hospital better equipped to deal with the issues of abuse than a busy ED. Additionally, when a file is pulled for a patient, multiple reports on this special colored paper are an easy visual cue that previous providers have suspected abuse. Share great examples like this of EMS making a difference to inspire creative problem solving in your students.

3. Researching Community Agencies That Aid the Abused. Have students research the agencies in their communities equipped to handle victims of abuse. They should include shelters, hospitals, clinics, and counseling programs. Require them to create a pocket card so that this information is at the ready should they need to refer a patient or abuser in the future.

4. Psychologist-Led Workshop on Communicating with Victims of Abuse. Ask a counselor or psychologist with expertise in victims of abuse to help you conduct a workshop on interviewing and communicating with these patients. Be sure it is not just a lecture but a real chance to practice the techniques taught by this professional during role-playing or scenarios. This is a difficult skill that often includes sensitive and embarrassing subject matter. The student will be woefully inept unless these skills are developed first in the classroom.

5. *Improving the Index of Suspicion.* Improve your students' index of suspicion for abuse by brainstorming physical and emotional findings that might suggest abuse. Ask students to give examples of contexts in which the finding would or would not be indicative of abuse. Being alert to the possibilities will increase the likelihood that students will assess for and report potential abuse.

6. *Newspaper Articles and Case Studies of Abuse.* Gather newspaper clippings and case studies of abuse and neglect for reading in class during this unit. Often providers cannot identify with the trauma of abuse until they meet a victim and realize the people are just like themselves or their family members. Gathering clippings lends realism to the topic.

The following strategy relates to Special Features in the student textbook and can be used to enhance the student's understanding:

Cultural Considerations: Medicinal Practices of the Hmong. While it is the responsibility of every health care practitioner to report suspected cases of abuse for further investigation, it is not the practitioner's responsibility to accuse anyone of abuse. Suspected abuse in one culture may be simply custom in another. Facilitate a discussion on various cultures and practices within your community that may be considered by some to be abuse.

The following strategies can be used at various points throughout the lesson or to help summarize and demonstrate what students have learned:

Learning Local Protocol for Reporting Abuse. Be sure students understand the reporting policy in your locale. EMS professionals are not mandatory reporters in every state. If the policy exists in your area, supply students with phone numbers, contact names, and timelines for reporting. This information is probably available from your Department of Health Services.

Guest Speakers. Seeing the faces behind the profiles: If you have appropriate contacts with a battered women's shelter, sexual assault nurse examiner (SANE), police officer, or public prosecutor, consider getting someone with extensive firsthand experience to speak to the students. Another possibility is someone who has recovered from a background of abuse or assault, preferably someone who had contact with EMS at some point in their background and could address what EMTs did in their case or did not do.

Role-Playing Abuse Scenarios. If your students feel comfortable doing so, ask them to take roles in different scenarios. One scenario might have parents involved in child abuse (as in You Make the Call for this chapter; see text page 235), the child, and an EMS provider; another may have an abused elder, an adult child caregiver who is abusive or neglectful, and an EMS provider.

Ask the students who watch each role-play to take notes of things the participants say or do (such as body posture, not making eye contact with provider) that give them insight into the situation and the provider's response to the medical, social, and legal aspects of the case.

Distinguishing Abuse from Medical Problems. Invite your students to brainstorm about situations (for partner, elder, child, and sexual abuse) that might be mistaken for abuse but are not. Then have them act out the roles and get feedback from participants and viewers about their feelings for the people suspected of abuse and the provider who feels there is real suspicion of an abuse situation in this case.

Practice in the Field. If possible, talk with the appropriate liaison individuals and consider sending students (one at a time or in pairs) to any of the following types of sites or groups:

- The sexual assault unit of the local police force or district attorney's office
- A correctional institute or community group for persons convicted of abuse or assault or undergoing therapy for anger management or abuse
- A meeting of SANEs
- A facility caring for children who have been abused
- A home that takes in elders who have been abused or provides day care for at-risk elders whose adult children work outside the home

TEACHING OUTLINE

Chapter 4 is the fourth lesson in Volume 5, *Special Considerations/Operations.* Distribute Handout 4-1 so that students can familiarize themselves with the learning goals for this chapter. If students have any questions about the objectives, answer them at this time.

Then present the chapter. One possible lecture outline follows. In the outline, the parenthetical references in regular type are references to text pages; those in bold type are to figures, tables, or procedures.

I. Introduction. Millions of children, adults, and elderly persons are abused and assaulted each year in the United States, and the EMS system is involved with many cases of abuse. It is crucial that EMS providers be prepared for all aspects of care involved in handling these patients. (p. 220)

A. Magnitude of the problem (p. 220)
   1. Nearly 3 million children are abused each year, with more than 1,000 deaths.
   2. Between 2 and 4 million women are battered each year by their partners.
   3. Between 700,000 and 1.1 million elders are abused each year.
B. Scope of the problem (p. 220)
   1. Abuse situations transcend gender, race, age, and socioeconomic status.
   2. Effects are serious and long-lasting and may form a cycle in which a victim of abuse later becomes an abuser.
C. Ramifications for EMS providers (p. 220)
   1. Cooperate with law enforcement personnel when they are present.
   2. Identify victims and initiate responsive action when law enforcement is not present.

II. Partner abuse. (pp. 220–223)

A. Introduction (p. 220)
   1. May occur in any type of domestic partnership.
   2. Both men and women may be victim or abuser.
   3. Abuse of women by men is the most widespread form of partner abuse.
   4. Characterizations of this form of abuse extend generally to most battery situations.
B. Reasons for not reporting abuse (pp. 220–221)
   1. Fear of reprisal
   2. Fear of humiliation
   3. Denial
   4. Lack of knowledge
   5. Lack of financial resources

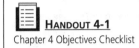
HANDOUT 4-1
Chapter 4 Objectives Checklist

POWERPOINT PRESENTATION
Volume 5, Chapter 4, PowerPoint slides 1–3

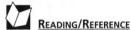
READING/REFERENCE
Lanzilotti, S., et al. "EMS and the Domestic Violence Patient," *JEMS*, June 1999.

POWERPOINT PRESENTATION
Volume 5, Chapter 4, PowerPoint slides 4–10

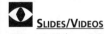
SLIDES/VIDEOS
"Domestic Violence." *Pulse: Emergency Medical Update*, Jan. 1997.

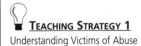
TEACHING STRATEGY 1
Understanding Victims of Abuse

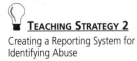
TEACHING STRATEGY 2
Creating a Reporting System for Identifying Abuse

C. Identification of partner abuse (10 generic risk factors) (p. 221)
  1. Male is unemployed.
  2. Male uses illegal drugs at least once a year.
  3. Partners have different religious backgrounds.
  4. Family income is below the poverty level.
  5. Partners are unmarried.
  6. Either partner is violent toward children at home.
  7. Male did not graduate from high school.
  8. Male is unemployed or has a blue-collar job.
  9. Male is between 18 and 30 years old.
  10. Male saw his father hit his mother.
D. Characteristics of partner abusers (pp. 221–222) **(Fig. 4-1)**
  1. History of family violence
  2. Two partners who do not know how to back down from conflict
  3. Overly aggressive personality in abusers
  4. Use of alcohol or drugs by abuser
  5. Cycle of feeling out of control then remorseful, then repetition of cycle by abuser
E. Characteristics of abused partners (pp. 222–223) **(Fig. 4-2)**
  1. Pregnancy
    a. Forty-five percent of abused women suffer some form of battery while pregnant.
  2. Substance abuse to seek a numbing effect
  3. Emotional disorders such as depression, anxiety, or suicidal behavior
  4. Tendency to protect attacker
F. Approaching the battered patient (p. 223)
  1. Use direct questioning techniques.
  2. Avoid judgmental comments and questions.
  3. Listen carefully, assuring patient of your respect and attention.
  4. Encourage victims to regain control of their lives.
  5. Advise patient to take all precautions.
    a. Be knowledgeable about local resources for assistance.

III. Elder abuse. (pp. 223–226) **(Fig. 4-3)**

A. Contributing factors (see also Chapter 3) (pp. 223–224)
  1. Increased life expectancy
  2. Increased dependency on others as a result of longevity
  3. Decreased productivity in later years
  4. Physical and mental impairments, especially among the very old
  5. Limited resources for long-term care of elderly
  6. Economic factors
  7. Stress on middle-aged caretakers responsible for two generations
B. Identification of elder abuse (p. 224)
  1. Domestic
    a. Elder in home-based setting
  2. Institutional
    a. Elder being cared for by a person paid to provide care
  3. Acts of commission
    a. Physical
    b. Sexual
    c. Emotional violence
  4. Acts of omission
    a. Neglect
C. Theories about causes of domestic elder abuse (p. 224)
  1. Stressed and overburdened caregivers
  2. Physical or mental impairment in elderly victim

READING/REFERENCE

Criss, E. "EMS—Resource for Battered Women," *JEMS,* July 2000.

TEACHING STRATEGY 3

Researching Community Agencies That Aid the Abused

TEACHING STRATEGY 4

Psychologist-Led Workshop on Communicating with Victims of Abuse

POWERPOINT PRESENTATION

Volume 5, Chapter 4, PowerPoint slides 11–16

3. Family history of violence
4. Personal problems for caregiver
D. Characteristics of abused elders (p. 225)
   1. If abuse
      a. Likely that elder is dependent upon another
   2. If neglect
      a. Likely elder lives alone and is afraid to ask for help
E. Characteristics of elder abusers (p. 225) (**Table 4-1**)

IV. **Child abuse.** (pp. 225–231) (**Fig. 4-4**)

A. Introduction (p. 225)
   1. One of most difficult situations paramedic will face
   2. Cases may range from neglect to violence resulting in emotional or physical impairment.
   3. Occurs among children of all ages (birth to 18 years)
   4. Can be inflicted by any caregiver, including a sibling or other child
   5. May be physical, emotional, or sexual
B. Characteristics of child abusers (p. 226)
   1. Any one or combination should raise index of suspicion
   2. Family history of abuse
   3. Use or abuse of drugs and/or alcohol
   4. Immaturity and preoccupation with self
   5. Lack of obvious feeling for the child, rarely looking at or touching the child
   6. Seemingly unconcerned about the child's injury, treatment, or prognosis
   7. Openly critical of the child, with little indication of guilt or remorse for involvement in the child's condition
   8. Little identification with the child's pain, whether it be physical or emotional
C. Characteristics of abused children (pp. 226–227)
   1. Any one or combination should raise index of suspicion
   2. Crying (often hopelessly) during treatment or not crying at all
   3. Avoiding parents or showing little concern for their absence
   4. Unusually wary or fearful of physical contact
   5. Apprehensive and/or constantly on the alert for danger
   6. Prone to sudden behavioral changes
   7. Absence of nearly all emotions
   8. Neediness, constantly requesting favors, food, or things
D. Identification of the abused child (pp. 227–230)
   1. Physical examination (**Table 4-2; Fig. 4-5**)
      a. Burns and scalds
      b. Fractures (**Fig. 4-6**)
      c. Head injuries
      d. Shaken baby syndrome
      e. Maternal drug abuse (**Fig. 4-7**)
         i. Fetal alcohol syndrome (FAS)
      f. Abdominal injuries
   2. Signs of neglect
      a. Malnutrition
         i. Sometimes as severely underweight as up to 30 percent
      b. Severe diaper rash
      c. Diarrhea and/or dehydration
      d. Hair loss
      e. Untreated medical conditions
      f. Inappropriate, dirty, or torn clothing
      g. Tired and listless attitudes
      h. Nearly constant demands for physical contact or attention

POWERPOINT PRESENTATION
Volume 5, Chapter 4, PowerPoint slides 17–30

READING/REFERENCE
Quirk, P., and P. D. Adelson. "Shaken-Baby Syndrome and the EMS Provider," *EMS*, Sept. 1997.

TEACHING STRATEGY 5
Improving the Index of Suspicion

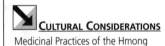

CULTURAL CONSIDERATIONS
Medicinal Practices of the Hmong

3. Signs of emotional abuse
   a. Caregiver ignoring child and showing indifference
   b. Caregiver rejecting, humiliating, or criticizing child
   c. Isolation of child with deprivation of normal human nurturing
   d. Terrorizing child with verbal bullying
   e. Caregiver encouraging destructive or antisocial behavior
   f. Overpressuring child with unrealistic expectations of success

E. Recording and reporting child abuse (pp. 230–231)
   1. You have a responsibility to report suspected cases of child abuse.
   2. Pay attention to requests for help or other signals from the abuser.
   3. Conduct examinations in suspected or known cases with a colleague present, if at all possible.
   4. Final documentation should be objective, legible, and written with the knowledge that it may be used in legal action.

V. Sexual assault. (pp. 231–235)

A. Sexual assault (p. 231)
   1. Unwanted oral, genital, rectal, or manual sexual contact
   2. Rape
      a. Penile penetration of genitalia or rectum without victim's consent
   3. The legal definition of rape varies from state to state.

B. Characteristics of victims of sexual assault/rape (pp. 231–232)
   1. Patterns
      a. Victim most likely to be a female adolescent under age 18
      b. Incidence most likely
         i. Between 6 P.M. and 6 A.M.
         ii. At victim's home or home of friend, relative, or acquaintance
      c. Assailant more likely to be someone known by victim
   2. Symptoms of sexual abuse (molestation)
      a. Nightmares
      b. Restlessness
      c. Withdrawal tendencies
      d. Hostility
      e. Phobias related to the offender
      f. Regressive behavior such as bed-wetting
      g. Truancy
      h. Promiscuity in older children and teens
      i. Drug and alcohol abuse

C. Characteristics of sexual assailants (p. 232)
   1. Assailants come from every background.
   2. Victimizers of children are more likely to have been abused themselves as children.
   3. Many, especially adolescents and abusive adults, believe domination is part of any relationship.
   4. Assaults often occur when assailant is under influence of alcohol or other drugs.
   5. Nearly 30 percent of rapists use weapons.
   6. Assailants may use date rape drugs.

D. Date rape drugs (predator drugs) (pp. 232–233)
   1. Occurring with increasing frequency
   2. Actions
      a. Render a person unresponsive
      b. Weakens person to a point where person is unable to resist an attacker
      c. Some of these medications cause amnesia, thus eliminating or distorting the victim's recall of the assault

---

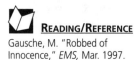

TEACHING STRATEGY 6
Newspaper Articles and Case Studies of Abuse

POWERPOINT PRESENTATION
Volume 5, Chapter 4, PowerPoint slides 31–48

READING/REFERENCE
Gausche, M. "Robbed of Innocence," *EMS,* Mar. 1997.

3. Rohypnol
    a. Characteristics
        i. Potent benzodiazepine
        ii. Colorless
        iii. Odorless
        iv. Tasteless
        v. Can be dissolved in a drink without being detected
        vi. Alcohol intensifies effects
    b. Body responses
        i. Sedative effect
        ii. Amnesia
        iii. Muscle relaxation
        iv. Slowing of the psychomotor response
    c. Street names
        i. Roofies
        ii. Rope
        iii. Ruffies
        iv. R2
        v. Ruffles
        vi. Roche
        vii. Forget-pill
        viii. Mexican valium
4. Gamma-hydroxybutyrate (GHB)
    a. Characteristics
        i. Liquid
        ii. Odorless
        iii. Colorless
        iv. Depressant with anesthetic-type qualities
        v. Used as an amino acid supplement by body builders
    b. Body responses
        i. Relaxation
        ii. Tranquility
        iii. Sensuality
        iv. Loss of inhibitions
    c. Street names
        i. Liquid ecstasy
        ii. Liquid X
        iii. Scoop
        iv. Easy lay
        v. Grievous Bodily Harm
5. Ketamine
    a. Characteristics
        i. Potent anesthetic agent
        ii. Widely used in veterinary practice
        iii. Used in human anesthesia
        iv. Chemically similar to the hallucinogenic LSD
    b. Body responses
        i. Hallucinations
        ii. Amnesia
        iii. Dissociation
    c. Street names
        i. K
        ii. Special K
        iii. Vitamin K
        iv. Jet
        v. Super acid

6. MDMA
   a. Characteristics
      i. Most commonly known as ecstasy
   b. Body responses
      i. Psychological difficulties
         • Confusion
         • Depression
         • Sleep problems
         • Drug craving
         • Severe anxiety
         • Paranoia
      ii. During and sometimes weeks after taking the drug
      iii. Physical symptoms
         • Muscle tension
         • Involuntary teeth clenching
         • Nausea
         • Blurred vision
         • Rapid eye movement
         • Faintness
         • Chills or sweating
   c. Street names for MDMA
      i. Ecstasy
      ii. Beans
      iii. Adam
      iv. XTC
      v. Roll
      vi. E
      vii. M
7. Precautions
   a. Persons attending parties and other events should be cautious in regard to predator drugs.
   b. It is best not to drink from a punch bowl or a bottle passed around.
   c. Notice the behavior of others at the party.
   d. If a person seems more intoxicated than the amount of alcohol consumed would warrant, then consider the possibility of predator drugs.
   e. If a rape victim thinks she has been drugged, a drug screen should be requested upon arrival at the emergency department.
   f. EMS personnel should note any suspicions or observations that may point to the use of a predator drug.
E. EMS responsibilities (p. 233)
   1. Ensure own and patient's safety foremost.
   2. Never enter a scene if you feel your safety is compromised; leave if you feel unsafe.
   3. Provide safety and privacy during patient care.
   4. Consider care by a same-sex provider. (Fig. 4-8)
   5. Give patient some feelings of control by offering choices wherever possible.
F. Legal considerations (pp. 234–235)
   1. Responsibility to report cases to appropriate law enforcement officials
   2. Obligation to know about available victim and witness protection programs
   3. Responsibility to know about specialized resources
      a. Shelters
      b. State agencies
      c. Nurses trained as SANEs

©2009 Pearson Education, Inc.
Paramedic Care: Principles & Practice, Vol. 5, 3rd. Ed.

4. Evidence
    a. Rules on obtaining possible evidence of crime
    b. Understanding of concept of chain of evidence
5. Familiarity with local protocols for abuse and assault

VI. Summary. (p. 235)

A. Incidence of abuse is widespread, and you will encounter it in your practice.

B. Learn the hallmarks of partner, elder, and child abuse, as well as sexual assault.

C. Recognize significant physical and emotional findings on assessment, as well as general characteristics of victims and assailants.

D. Remember that proper treatment includes fulfilling legal requirements.

SKILLS DEMONSTRATION AND PRACTICE

Students can practice skills discussed in the chapter in the following role-play.

Form groups of students and have each write a role-play scenario for partner, child, or elder abuse or for sexual assault. Have each writing group come up with a list of items that are present in the script (or should be present in the acting) that are historical, environmental, or behavioral clues to the type of abuse or assault being presented. They may wish to do this before or after writing the script itself.

Have another group present the scenario, and then have the class as a whole discuss what they have seen. See if class members find all of the clues that the writing group listed or if they come up with different or additional clues.

If you have had speakers come to the group or students have made field visits, have the students with firsthand experience compare and contrast their actual experience with what they saw in the scenario and heard in the group discussion.

YOU MAKE THE CALL

Review student responses to the You Make the Call scenario on text page 235. Suggested responses to the questions that follow the scenario are given below. Point out to students that these are acceptable answers but not necessarily the only ones. Discuss with students the pros and cons of points where their responses differ from these.

1. What do you suspect is taking place?
(You suspect that the patient is a victim of child abuse.)
2. What physical evidence do you have to support this suspicion?
(The boy has bruises to both his upper arms and his back, all at different stages of healing.)
3. What emotional evidence do you have to support this suspicion?
(The boy is unusually quiet for his age and does not make any effort to contact his parents.)
4. What other clues lead you to believe that abuse might be taking place?
(The boy is in the care of parents involved in a domestic dispute and is dressed inappropriately for the circumstances.)
5. What are your priorities in this case?
(Your priorities are to assess the patient for physical injuries requiring immediate treatment, to alert the police officers to the possible abuse situation, to remove the patient to a medical facility appropriate for abused children, and to document your findings.)

POWERPOINT PRESENTATION
Volume 5, Chapter 4, PowerPoint slide 49

READING/REFERENCE
Hunt, R., et al. "Educating EMS on Domestic Violence," *JEMS*, August 2000.

WORKBOOK
Chapter 4 Activities

READING/REFERENCE
Textbook Chapter 5, pp. 238–262

HANDOUT 4-2
Chapter 4 Quiz

HANDOUT 4-3
Chapter 4 Scenario

PARAMEDIC STUDENT CD
Student Activities

COMPANION WEBSITE
http://www.prenhall.com/bledsoe

TestGen
Volume 5, Chapter 4

EMT Achieve:
Paramedic Test Preparation
Mistovich & Beasley. *EMT Achieve:*
Paramedic Test Preparation,
http://www.prenhall.com/emtachieve

Success! for the
Paramedic
Cherry. *SUCCESS! for the Paramedic,*
4th edition

Handouts 4-4 to 4-5
Reinforcement Activities

Paramedic Student CD
Student Activities

PowerPoint
Presentation
Volume 5

Companion Website
http://www.prenhall.com/bledsoe

OneKey
Volume 5, Chapter 4

Advanced Life
Support Skills
Larmon & Davis. *Advanced Life*
Support Skills

Advanced Life
Skills Review
Larmon & Davis. *Advanced Life Skills*
Review

Brady Skills
Series: ALS
Larmon & Davis. *Brady Skills Series:*
ALS

Paramedic National
Standards Self-Test
Miller. *Paramedic National Standards*
Self-Test, 5th edition

ASSIGNMENTS

Assign students to complete Chapter 4 of the Workbook. Also assign them to read Chapter 5, "The Challenged Patient," before the next class.

EVALUATION

Chapter Quiz and Scenario   Distribute copies of the Chapter Quiz and scenario provided in Handouts 4-2 and 4-3 to evaluate student understanding of this chapter. Make sure each student reads the scenario to reinforce critical thinking on the scene. Remind students not to use their notes or textbooks while taking the quiz.

Student CD   Quizzes for every chapter are contained on the dynamic and highly visual in-text student CD.

Companion Website   Additional quizzes for every chapter are contained on this exciting website.

TestGen   You may wish to create a custom-tailored test using *Prentice Hall TestGen for Paramedic Care: Principles & Practice,* 3rd edition, to evaluate student understanding of this chapter.

Online Test Preparation (for students and instructors)   Additional test preparation is available through Brady's new online product, EMT Achieve: Paramedic Test Preparation, at *http://www.prenhall.com/emtachieve.* Instructors can also monitor student mastery online.

Success! for the Paramedic   Keyed to *Paramedic Care: Principles & Practice* and *Essentials of Paramedic Care,* this comprehensive exam review contains hundreds of test questions and rationales.

REINFORCEMENT

Handouts   If classroom discussion or performance on the quiz indicates that some students have not fully mastered the chapter content, you may wish to assign some or all of the Reinforcement Handouts for this chapter.

Student CD (for students)   A wide variety of material on this CD-ROM will reinforce and also expand student knowledge and skills.

PowerPoint Presentation (for instructors)   The PowerPoint material developed for this chapter offers useful reinforcement of chapter content.

Companion Website (for students)   Additional review quizzes and links to EMS resources will contribute to further reinforcement of the chapter.

OneKey   Online support is offered for this course on one of three platforms: CourseCompass, Blackboard, or WebCT. Includes the IRM, PowerPoints, Test Manager, and Companion Website for instruction. Ask your local sales representative for more information.

Brady Skills Series: Advanced Life Skills (Video or CD)   Have your students watch the skills come to life on VHS or CD-ROM, or they can purchase the highly visual, full-color text with step-by-step procedures with rationales.

Paramedic National Standards Self-Test   Another comprehensive review manual containing hundreds of review questions with page references keyed to several Brady texts.

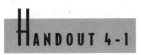 ANDOUT 4-1

CHAPTER 4 OBJECTIVES CHECKLIST

Knowledge Objective	Date Mastered
1. Discuss the incidence of abuse and assault.	
2. Describe the categories of abuse.	
3. Discuss examples of spouse, elder, child, and sexual abuse.	
4. Describe the characteristics associated with the profile of a typical spouse, elder, or child abuser and the typical assailant of sexual abuse.	
5. Identify the profile of the "at-risk" spouse, elder, and child.	
6. Discuss the assessment and management of the abused patient.	
7. Discuss the legal aspects associated with abuse situations.	
8. Identify community resources that are able to assist victims of abuse and assault.	
9. Discuss the documentation necessary when caring for abused and assaulted patients.	

Student's Name _____

CHAPTER 4 QUIZ

Write the letter of the best answer in the space provided.

_____ 1. Which of the following is NOT one of the several common reasons why a domestic partner does not report that he or she is being abused?
A. fear of reprisal by the abusing partner
B. lack of knowledge of how to report abuse or seek help
C. fear that he or she will not be believed
D. denial that the situation is one of abuse

_____ 2. Characteristics of abused partners include all of the following EXCEPT:
A. pregnancy in a female partner.
B. chronic physical condition.
C. substance abuse.
D. emotional disorders.

_____ 3. Elder abusers are often all EXCEPT which of the following individuals?
A. a grandchild
B. an adult child
C. a spouse
D. a different kind of familial relative

_____ 4. All of the following injuries in a child should give you a high level of suspicion that child abuse is involved, EXCEPT:
A. burns on the soles of the feet, palms of the hands, back, or buttocks.
B. head injuries.
C. fractures of the skull, nose, or ribs.
D. burns in a "splash" pattern.

_____ 5. All of the following are common clues that a child is being neglected EXCEPT:
A. severe diaper rash.
B. malnutrition and underweight condition.
C. a child patient ignoring and avoiding physical contact with EMS provider.
D. untreated medical conditions.

_____ 6. Common characteristics of victims of sexual assault include all of the following EXCEPT:
A. celibacy and denial of own sexuality.
B. phobias related to the offender.
C. regressive behavior such as bed-wetting.
D. withdrawal tendencies.

_____ 7. Which of the following medical conditions is NOT easily mistaken for a sign of abuse?
A. chickenpox
B. car seat burns
C. blood disorders that cause easy bruising
D. measles

_____ 8. All of the following are correct correlations between the age of a bruise and its skin appearance, EXCEPT:
A. 0 to 2 days and a reddened, swollen, tender appearance.
B. 10 or more days and a yellow color.
C. 0 to 5 days and blue or purple color.
D. 5 to 7 days and a green color.

_____ 9. Which of the following is NOT one of the common characteristics of child abusers?
A. history of having been abused themselves
B. overly concerned with child's welfare and severity of any injury during interview
C. pattern over time of becoming more frequently and more severely abusive
D. immaturity and preoccupation with self

_____ **10.** All of the following are common characteristics of abused children EXCEPT:
   A. constant crying or no crying during treatment.
   B. absence of emotion or constant neediness for attention from the EMS provider.
   C. avoiding parents or constantly asking for parents' attention.
   D. sudden behavioral changes during interview and treatment.

_____ **11.** All of the following are characteristic of abusers of women EXCEPT:
   A. unemployment.
   B. use of illegal drugs at least once a year.
   C. family income over $95,000 a year.
   D. different religious background from the woman.

_____ **12.** In cases of neglect, the elders most commonly:
   A. have incomes less than $75,000 a year.
   B. live alone.
   C. live with grandchildren.
   D. have a chronic medical condition requiring medication.

_____ **13.** The physical or emotional violence or neglect that is carried out when an elder is being cared for by a person paid to provide care is:
   A. professional elder abuse.   **C.** common elder abuse.
   B. institutional elder abuse.   **D.** mercenary elder abuse.

_____ **14.** The number of states that require health care workers to report suspected cases of child abuse is:
   A. 35.   **C.** 45.
   B. 40.   **D.** 50.

_____ **15.** Your primary responsibility at a call to a scene of suspected abuse is:
   A. preserving the chain of evidence.
   B. discovering the identity of the abuser.
   C. your safety and that of the patient.
   D. psychological support.

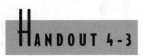

Student's Name _____

CHAPTER 4 SCENARIO

Review the following real-life situation. Then answer the questions that follow.

A team is called to a neighborhood nursing home to check "an elderly woman who fell." On arrival, the team waits in the lobby until an aide comes for them.

They walk down the hall and find an elderly lady sitting up in bed, clutching the side rails with both hands. Her hair is uncombed, and she looks vacantly out before her. The aide says she is busy and cannot stay and then leaves them with the patient.

They introduce themselves, and the lady says her name is Lillian Good and that she is 84 years old. Kerry starts to ask her whether she fell when a nurse comes into the room and answers the question by saying, "Lillian knew she shouldn't get out of bed without help, but she tried anyway." Lillian is quiet. Kerry says she needs to examine the patient, but then has to squeeze past the nurse to get to the bedside. Kerry asks Mrs. Good about the fall as she gently takes a hand to check a pulse and looks closely at the patient.

Kerry notes that the lady looks and smells as if she has not bathed recently, and there is a clear odor of urine. The bottom sheet is crisp and white in contrast to the top sheet, which has a variety of food stains on it. As Kerry gently asks her question about the fall again, the nurse interrupts to say that Mrs. Good falls often and a new aide called the paramedics. "It was really a mistake," she says. "We don't need your help. If you just want to check her vital signs, you can leave."

1. Based on initial impressions, what, if any, problems do you suspect in addition to your need to work up the alleged fall?

2. Does the nurse's behavior arouse your index of suspicion? Why or why not?

3. Based on this impression, are there any signs you should look for while conducting a physical examination of the patient?

4. If your physical is within normal limits, the patient does not supply any information, and there is no evidence of injury from the (alleged) fall, is there anything more you should do before discussing the case with medical direction?

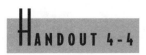

CHAPTER 4 REVIEW

Write the word or words that best complete each sentence in the space(s) provided.

1. The pattern of abuse and assault forms a(n) _____ that is difficult to break.

2. Victims of partner abuse hesitate or fail to report the problem because of fear of _____, fear of humiliation, denial, lack of knowledge, and lack of _____ _____.

3. Partner abuse may be categorized as _____ abuse, the most obvious form, _____ abuse, which damages self-esteem, and _____ abuse, a form of physical abuse.

4. A history of _____ _____ makes a person more likely to repeat the pattern of partner abuse as an adult.

5. The three characteristics of abused partners are _____ (45 percent of abused women), _____ _____, and emotional disorders such as _____, evasiveness, anxiety, and suicidal behavior.

6. When speaking with an abused partner, be prepared to share your knowledge of _____ _____.

7. _____ _____ _____ takes place when an elder is being cared for in a home situation; _____ elder abuse occurs when an elder is being cared for by a person who is paid for such care.

8. One of the four main theories about the causes of elder abuse is that caregivers feel _____ or _____.

9. Elder abuse can be either acts of _____ (physical, sexual, or emotional violence) or acts of _____ (neglect).

10. _____ _____ make up the largest group of perpetrators of domestic elder abuse.

11. Most _____ _____ were physically or emotionally abused as children.

12. In cases of reported physical child abuse, perpetrators tend to be _____.

13. Abused children may be unusually wary and fearful of _____ _____.

14. Abused children under age 6 usually appear excessively _____, while those over age 6 appear _____.

15. Frequent behavioral traits of child abusers include immaturity and preoccupation with _____; seeming _____ about a child's injury, treatment, or prognosis; and little indication of _____ or _____ for involvement in the child's condition.

16. A green bruise on a child who has been abused is _____ to _____ days old.

17. The paramedic can frequently recognize the source of intentional burns to children by their _____ and/or _____.

18. _____ _____ _____ may occur when a parent or caregiver becomes frustrated with a crying child.

19. Neglected children are frequently _____, causing them to be underweight, sometimes by up to 30 percent.

REINFORCEMENT

20. Neglected children may also exhibit _____ or _____ attitudes or make near constant demands for _____ _____.

21. _____ _____ is unwanted sexual contact, while _____ is generally defined as penile penetration of the genitalia or rectum.

22. The group most likely to be the victims of sexual assault/rape are _____ younger than age _____.

23. Government figures show that approximately one-third of all juvenile victims of assault/rape are younger than _____ years of age.

24. In cases of date rape, the assailant may have drugged the victim with _____, known by the street names of roofie, roche, rib, and rope.

25. As well as physical care, the paramedic is responsible for providing proper _____ care for the victims of assault and rape.

©2009 Pearson Education, Inc.
Paramedic Care: Principles & Practice, Vol. 5, 3rd. Ed.

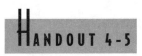
ABUSE AND ASSAULT TRUE OR FALSE

Indicate whether the following statements are true or false by writing T or F in the space provided.

_____ 1. Abuse and assault in the United States involve persons of each gender and of every race, age, and socioeconomic status.

_____ 2. Partner abuse can involve heterosexual couples or same-sex couples, but men are the abusers in relationships that involve a man.

_____ 3. You may find that an abuse victim who is a patient of yours has both direct injury and indirect injury, with the latter represented by aggravation of an existing medical condition such as asthma or diabetes.

_____ 4. When you are talking with a patient who has been physically battered, you will find that direct, nonjudgmental questioning generally works best.

_____ 5. Elder abuse commonly takes place in homes, but not in institutional settings such as a nursing home.

_____ 6. Approximately 1 million women in the United States are battered by their spouses each year.

_____ 7. Nearly 3 million children in the United States suffer abuse each year.

_____ 8. Battery is not a problem between same-sex couples.

_____ 9. Forty-five percent of women suffer some form of battery during pregnancy.

_____ 10. One of the most common theories holds that caregivers in cases of elder abuse feel stressed and overburdened.

_____ 11. A child's behavior is one of the most important indicators of abuse.

_____ 12. Because rib fractures are common in children, they are not a good indicator of abuse.

_____ 13. When confronted with a case of child abuse, try to conduct the examination with another colleague present.

_____ 14. One in two rape victims in the United States is under age 18.

_____ 15. In a case of rape, allow the victim to urinate or defecate if it will calm her.

Chapter 4 Answer Key

Handout 4-2: Chapter 4 Quiz

1. C	5. C	9. B	13. B
2. B	6. A	10. C	14. D
3. A	7. D	11. C	15. C
4. D	8. B	12. B	

Handout 4-3: Chapter 4 Scenario

1. There should be a high level of suspicion of institutional elder neglect or abuse. There are signs that the patient's personal hygiene has not been adequately addressed (uncombed hair, indications that she hasn't bathed or been bathed), her environment has not been adequately cared for (top sheet with old and new food stains, indicating it hasn't been changed), and that she hasn't had needed care (the clear smell of urine and signs that the bottom sheet has just been changed).

2. The nurse is excluding the patient from conversation with the paramedics and is dismissive of the incident. She clearly wants the team to leave as soon as possible.

3. There may be signs of direct abuse or further evidence of neglect. Signs of abuse might include bruises of various ages. Signs of neglect might include bedsores on the buttocks, heels, or elbows or evidence of urine or fecal material on the bedding, clothing, or patient. Other potential signs of abuse or neglect would include any indications of dehydration or malnutrition.

4. You must organize the reasons for your suspicion of elder abuse or neglect for yourself, as well as document them thoroughly. You must further evaluate your impressions of the nurse as well as any other staff you encounter while on-scene and appraise medical direction of any concerns you may have for the patient's safety if she is not transported to a facility for evaluation. You should also ask (if it is not clear per local protocol) whether the nurse or another member of the nursing home staff can refuse transport of the patient.

Handout 4-4: Chapter 4 Review

1. cycle
2. reprisal, financial resources
3. physical, verbal, sexual
4. family abuse
5. pregnancy, substance abuse, depression
6. community resources
7. Domestic elder abuse, Institutional
8. stressed, overburdened
9. commission, omission
10. Adult children
11. child abusers
12. men
13. physical contact
14. passive, aggressive
15. self, unconcerned, guilt, remorse
16. 5, 7
17. shape, pattern
18. Shaken baby syndrome
19. malnourished
20. tired, listless, physical contact
21. Sexual assault, rape
22. females, 18
23. 6
24. flunitrazepam (Rohypnol)
25. psychosocial

Handout 4-5: Abuse and Assault True or False

1. T	5. F	9. T	13. T
2. F	6. F	10. T	14. T
3. T	7. T	11. T	15. F
4. T	8. F	12. F	

©2009 Pearson Education, Inc.
Paramedic Care: Principles & Practice, Vol. 5, 3rd. Ed.

Chapter 5

The Challenged Patient

INTRODUCTION

Throughout your students' careers, they will encounter patients who live with a challenge, who may present special needs. The challenges that these patients face may be obvious to the EMS provider (such as complete blindness, cerebral palsy, or paraplegia). In other cases, they may be so subtle that they are not identified readily in initial conversation with the patient (such as slight mental retardation or some degree of traumatic brain injury, some degree of hearing impairment, some forms of mental illness). In still other cases, the challenges are not medical at all—the patient might speak a different language than the provider's, live in a community culture with very different expectations for health care, or be a foreign citizen in the United States. In all of these and in many other cases, it is important for the provider to realize that individuals with challenges, "challenged patients," exist and may require some level of accommodation for proper patient care to be given.

CHAPTER OBJECTIVES

Knowledge Objectives

1. Describe the various etiologies and types of hearing impairments. (pp. 241–242)
2. Recognize the patient with a hearing impairment. (p. 242)
3. Anticipate accommodations that may be needed in order to properly manage the patient with a hearing impairment. (pp. 242–243)
4. Describe the various etiologies and types, recognize patients with, and anticipate accommodations that may be needed in order to properly manage each of the following conditions:

   a. visual impairments (pp. 243–245)
   b. speech impairments (pp. 245–246)
   c. obesity (pp. 246–248)
   d. paraplegia/quadriplegia (p. 249)
   e. mental illness (pp. 249–250)
   f. developmentally disabled (pp. 250–252)
   g. Down syndrome (p. 251)
   h. emotional/mental impairment (pp. 249–250)

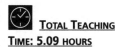

TOTAL TEACHING TIME: 5.09 HOURS
The total teaching time is only a guideline based on the didactic and practical lab averages in the National Standard Curriculum. Instructors should take into consideration such factors as: the pace at which students learn, the size of the class, and breaks. The actual time devoted to teaching objectives is the responsibility of the instructor.

5. Describe, identify possible presenting signs, and anticipate accommodations for the following diseases/illnesses:

    a. arthritis (p. 253)
    b. cancer (pp. 253–255)
    c. cerebral palsy (p. 255)
    d. cystic fibrosis (pp. 255–256)
    e. multiple sclerosis (p. 256)
    f. muscular dystrophy (pp. 256–257)
    g. myasthenia gravis (p. 258)
    h. poliomyelitis (p. 257)
    i. spina bifida (p. 258)
    j. patients with a previous head injury (pp. 257–258)

6. Define, recognize, and anticipate accommodations needed to properly manage patients who:

    a. are culturally diverse (pp. 258–259)
    b. are terminally ill (pp. 259–260)
    c. have a communicable disease (p. 260)
    d. have a financial impairment (p. 260)

Skill Objective

7. Given several challenged patients, provide the appropriate assessment, management, and transportation. (pp. 240–260)

FRAMING THE LESSON

Begin teaching the lesson by splitting students into groups and assigning each group a general type of challenge: Ask them to name as many examples as they can. For example, types might include congenital conditions, changes resulting from aging, permanent disabilities, short-term disabilities, chronic conditions, and nonmedical challenges. As the students develop their list, have them think about the way in which a patient would manifest or try to hide each example and how they, as providers, might recognize and respond to that challenge.

    For example, a patient might be a foreign citizen in the United States. A tourist might be concerned about her ability to express herself in the English language or be unclear about the structure and funding of American health care. If the EMS provider raised the concern and asked if the person or her family had any questions, a constructive conversation might follow. However, if the patient were an unregistered alien living in the United States, her ability to voice her concerns might be much less and the provider might not realize the level of the patient's anxiety over getting involved in the EMS system.

- Congenital conditions might involve sensory impairment (blindness or deafness), motor and speech ability (cerebral palsy), appearance (cleft lip or palate, hare lip, birthmarks), or even immune function (in a child born with immune deficiency resulting from HIV/AIDS or a genetic immune deficiency syndrome).
- Changes caused by aging might be as subtle as poor flexibility and balance while on steps or uneven ground or as obvious as nearly total sensory loss. Severe osteoarthritis or osteoporosis may cause chronic pain or disfigurement. Macular degeneration may cause partial or total loss of vision.
- Permanent disabilities include motor loss (paraplegia, quadriplegia, amputation of a limb), sensory loss, and visible scarring from a burn or

©2009 Pearson Education, Inc.
Paramedic Care: Principles & Practice, Vol. 5, 3rd. Ed.

other injury. One type of long-term disability that requires accommodation is immune compromise resulting from either therapy for cancer or diseases such as AIDS.

- Short-term disabilities might include pregnancy, anxiety over health in someone who had a recent MI or other major medical condition, impaired mobility in someone who had recent major surgery, or even the confusion and fatigue of someone with a high fever caused by the flu or other infectious illness. One common instance providers might see is a patient with vomiting or diarrhea who feels uncomfortable saying "excuse me" and running to the bathroom.
- Chronic conditions are numerous and include impairment secondary to stroke or head injury, asthma, COPD, heart failure, diabetes, epilepsy, inflammatory bowel disease, and different forms of anemia.
- Nonmedical challenges other than the citizenship example already given include poor finances, difficulties with English as a communication language, and membership in a community culture with possible differences in expectations about health care and interaction between men and women (for example, Asian health beliefs, or membership in Hasidic Judaism or Amish culture).

CONSIDERING THE CASE STUDY

Ask a volunteer to read aloud the Case Study that begins on text page 239. Suggest that students close their eyes as the scenario is read to help them visualize the events described in it. You can use the following questions as a starting point for teaching the chapter—a sort of chapter preview in a functional setting.

When the chapter is completed, you may wish to return to the Case Study and encourage further discussion aimed at answering the questions.

CASE STUDY DISCUSSION QUESTIONS (AND ANSWERS)

1. What thoughts might the providers have en route about possible special needs on the part of the patient based on the description of the fall as "out of her wheelchair?"
   (Some examples of responses: The providers might wonder if the patient is a long-term user of a wheelchair or is using it on a short-term basis because of a recent injury or illness and how they might get that information while taking the history. They might think about accommodations needed to transport a patient in a wheelchair in their specific vehicle.)
2. How would you characterize Mrs. Wade's attitude toward her wheelchair use and her impairments secondary to polio?
   (She is matter-of-fact about her impairment, articulate in describing it, and shows that she has adapted it into her style of living.)
3. Do you think Mrs. Wade's attitude toward her challenges makes the providers' job easier or more difficult? Why?
   (Her ability to talk easily about her challenges and take them into account in terms of the providers' responsibilities toward her make it easy for them to discuss her history, her current condition, and her needs in terms of any accommodations necessary to keep her comfortable and in a position of some control. Later, because the providers know her left arm is weak, they could allow her to position herself so she can use her

right arm easily; they could also note this on the chart so that hospital staff could ask her in which arm she would like an IV placed, if IV access is required.)

TEACHING STRATEGIES

People learn in a variety of ways. Some do better with the spoken word, while others prefer the written. Some prefer to work alone, whereas others profit from working in groups. Recognizing these different ways of acquiring knowledge, the authors of this *Instructor's Resource Manual* have provided a variety of teaching strategies for the different types of learners. These strategies are intended to foster higher-level cognitive skills and encourage creative learning and problem solving.

For greatest effectiveness, incorporate these strategies into your class lecture. Marginal notes in the Teaching Outline indicate the points at which various exercises might be most appropriate. Other strategies can be used to preview the lesson or to summarize it.

The following strategies are keyed to specific sections of the lesson:

1. Creating a Device to Improve Communication. Have students work in groups to create a device or implement to improve communication with a challenged patient. This could be hearing or visually impaired, wheelchair bound, and so on. Give them plenty of time, then have them present their ideas to the group. Some might be good enough to install in your local emergency vehicles. This activity is kinesthetic and improves problem-solving skills.

2. Simulated Deafness. Simulate deafness in your classroom for an entire session by having everyone wear disposable earplugs. Be sure the students attend lectures, ask questions, and socialize, all while wearing their earplugs. At the end of the day, note how much longer it took to accomplish the same amount of material you normally cover. Ask students to record their feelings about the challenge by writing a paragraph at the end of the day. This empathy exercise is an affective domain activity.

3. Learning to Communicate through an Interpreter. Assessment and treatment of a patient using an interpreter is extremely challenging. Set up scenarios in your class that require the use of an interpreter or other means of communication. Consider using family members of students, community members, members of cultural groups, or foreign-language students to act as your patients and interpreters. Emphasize that a paramedic cannot give up on obtaining the assessment or fail to communicate altogether simply because of a language barrier.

4. Teacher's Aide Assignment. Many students with special challenges are being mainstreamed into regular schools and classrooms. Assign students to assist the teachers and caregivers in these classrooms in order to better understand the physical and mental abilities and limitations of these people. Additionally, the often overworked teachers will appreciate the extra set of hands.

5. Speaker from Arthritis Foundation. A speaker from the Arthritis Foundation is probably available in your area. He or she can teach students about the disease, including current pharmacology, special challenges for arthritis patients, and accommodations that health care providers could make to improve the care provided to arthritis patients. Most of us could modify our handling and positioning of patients to make emergency procedures less painful and improve cooperation of patients suffering from this disease.

6. Diversity Exercise. To help students appreciate their differences and discover how easily one can be labeled "different," have them write on a sticky note one thing that makes them different, insecure, or afraid. Then, have the class guess who belongs to each of the differences. Discuss how it feels to be vulnerable. Emphasize the importance of tolerance and impartiality in health care providers.

The following strategy relates to Special Features in the student textbook and can be used to enhance the student's understanding:

Patho Pearls: Dealing with the Morbidly Obese Patient. Fill the pockets of a fishing-type vest and a pair of oversized cargo pants with bags of sand. While one student wears these items to simulate obesity, the others can work through a variety of patient simulations to evaluate how obesity can change patient management and handling.

The following strategies can be used at various points throughout the lesson or to help summarize and demonstrate what students have learned:

Understanding Both Sides of the Problem. For one or more medical challenges (hearing impairment, visual impairment, obesity, requirement for a wheelchair), split students into small groups. Ask one student to simulate a patient with that challenge (through placement of earplugs, use of blindfold, wearing multiple jackets and pants, being confined to a wheelchair) while the others act as the EMS team. Afterward, have the students discuss their experiences: What discomforts did the patients feel? What actions by the EMS team eased or worsened the experience for them? For the EMS providers, what actions by the patients or themselves did they feel improved the quality of communication or the ease of patient care?

Repeat this exercise after the chapter is completed to reinforce the chapter content regarding approach to the challenged patient.

Listening to Firsthand Experience. Ask individuals with a variety of challenges who have had experience with EMS to talk to the students about their interactions with EMS providers and what recommendations they have for the students.

In the Field. Take the students to an EMS unit that is off duty and have them ask the team what equipment/procedural accommodations they can make readily for patients with a variety of challenges (blind or deaf, wheelchair-bound, obese, spastic limbs, and so on).

TEACHING OUTLINE

HANDOUT 5-1
Chapter 5 Objectives Checklist

Chapter 5 is the fifth lesson in Volume 5, *Special Considerations/Operations*. Distribute Handout 5-1 so that students can familiarize themselves with the learning goals for this chapter. If students have any questions about the objectives, answer them at this time.

Then present the chapter. One possible lecture outline follows. In the outline, the parenthetical references in regular type are references to text pages; those in bold type are to figures, tables, or procedures.

READING/REFERENCE
Deschamp, C., and R. C. Sneed. "EMS for Children with Special Healthcare Needs," *EMS*, Nov. 1999.

I. Introduction. A wide variety of challenges and impairments may be present in the patients that paramedics encounter. Thus, they will need to understand and recognize these special conditions and make accommodations needed for proper patient care. (p. 240)

POWERPOINT
PRESENTATION
Volume 5, Chapter 5, PowerPoint slides 1–3

II. Physical challenges. (pp. 240–249)

A. Hearing impairments (pp. 241–243)
 1. Decrease in or loss of ability to hear or distinguish sounds, especially speech

POWERPOINT
PRESENTATION
Volume 5, Chapter 5, PowerPoint slides 4–17

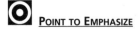

TEACHING STRATEGY 1
Creating a Device to Improve
Communication

TEACHING STRATEGY 2
Simulated Deafness

2. Conductive deafness
   a. Blockage of sound wave transmission through external ear canal to middle or inner ear
   b. May be treated or cured
   c. In children, rule out congenital deafness and consider otitis media.
   d. In all, consider impacted cerumen, water, or another irritant.
   e. In trauma cases, consider trauma-related causes such as hematoma.
3. Sensorineural deafness
   a. Inability of nerve impulses to reach auditory center in brain because of nerve damage to either inner ear or the brain
   b. Is usually permanent
   c. At-risk infants and children include
      i. Preterm infants
      ii. Those treated with ototoxic drugs
      iii. Those exposed in utero to rubella or cytomegalovirus
   d. Impairment may be secondary to infection.
      i. Bacterial meningitis or viruses
   e. Impairment may be temporary.
      i. Aspirin toxicity
         • Manifested as ringing in the ears, tinnitus
   f. Among elderly, presbycusis (progressive age-related impairment) becomes significant in persons over age 65 years.
4. Recognition of deafness
   a. Typical behaviors that may be mistaken for evidence of head injury
      i. Asking questions repeatedly
      ii. Misunderstanding questions or answers to their questions
      iii. Responding inappropriately to questions or requests
   b. Clues that may aid recognition
      i. Presence of hearing aid (**Fig. 5-1**)
      ii. Use of sign language
      iii. Continual positioning to be squarely in front of your face (so patient can lip read)
5. Accommodations for deaf patients
   a. Address patient face to face and make sure patient understands each question or request.
   b. Speak slowly and in low-pitched voice; do not yell or overtly gesture, as these may be perceived as threatening.
   c. Reduce background noise to a minimum.
   d. On night calls, consider the following:
      i. Looking for hearing aid
      ii. Placing stethoscope on patient and speaking into it
      iii. Using pen and paper
      iv. Trying to find an American Sign Language (ASL) interpreter
         • Call ahead if one will be needed at hospital

B. Visual impairments (pp. 243–245)
   1. Etiologies (**Fig. 5-2**)
      a. Injury
         i. Previous injury usually includes eye and tissue around orbit.
         ii. Penetrating injury often results in enucleation, removal of the eyeball.
         iii. Permanent injury may be caused by chemical and thermal burns.
         iv. Causes of temporary impairment includes
            • Deployment of an airbag
            • Corneal abrasion

TEACHING STRATEGY 3
Learning to Communicate through
an Interpreter

POINT TO EMPHASIZE
Address deaf patients face to face to
give them the opportunity to read
lips and interpret expressions.

b. Disease
  i. Glaucoma
  ii. Diabetic retinopathy
c. Congenital conditions
  i. Cerebral palsy
  ii. Premature birth
d. Infection
  i. Cytomegalovirus infection in AIDS patients can lead to blindness via retinitis.
e. Degeneration of retina, optic nerve, or nerve pathways
2. Recognizing and accommodating visual impairments
  a. Identify yourself on approach.
  b. Describe everything you do before/as you do it.
  c. Do not touch or disturb a guide dog without patient's permission.
  d. Refer to local protocol regarding transportation of a guide dog.
  e. If there is no guide dog, ask if there are any tools (such as a white cane) that the patient wants to have transported with him.
  f. Allow patient to take your arm rather than taking patient's arm if you are guiding him.
C. Speech impairments (pp. 245–246)
  1. Language disorders
    a. Impaired ability to understand spoken or written word
    b. Aphasia
      i. Loss of ability to communicate in speech, writing, or signs
    c. Sensory aphasia
      i. Patient cannot understand the spoken word, what you are saying
    d. Motor aphasia (expressive aphasia)
      i. Patient understands what is said but cannot speak
    e. Global aphasia
      i. Patient has both sensory and motor aphasia.
      ii. Brain tumor in Broca's region is one cause
  2. Articulation disorders (dysarthria)
    a. Occur when sounds are produced or put together incorrectly in a way that makes it difficult for the listener to understand
    b. Can occur in children or adults
  3. Voice production disorders
    a. Affect the quality of the person's voice
    b. Patients will show
      i. Hoarseness
      ii. Harshness
      iii. Inappropriate pitch
      iv. Abnormal nasal resonance
    c. Causes
      i. Trauma to the vocal cords
      ii. Infection of the vocal cords
      iii. Cancer of the larynx is a cause in adults
  4. Fluency disorders
    a. Present as a form of stuttering
    b. More common in males than females
  5. Accommodations for speech impairments (**Fig. 5-3**)
    a. Listen to what is said, not how it's said.
    b. Listen carefully and wait for complete responses.
    c. Never assume that the patient's intelligence is affected.
      i. Use normal phrasing of questions.
    d. Do not rush patient or finish responses.
    e. Use question phrasing that invites short, direct answers.

 POINT TO EMPHASIZE
When speaking to a patient with a speech impairment, try to form questions that require short, direct answers.

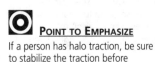

PATHO PEARLS

Dealing with the Morbidly Obese
Patient, p. 247

f. Be prepared that the interview may take longer than usual.

g. Look directly at the patient when asking questions.

h. Ask for a repeated response if you didn't understand the first time.

i. Never pretend to understand when you do not.

j. Be prepared to offer pen/paper or alternative means of communication.

D. Obesity (pp. 246–249)

    1. Over 40 percent of Americans are obese.

    2. Complicates EMS care

        a. Directly

            i. Making lifting and moving more difficult

        b. Indirectly

            i. Aggravating medical conditions

                • Hypertension

                • Heart disease

                • Strokes

                • Diabetes

                • Musculoskeletal problems

    3. Etiologies

        a. Defined as 20 to 30 percent or more over ideal weight

        b. Causes

            i. Improper diet

            ii. Lack of exercise

            iii. Genetic factors or medical conditions that lower metabolism

                • Usually hypothyroidism

    4. Accommodations for obese patients (**Fig. 5-4a; Fig. 5-4b; Fig. 5-4c**)

        a. Obtain a complete history.

        b. Don't allow patient to dismiss a complaint (such as shortness of breath) as related to obesity.

        c. Make necessary accommodations during assessment.

            i. ECG electrode placement on the arms and thighs if chest is unavailable

            ii. Lung auscultation on anterior surface if patient cannot lean forward

        d. Before transporting, ensure that your equipment is rated for the patient's weight.

        e. Call for transportation assistance if necessary from another EMS crew or the fire department.

        f. Be sure to let receiving facility know the patient's weight.

        g. Try not to bring unneeded attention to patient to protect his dignity.

E. Paralysis (including paraplegia and quadriplegia) (p. 249)

    1. Ventilators

        a. If patient requires a ventilator, be sure you maintain airway (suction may be needed) and keep ventilator functioning.

        b. If ventilator isn't easily portable, use a bag-valve-mask (BVM) device while transporting patient to ambulance.

        c. When possible, use onboard ventilator to minimize strain on patient's battery-powered unit.

        d. Reassure patient before making any changes in life-support system.

    2. Halo traction

        a. Stabilize traction before transport.

        b. Ask patient, and check with physician if there is any question.

    3. Colostomy

        a. Be sure not to disturb external bag or stoma site.

POINT TO EMPHASIZE

If a person has halo traction, be sure to stabilize the traction before transport.

4. Assistance devices
   a. Be sure to ask patient what devices (for example, canes, walkers, wheelchairs) should be transported to give patient some autonomy after arrival at receiving facility.

III. Mental challenges and emotional impairments. (pp. 249–250)

A. Wide range, from psychotic states and mood disorders to emotional responses to a recent or ongoing traumatic experience (pp. 249–250)

B. Review Volume 3, Chapter 12, for details on assessment, management, and treatment of patients with these types of disorders. (pp. 249–250)

IV. Developmental disabilities. (pp. 250–252)

A. Impaired or insufficient brain development that causes learning disabilities (p. 250)

B. Accommodations for developmental disabilities (pp. 250–251)
   1. Many will be fully competent on interview, and no accommodation is required.
   2. Some may require help in history and physical from a familiar caregiver. (**Fig. 5-5**)
   3. Remember that patients will recognize your body language and verbal tone, so it is especially important that they see your respect for them.
   4. Establish trust and explain what you need from the patient during the interview, physical, or treatment, and keep in mind that patients may be confused or anxious, especially the severely impaired.
   5. It may be necessary to keep primary caregiver with patient at all times, depending on age and degree of disability.
   6. Be sure to assess level of impairment for the individual patient before establishing the treatment plan.

C. Down syndrome (p. 251) (**Fig. 5-6**)
   1. Typical physical features
      a. Eyes sloped upward at outer corners
      b. Folds of skin on either side of the nose that cover the inner corner of the eye
      c. Small face and features
      d. Large and protruding tongue
      e. Flattening on back of head
      f. Short, broad hands
   2. Medical associations
      a. Heart or intestinal defects and chronic lung problems
      b. At high risk for development of cataracts and early-onset Alzheimer's disease

D. Fetal alcohol syndrome (pp. 251–252)
   1. May physically resemble Down syndrome, but is due to excessive alcohol consumption during pregnancy
   2. Typical physical features (**Fig. 5-7**)
      a. Small head with multiple facial abnormalities
      b. Small eyes with short slits
      c. Wide, flat nose bridge
      d. Lack of a groove between nose and upper lip
      e. Small jaw
   3. Developmental associations
      a. Delayed physical growth
      b. Mental disabilities
      c. Hyperactivity

V. Pathological challenges. (pp. 252–258)

A. Arthritis (p. 253)

POWERPOINT PRESENTATION
Volume 5, Chapter 5, PowerPoint slides 18–22

TEACHING STRATEGY 4
Teacher's Aide Assignment

POINT TO EMPHASIZE
Patients with Down syndrome are often loving and trusting. Be sure to treat them with respect and patience.

POWERPOINT PRESENTATION
Volume 5, Chapter 5, PowerPoint slides 23–39

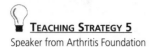
1. Three most common types
   a. Juvenile rheumatoid arthritis (JRA)
      i. Connective tissue disorder that presents before age 16 years
   b. Rheumatoid arthritis
      i. Autoimmune disorder
   c. Osteoarthritis
      i. Degenerative joint disease that is the most common arthritis seen in elderly patients
2. Common characteristics
   a. Painful swelling and irritation of joints
   b. Joint stiffness
   c. Limited range of motion
   d. Sometimes deformity of smaller joints of hands and feet (**Fig. 5-8**)
   e. Children with JRA may have liver or spleen complications.
3. Treatment
   a. Includes use of aspirin and nonsteroidal anti-inflammatory drugs (NSAIDs), and/or corticosteroids
   b. Side effects of these drugs to distinguish symptoms from those of a disease
      i. NSAIDs
         • Can cause stomach upset and vomiting, with or without blood emesis
      ii. Corticosteroids
         • Can cause hyperglycemia, bloody emesis, and decreased immune function
4. Management
   a. Be sure you get complete list of medications to avoid inadvertently giving something that will interact with a medication.
   b. Keep the physical discomfort of the patient in mind when examining and transporting; special padding may be required.
B. Cancer (pp. 253–255)
   1. All cancers are caused by abnormal growth of cells.
   2. Type of cancer determined by site of origin of malignant cells
      a. Carcinomas arise in epithelial tissue.
      b. Sarcomas arise in connective tissue.
   3. Sometimes most obvious sign is not of disease but rather of treatment.
      a. Anorexia and weight loss
      b. Hair loss (alopecia)
      c. Skin markings to show radiation therapy portals
      d. Evidence of surgery such as mastectomy
   4. Effects of cancer treatment on EMS care
      a. Poor immune function and high vulnerability to infection secondary to chemotherapy-induced neutropenia
         i. Loss of neutrophilic white blood cells
         ii. Keep a mask on the patient during transport and in emergency department. (**Fig. 5-9**)
      b. Poor veins for establishing IV access
         i. Look for possible implanted infusion port, but do NOT use such a port unless you have the specific training to do so.
         ii. If patient requests that you not start a peripheral IV, consider whether you can do so (Is IV a life-saving necessity or not?).
         iii. If patient has a peripheral access device such as a Groshong or Hickman catheter, consider using it if IV access is needed.
   5. Remember, whenever possible, to involve patient in decision making and defer to his requests.
C. Cerebral palsy (p. 255)
   1. Group of disorders caused by cerebral damage in utero or during birth

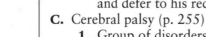

POINT TO EMPHASIZE

If a patient has been undergoing chemotherapy, assume he is neutropenic and keep a mask on the patient to reduce risk of infection.

2. Causes include:
  a. Prenatal rubella exposure
  b. Hypoxia during birth
  c. Postnatal infections or trauma
3. General characteristics
  a. Difficulty with motor control
    i. Spasticity of single limb or full body
  b. About two-thirds of persons affected have below-normal intellectual capacity.
  c. About half of persons affected have seizures.
4. Types
  a. Spastic paralysis
    i. Most common
    ii. Forces muscles into state of permanent contracture
  b. Athetosis
    i. Involuntary writhing movement
    ii. Usually affects upper and lower extremities
    iii. If face affected, drooling or grimacing common
  c. Ataxia
    i. Least common
    ii. Causes uncoordinated gait and balance
5. Management
  a. Don't assume below-normal intelligence.
    i. Many people with cerebral palsy are highly intelligent and can communicate if special devices allow them to do so.
  b. Be sure to recognize, use, and transport all necessary communication and mobility special devices.
  c. Make accommodations for transport to prevent further injury.
    i. Pillows and extra blankets to pad extremities that are not in proper alignment
    ii. Ready suction if drool is a concern
  d. If there is a caregiver, get his help during assessment.
  e. If the patient uses sign language, call ahead for an interpreter if one will be needed at the receiving facility.
D. Cystic fibrosis (CF) (or mucoviscidosis) (pp. 255–256)
  1. Genetic disease that involves mucus glands, primarily in the lungs and digestive system
  2. Pathology
    a. Thick, abnormal mucus causes bronchial obstruction and atelectasis in the lungs.
    b. Blockages in the exocrine ducts of the pancreas, leading to decrease in pancreatic enzymes and malnutrition
  3. Complete medical history important in detecting CF
    a. "Sweat test" detects high chloride concentration in sweat
    b. Disease present from birth with typical prognosis of death by early adulthood
      i. With late outliers extending life span into the thirties
  4. Medical characteristics
    a. High chloride concentration in sweat
    b. Frequent lung infections
    c. Clay-colored stool
    d. Clubbing of fingers and toes
  5. Management
    a. Transport issues may be difficult for both patient and family because most patients you will see are children or adolescents who do not want another trip to the hospital.

 POINT TO EMPHASIZE

CF patients may have been chronically ill all their lives. The last thing they want is another trip to the hospital.

        b. Be prepared to give oxygen therapy to all CF patients, either by mask or as blow-by oxygen, with patient or family member holding source if patient won't tolerate mask.

        c. Be prepared to suction airway secretions.

        d. Be sure to get list of medications (antibiotics and Mucomyst are typical) and bring all along to the hospital.

E. Multiple sclerosis (MS) (p. 256)

    1. Disorder of the CNS

    2. Perhaps autoimmune in origin

    3. Pathology

        a. Centers on inflammation and damage to myelin sheaths of neurons

        b. Causes formation of scar tissue that blocks impulses to affected area

    4. Most often affects persons ages 20 to 40, women more than men

    5. Symptoms and progression

        a. Typical onset is slow, with slight strength change in muscle associated with numbness or tingling.

        b. Disease may progress till gait unsteady or wheelchair is necessary.

        c. Speech may slur.

        d. Double vision or eye pain common

        e. Symptoms often have a come-and-go pattern and become more frequent, more severe, and longer lasting over time.

        f. Patients may eventually be bedridden and lose bladder control.

        g. Death often results from infection.

    6. Management

        a. Know that, as with other patients with chronic illness, persons may experience mood swings and sometimes seek medical care for their feelings.

        b. Transport may require oxygen therapy and other supportive care.

        c. Position for comfort and safety and do not expect patient to walk to ambulance.

        d. Be sure to transport all assistive devices (e.g., wheelchair or cane) with patient. **(Fig. 5-10)**

F. Muscular dystrophy (MD) (pp. 256–257)

    1. Group of genetic diseases characterized by progressive weakness and wasting of muscle tissue

    2. Multiple forms, most classified by age of onset, muscles affected, and history

    3. Most common type is Duchenne MD

        a. Typically develops in boys ages 3 to 6 and leads to progressive muscle weakness, paralysis, and death by age 12 or so

    4. Death is often due to involvement of respiratory muscles and/or heart.

    5. Management

        a. Be sure to get full family history, if possible.

        b. Be sure to note which muscles are affected and any muscle groups that the patient cannot move.

        c. Because most of the patients you will see are children, use age-appropriate language.

        d. Supportive therapy, particularly oxygen, may be needed, especially late in course of disease.

G. Poliomyelitis (p. 257)

    1. Viral communicable disease that affects brain gray matter and the spinal cord

    2. Now rare in developed nations because of immunization

    3. Although polio is now rare in the United States, there are many people born before the 1950s who are affected by the disease (recall Case Study at opening of chapter).

4. Pathology

    a. Initial attack centers on virus entering body through GI tract, entering bloodstream, and then traveling to the CNS, where the virus enters nerve cells and alters them.

5. Paralytic polio

    a. Patients experience asymmetrical muscle weakness that leads to permanent paralysis.

6. Most patients recover from initial attack, but are left with permanent paralysis in affected muscles.

    a. Look for assistive devices, muscle atrophy of affected limb, or even ventilator if respiratory muscles are involved.

7. Post-polio syndrome

    a. Affects persons who suffered severely more than 30 years ago and who currently have syndrome constellation of easy fatiguing, especially after exercise, and develop cold intolerance in extremities

8. Management

    a. Make appropriate accommodations for patients on long-term ventilator assistance who may have tracheotomies.

    b. Know that because many patients pride themselves on their independence, transport may be frustrating.

    c. Transport all assistive devices with the patient.

    d. Encourage the patient not to get fatigued by walking to ambulance.

    e. Try to alleviate the patient's anxiety as much as possible.

H. Previous head injury (pp. 257–258)

    1. Wide range of presentations, depending on site and severity of brain injury

    2. Patients may have strokelike symptoms.

        a. Aphasia

        b. Slurred speech

        c. Loss of vision or hearing

        d. Learning disabled

        e. Affected by frequent seizures

    3. A complete history of preexisting deficits is crucial to assessment, but some patients may not remember or be able to give historical information.

    4. Where possible, document symptoms known to be new or recurrent.

    5. Conduct physical slowly and look carefully for signs of trauma or responses typical of pain, especially if patient cannot talk.

    6. Transport depends on current complaint.

    7. Regardless of complaint, give as much information as possible to receiving facility about the previous head injury.

I. Spina bifida (p. 258)

    1. Congenital anomaly within the group called neural tube defects in which the spinal canal and spinal column did not close properly

    2. Types

        a. Spina bifida occulta

            i. Condition may be nearly invisible and asymptomatic.

            ii. Bone underneath skin did not close properly.

        b. Spina bifida cystica

            i. Either bone of vertebra(e), the bone and meninges surrounding the spinal cord, or all three types of tissue protrude from the back with obvious deformity.

    3. Symptoms

        a. Depend on degree of tissue protrusion and vertebral level of deformity

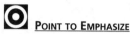 **POINT TO EMPHASIZE**

For safety, assume all spina bifida patients have a latex allergy.

      b. Paralysis of lower extremities and lack of bowel or bladder control common

      c. Hydrocephalus, accumulated fluid within brain, common in children born with spina bifida cystica

         i. Requires surgical implantation of a shunt

    4. Management

      a. Because a significant proportion of affected children and adolescents have latex allergy, assume that all spina bifida patients have the allergy.

      b. Be sure to transport all assistive devices with patient.

      c. Transport infants in car seat unless contraindicated.

J. Myasthenia gravis (p. 258)

    1. Autoimmune disease characterized by chronic weakness of voluntary muscles and progressive fatigue.

    2. Develops most frequently in women between ages 20 and 50

    3. Pathology centers on blockage of neural impulse from nerve cell to nerve cell.

    4. Symptoms commonly include

      a. Double vision

      b. Complete lack of energy

         i. Especially in evening

         ii. Often involving facial muscles

            • Drooping eyelid

            • Difficulty in chewing or swallowing

    5. In severe cases, respiratory muscles may be affected, leading to respiratory arrest, and these patients may require assisted ventilation en route to receiving facility.

    6. Other accommodations are specific to the individual patient's needs.

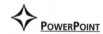 **POWERPOINT PRESENTATION**

Volume 5, Chapter 5, PowerPoint slides 40–44

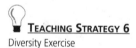 **TEACHING STRATEGY 6**

Diversity Exercise

VI. Other challenges. (pp. 258–260)

A. Cultural diversity (pp. 258–259) (**Fig. 5-11**)

    1. It is your ethical responsibility to treat all patients in the same manner.

    2. Respect the folk medicine beliefs of ethnic groups.

    3. Respect a patient's right to refuse treatment even after you fully explain the need and possible consequences.

    4. Always make sure you obtain a signed refusal of treatment and transportation form for your records. (**Fig. 5-12**)

    5. Be familiar with any foreign language spoken by a significant number of residents in your area and look for translation help from family or through use of a translator device or telephone language line.

      a. Always let receiving facility know if they will need a translator.

B. Terminally ill patients (pp. 259–260)

    1. Paramedic may be called when a patient has decided to die at home but the family gets to a crisis point in management and calls an ambulance or when a new medical condition has developed that (in the patient's or family's view) merits EMS evaluation.

    2. Review Chapter 6 of the text for guidelines on caring for the terminally ill patient either at home or in a hospice setting.

C. Patients with communicable diseases (p. 260)

    1. Take all appropriate standard precautions while refraining from any judgments and keeping the patient's sensitivities in mind.

    2. Explain that standard precautions are specific to the disease, not the patient; all patients with a similar disease are treated similarly.

    3. Refer to Volume 3, Chapter 11 for details on communicable diseases.

D. Patients with financial challenges (p. 260)

    1. Always treat the patient, not his financial situation.

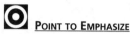 **POINT TO EMPHASIZE**

Treat the patient, not the patient's financial situation.

2. Become familiar with public hospitals and clinics that provide services to patients who do not have adequate funds or insurance.
3. Calm the patient while discussing this information. (Fig. 5-13)

VII. Summary. It is as important to understand the challenges that patients face and that may complicate your job (such as physical or mental impairments or the presence of certain chronic conditions) as it is to understand the pathophysiology of the diseases or injuries that you are treating. (p. 260)

POWERPOINT PRESENTATION
Volume 5, Chapter 5, PowerPoint slide 45

YOU MAKE THE CALL

Review student responses to the You Make the Call scenario on text pages 260–261. Suggested responses to the questions that follow the scenario are given below. Point out to students that these are acceptable answers but not necessarily the only ones. Discuss with students the pros and cons of points where their responses differ from these.

1. Why did the patient's doctor tell her that she has an increased risk of infection from communicable diseases?
(Cancer patients are at a high risk for infection if they have recently undergone chemotherapy. Chemotherapy can lead to neutropenia, which is a decrease in the white blood cells that help fight infection. For this reason, patients on chemotherapy do not have the ability to fight infection as well as a person with a normal neutrophil count.)

2. What signs indicate that this patient has cancer?
(The patient usually wears a wig to cover her head because of alopecia, she has lost her appetite, and she is vomiting. All of these conditions are side effects of chemotherapy. The patient has also recently had a mastectomy, which is a treatment for breast cancer.)

3. Is it necessary for all three of you to wear a mask? Explain.
(It is important for your partner to wear a mask because he has an illness that is spread through the respiratory tract. It is important for your patient to wear a mask so she is not exposed to your germs or to any droplets that may have been left in the ambulance from the previous patient. Since you are healthy and you are not at risk for contracting a communicable disease from your patient, it is not necessary for you to wear a mask, but you may do so to reassure your patient.)

4. Will you start a peripheral IV on this patient? Explain.
(You will probably not start a peripheral IV on this patient. She most likely has a subcutaneous port because she is currently undergoing chemotherapy treatment. It will be accessed when she gets to the emergency department, based on the lack of a life-threatening emergency when presenting to you.)

5. What information will you include in your patient report so the emergency department is prepared for this patient?
(It is important to relay the neutropenic status of your patient to the emergency department so they can have a private room ready to decrease her exposure to other illnesses.)

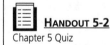
WORKBOOK
Chapter 5 Activities

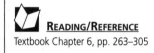
READING/REFERENCE
Textbook Chapter 6, pp. 263–305

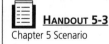
HANDOUT 5-2
Chapter 5 Quiz

HANDOUT 5-3
Chapter 5 Scenario

ASSIGNMENTS

Assign students to complete Chapter 5 of the Workbook. Also assign them to read Chapter 6, "Acute Interventions for the Chronic Care Patient," before the next class.

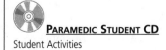
PARAMEDIC STUDENT CD
Student Activities

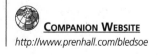
COMPANION WEBSITE
http://www.prenhall.com/bledsoe

TestGen
Volume 5, Chapter 5

EMT Achieve:
Paramedic Test Preparation
Mistovich & Beasley. *EMT Achieve: Paramedic Test Preparation,* http://prenhall.com/emtachieve

Success! for the
Paramedic
Cherry. *SUCCESS! for the Paramedic,* 4th edition

Handouts 5-4 to 5-5
Reinforcement Activities

Paramedic Student CD
Student Activities

PowerPoint
Presentation
Volume 5

Companion Website
http://www.prenhall.com/bledsoe

OneKey
Volume 5, Chapter 5

Advanced Life
Support Skills
Larmon & Davis. *Advanced Life Support Skills*

Advanced Life
Skills Review
Larmon & Davis. *Advanced Life Skills Review*

Brady Skills
Series: ALS
Larmon & Davis. *Brady Skills Series: ALS*

Paramedic National
Standards Self-Test
Miller. *Paramedic National Standards Self-Test,* 5th edition

EVALUATION

Chapter Quiz and Scenario   Distribute copies of the Chapter Quiz provided in Handout 5-2 to evaluate student understanding of this chapter. Make sure each student reads the scenario to reinforce critical thinking on the scene. Remind students not to use their notes or textbooks while taking the quiz.

Student CD   Quizzes for every chapter are contained on the dynamic and highly visual in-text student CD.

Companion Website   Additional quizzes for every chapter are contained on this exciting website.

TestGen   You may wish to create a custom-tailored test using *Prentice Hall TestGen for Paramedic Care: Principles & Practice,* 3rd edition, to evaluate student understanding of this chapter.

Online Test Preparation (for students and instructors)   Additional test preparation is available through Brady's new online product, EMT Achieve: Paramedic Test Preparation, at *http://www.prenhall.com/emtachieve.* Instructors can also monitor student mastery online.

Success! for the Paramedic   Keyed to *Paramedic Care: Principles & Practice* and *Essentials of Paramedic Care,* this comprehensive exam review contains hundreds of test questions and rationales.

REINFORCEMENT

Handouts   If classroom discussion or performance on the quiz indicates that some students have not fully mastered the chapter content, you may wish to assign some or all of the Reinforcement Handouts for this chapter.

Student CD (for students)   A wide variety of material on this CD-ROM will reinforce and also expand student knowledge and skills.

PowerPoint Presentation (for instructors)   The PowerPoint material developed for this chapter offers useful reinforcement of chapter content.

Companion Website (for students)   Additional review quizzes and links to EMS resources will contribute to further reinforcement of the chapter.

OneKey   Online support is offered for this course on one of three platforms: CourseCompass, Blackboard, or WebCT. Includes the IRM, PowerPoints, Test Manager, and Companion Website for Instruction. Ask your local sales representative for more information.

Brady Skills Series: Advanced Life Skills (Video or CD)   Have your students watch the skills come to life on VHS or CD-ROM, or they can purchase the highly visual, full-color text with step-by-step procedures with rationales.

Paramedic National Standards Self-Test   Another comprehensive review manual containing hundreds of review questions with page references keyed to several Brady texts.

©2009 Pearson Education, Inc.
Paramedic Care: Principles & Practice, Vol. 5, 3rd. Ed.

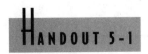

Student's Name _____

OBJECTIVES

CHAPTER 5 OBJECTIVES CHECKLIST

Knowledge Objective	Date Mastered
1. Describe the various etiologies and types of hearing impairments.	
2. Recognize the patient with a hearing impairment.	
3. Anticipate accommodations that may be needed to properly manage the patient with a hearing impairment.	
4. Describe the various etiologies and types, recognize patients with, and anticipate accommodations that may be needed in order to properly manage each of the following conditions:	
a. visual impairments	
b. speech impairments	
c. obesity	
d. paraplegia/quadriplegia	
e. mental illness	
f. developmentally disabled	
g. Down syndrome	
h. emotional/mental impairment	
5. Describe, identify possible presenting signs, and anticipate accommodations for the following diseases/illnesses:	
a. arthritis	
b. cancer	
c. cerebral palsy	
d. cystic fibrosis	
e. multiple sclerosis	
f. muscular dystrophy	
g. myasthenia gravis	
h. poliomyelitis	

OBJECTIVES

Knowledge Objective	Date Mastered
i. spina bifida	
j. patients with a previous head injury	
6. Define, recognize, and anticipate accommodations needed to properly manage patients who:	
a. are culturally diverse	
b. are terminally ill	
c. have a communicable disease	
d. have a financial impairment	

Skill Objective	Date Mastered
7. Given several challenged patients, provide the appropriate assessment, management, and transportation.	

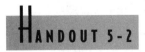

CHAPTER 5 QUIZ

Write the letter of the best answer in the space provided.

_____ 1. Persons with impaired maturation of the brain who are unable to learn at the usual rate are considered to have what type of challenge?
A. physical challenge
B. developmental challenge
C. mental challenge
D. pathological challenge

_____ 2. Which one of the following is NOT a cause of conductive hearing impairment?
A. neonatal asphyxia
B. childhood otitis media
C. impacted cerumen
D. trauma to the mandible or ear

_____ 3. The types of speech impairments are called:
A. articulation disorders.
B. language disorders.
C. fluency disorders.
D. aphasia disorders.

_____ 4. Patients with _____ have been ill for their entire lives, and you need to remember that the last thing they want is another exposure to the medical system or another hospitalization.
A. multiple sclerosis
B. cystic fibrosis
C. muscular dystrophy
D. spina bifida

_____ 5. Always assume that patients with this condition have a latex allergy.
A. cerebral palsy
B. cancer
C. cystic fibrosis
D. spina bifida

_____ 6. Clues that a person may have cancer include all of the following EXCEPT:
A. alopecia (hair loss).
B. significant weight loss.
C. thirstiness and frequent urination.
D. implanted infusion port.

_____ 7. Assume that a person who has recently undergone chemotherapy as a form of cancer therapy is neutropenic and thus vulnerable to:
A. infection.
B. hypoglycemia.
C. bradycardia.
D. tachypnea.

_____ 8. Common accommodations you should make for persons with severe hearing impairment do NOT include which of the following?
A. Make initial connection with the patient via movement or by gentle touch.
B. Maintain a face-to-face position.
C. Exaggerate facial and body language to make points more clear.
D. Reduce background noise to lowest possible level.

_____ 9. One cause of temporary vision loss is:
A. injury.
B. deployment of vehicle air bag.
C. infection.
D. disease.

_____ 10. Individuals who may need to be transported with the patient for medical reasons include all of the following EXCEPT a(n):
A. home nurse.
B. interpreter (either sign language or spoken language).
C. caregiver for the severely mentally impaired.
D. assistance dog.

_____ 11. A large proportion of persons with cerebral palsy are:
A. developmentally challenged.
B. highly intelligent.
C. unable to communicate in any way.
D. mentally challenged.

EVALUATION

_____ **12.** Persons who may have difficulty walking to the ambulance when ill do NOT include patients with:
   A. myasthenia gravis.   **C.** post-polio syndrome.
   B. multiple sclerosis.   **D.** spina bifida.

_____ **13.** Whenever possible when dealing with a culturally diverse patient, you should:
   A. maintain face-to-face positioning.
   B. remember that some folk remedies may interact with medical therapies.
   C. work through an interpreter.
   D. document the fact that the patient is culturally diverse.

_____ **14.** It is particularly important to explain all standard precautionary procedures as they arise with patients who:
   A. have a communicable disease.   **C.** have cystic fibrosis.
   B. have had recent chemotherapy.   **D.** are terminally ill.

_____ **15.** Causes of permanent vision loss include all of the following EXCEPT:
   A. glaucoma.   **C.** CMV infection.
   B. diabetic retinopathy.   **D.** corneal abrasion.

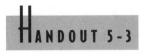
CHAPTER 5 SCENARIO

Review the following situation, and then answer the questions that follow.

You and your partner are called out shortly after 1:00 A.M. to the site of a single-vehicle collision. When you arrive at the scene, you see a fair amount of debris in the right lane that looks like cardboard or paneling and an apparently undamaged car on the shoulder. A police officer is talking with an older man who appears to be physically unhurt. As you walk toward them, you see an older woman standing quietly on the far side of the car.

The two men explain that the couple, Mr. and Mrs. Barrett, had been awakened by a phone call that their daughter had gone into labor with her first child. The couple dressed quickly and set out for the hospital. Unfortunately, Mr. Barrett did not see the debris in his lane until too late, and the car went over some of the cardboard as he tried to swerve away into another lane. Mr. Barrett tells you that both he and his wife were wearing their seat belts, and he thinks they were "just a bit shaken up."

Your partner, who is standing near Mrs. Barrett, gestures, and you walk over to them. He tells you in a quiet voice that she only shook her head in response to his questions and, although he can't see any blood or bruises in the darkness, he is worried about head injury.

You touch Mrs. Barrett gently on her arm, and she looks up, almost surprised to see you. She doesn't say anything when you ask her if she has any discomfort anywhere, but she continues to watch your face. Suddenly, you get an idea, and you tell her you'd like to walk over to the ambulance and talk there. As you take her arm gently, she says "all right" and willingly walks with you toward the lights of the ambulance. As you glance at her, you see no sign of injury.

1. What clues, if any, suggest that Mrs. Barrett may have a type of challenge rather than head trauma? What type of challenge do you suspect?

2. When you reach the relatively well-lit area beside the ambulance, what accommodations should you make, on the assumption Mrs. Barrett may be hearing impaired, as you try to begin an interview with her?

3. When you ask Mrs. Barrett whether she can hear you all right, she reaches up to touch her ears and says "Oh, my. I forgot to put my hearing aids in." What question should you ask next?

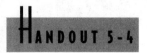

CHAPTER 5 REVIEW

Write the word or words that best complete each sentence in the space(s) provided.

1. Physical challenges include sensory impairments such as visual or hearing loss, as well as speech impairments and physical states such as _____ or _____.

2. When obesity complicates positioning of ECG electrodes, remember that you can place electrodes on the _____ and _____ instead of on the chest.

3. A person with _____ aphasia cannot understand the spoken word, whereas a person with _____ aphasia cannot clearly articulate a response to what you say.

4. When speaking with a person who has a speech impairment, try to phrase questions so that they can be answered with _____, direct responses.

5. An individual with paralysis due to an injury of the cervical vertebrae may have compromise of _____ muscles and require use of a home _____.

6. Be sure to have _____ ready when you treat quadriplegic patients in case there are excess secretions in the airway.

7. If a patient is wearing a halo device, be sure to _____ _____ before transport.

8. It may be necessary to spend extra time on the physical examination of an adult with a(n) _____ disability if the person does not have sufficient cognitive or communicative skills to give you history information.

9. Remember that individuals with Down syndrome may have other physical conditions involving one or more of these three organs: _____, _____, and _____.

10. _____ _____ syndrome is sometimes confused with Down syndrome because of similar facial characteristics, even though it is due to a form of toxic injury during pregnancy.

11. Because _____ distress is highly probable in patients with cystic fibrosis, be prepared to give oxygen therapy.

12. If you use an interpreter for any reason, be sure to document the _____ _____ and the _____ _____ _____ _____.

13. Remember that every patient who has decision-making ability has the right to _____ _____; if this occurs, be sure it is documented properly.

14. One axiom about caring for patients with monetary challenges is to care for the _____, not the _____ _____.

15. Signs of myasthenia gravis that are readily observed in the face are _____ _____ and difficulty with _____ or _____.

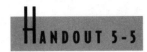

Student's Name _____

THE MANY TYPES OF CHALLENGED PATIENTS

Fill in the blanks to complete the information on different types of challenged patients.

1. Examples of physical challenges:

   A. _____ impairment with _____ deafness and _____ deafness

   B. _____ impairment

   C. _____ impairment with _____ aphasia, _____ aphasia, and _____ aphasia

   D. _____

   E. _____ with possible paraplegia or quadriplegia

2. _____ challenges and _____ impairment (including the psychoses, mood disorders, personality disorders, and responses to a traumatic experience)

3. _____ disabilities (including patients with Down syndrome, fetal alcohol syndrome, and disabilities of many other origins)

4. Examples of _____ challenges (chronic conditions):

   A. Arthritis

   B. _____

   C. _____ palsy

   D. _____ _____ (mucoviscidosis)

   E. _____ _____ (MS)

   F. _____ _____ (MD)

   G. _____ and post- _____ syndrome

   H. Previous _____ _____

   I. _____ _____ with _____ _____ occulta or _____ _____ cystica

   J. _____ gravis

5. Other challenges include:

   A. _____ _____ patients

   B. _____ _____ patients

   C. Patients with _____ diseases

   D. Patients with _____ challenges

Chapter 5 Answer Key

Handout 5-2: Chapter 5 Quiz

1. B	5. D	9. B	13. B
2. A	6. C	10. A	14. A
3. D	7. A	11. B	15. D
4. B	8. C	12. D	

Handout 5-3: Chapter 5 Scenario

1. The undamaged appearance of the car, the uninjured appearance and settled voice of Mr. Barrett, as well as the information that the couple were both wearing seat belts by no means rule out head injury in Mrs. Barrett, but they do not raise your level of concern, either.
   Her surprise when you walk close to her and her fixing on your face in the darkness are clues that she might be hearing impaired. It is difficult to assess her status in the darkness. You realize that the poor light—if she has a hearing impairment—is making it harder for her, especially after the news of her daughter's labor and the minor car accident, to focus on and respond to what you say.
   The fact that she said "all right" clearly when you asked her to walk over to the ambulance does not rule out a speech impairment, but it does make it somewhat less likely than hearing impairment.
2. You should assume a directly face-to-face position. Speak clearly in a low-pitched voice and without exaggeration. Look for a hearing aid. Ask her directly if she can hear you properly because you need to ask her a few questions about how she feels. Reduce background noise as much as possible. (For example, make sure radio is turned down or partner sits in ambulance to listen to any incoming calls. Stand at the side farther from the highway to muffle any road noise.)
3. Any question that directly calls for a response on whether she can hear you well enough to answer a few questions is proper. If she can't hear well enough, ask her husband to stand with her and ask them questions jointly to ascertain whether either has been injured sufficiently to require intervention. Be matter-of-fact. Hearing impairment is a complication to patient interview but not a problem itself.

Handout 5-4: Chapter 5 Review

1. obesity, paralysis
2. arms, thighs
3. sensory, motor (expressive)
4. short
5. respiratory, ventilator
6. suction
7. stabilize traction
8. developmental
9. heart, intestines, lungs
10. Fetal alcohol
11. respiratory
12. person's name, information the person provided
13. refuse treatment
14. patient, financial condition
15. drooping eyelid, swallowing, chewing

Handout 5-5: The Many Types of Challenged Patients

1. a. Hearing, conductive, sensorineural
   b. Visual
   c. Speech, sensory, motor (expressive), global
   d. Obesity
   e. Paralysis

2. Mental, emotional
3. Developmental
4. pathological
   a. Arthritis
   b. Cancer
   c. Cerebral
   d. Cystic fibrosis
   e. Multiple sclerosis
   f. Muscular dystrophy
   g. Poliomyelitis, polio
   h. head injury
   i. Spina bifida, spina bifida, spina bifida
   j. Myasthenia

5. a. Culturally diverse
   b. Terminally ill
   c. communicable
   d. financial

©2009 Pearson Education, Inc.
Paramedic Care: Principles & Practice, Vol. 5, 3rd. Ed.

Chapter 6

Acute Interventions for the Chronic Care Patient

INTRODUCTION

Because of the movement toward early hospital discharge followed by home care, there has been a huge increase in home health care needs and services over the past 30 to 40 years. Currently, more than 665,000 caregivers—nurses, home health aides, physical therapists, occupational therapists, and other health care professionals—support patients who receive home care. Experts expect this trend to continue. Thus, an increasingly large number of patients will receive treatment, even for terminal illness, in a prehospital setting. Your students will receive calls to assess and treat patients with chronic conditions who are receiving care at home. This chapter will teach them how to assess whether the EMS call is for an acute problem unrelated to the chronic condition, reflects an exacerbation of the chronic condition, is related to home care equipment, or is due to another reason. This chapter covers the epidemiology of home care, reasons for ALS intervention in home care cases, and pertinent general system pathophysiology, assessment, and management.

CHAPTER OBJECTIVES

Knowledge Objectives

1. Compare and contrast the primary objectives of the paramedic and the home care provider. (pp. 267–268, 273)
2. Identify the importance of home health care medicine as it relates to emergency medical services. (pp. 266–268)
3. Differentiate between the role of the paramedic and the role of the home care provider. (pp. 267–268, 273)
4. Compare and contrast the primary objectives of acute care, home care, and hospice care. (pp. 266–267, 273, 300–302)
5. Discuss aspects of home care that enhance the quality of patient care and aspects that have the potential to become detrimental. (pp. 268–272)
6. List pathologies and complications in home care patients that commonly result in ALS intervention. (pp. 267–272, 280–300)
7. Compare the cost, mortality, and quality of care for a given patient in the hospital vs. the home care setting. (pp. 266–267)

 TOTAL TEACHING TIME: 5.69 HOURS
The total teaching time is only a guideline based on the didactic and practical lab averages in the National Standard Curriculum. Instructors should take into consideration such factors as: the pace at which students learn, the size of the class, and breaks. The actual time devoted to teaching objectives is the responsibility of the instructor.

8. Discuss the significance of palliative care programs as related to a patient in a home health care or hospice setting. (pp. 273, 300–302)

9. Define hospice care, comfort care, and DNR/DNAR as they relate to local practice, law, and policy. (pp. 267, 273, 279, 300–302)

10. List and describe the characteristics of typical home care devices related to airway maintenance, artificial and alveolar ventilation, vascular access, drug administration, and the GI/GU tract. (pp. 272–273, 280–282, 284–298)

11. Discuss the complications of assessing each of the devices described in objective 10. (pp. 287–288, 290–291, 293, 294–295, 296–297)

12. Describe indications, contraindications, and techniques for urinary catheter insertion in the male and female patient in an out-of-hospital setting. (p. 294)

13. Identify failure of GI/GU, ventilatory, vascular access, and drain devices found in the home care setting. (pp. 287–288, 290–291, 293, 294–295, 296–297)

14. Discuss the relationship between local home care treatment protocols/SOPs and local EMS protocols/SOPs. (p. 273)

15. Discuss differences in the ability of individuals to accept and cope with their own impending death. (p. 302)

16. List the stages of the grief process and relate them to an individual in hospice care. (p. 302)

17. Discuss the rights of the terminally ill patient. (pp. 300–302)

18. Summarize the types of home health care available in your area and the services provided. (pp. 266, 273–274)

Skill Objectives

19. Given a series of home care scenarios, determine which patients should receive follow-up home care and which should be transported to an emergency care facility. (pp. 266–302)

20. Given a series of scenarios, demonstrate interaction and support with the family members/support persons for a patient who has died. (p. 302)

FRAMING THE LESSON

Break students into groups to brainstorm examples of patients who receive home care. You may wish to use categories based on age or health condition. For example, a group asked to think about age-related reasons for home care might think of the following examples:

- A premature infant who needs follow-up care after hospital discharge
- A small child with a serious, chronic disorder requiring special respiratory, GI, or other care
- Elderly individuals who require monitoring of blood glucose, blood pressure, or another variable or who require in-home care because of physical disability, dementia, or another medical problem

A group challenged to think of short-term or temporary conditions requiring home care might come up with examples such as the following:

- A new mother who had significant delivery complications and needs follow-up home care
- A patient returning home from a rehab center who requires in-home personal care and support with exercises and other rehabilitation measures

©2009 Pearson Education, Inc.
Paramedic Care: Principles & Practice, Vol. 5, 3rd. Ed.

- A patient who has had transplant surgery and requires at-home health care to recuperate from surgery and learn how to handle the medications and other needs associated with post-transplantation living
- A patient who is terminally ill and has come home to die

Students asked to think of long-term examples of home care will probably focus on the major chronic conditions that affect North Americans, especially elderly persons:

- A patient with diabetes and complications such as diabetic retinopathy and/or extremity amputation who requires medical monitoring and personal care
- A person with a developmental disability and a chronic condition such as inflammatory bowel disease who needs personal and medical support
- A patient with paraplegia or quadriplegia who requires intensive medical support on a constant basis
- A patient with severe atherosclerosis who has had previous MIs and amputation because of vascular insufficiency

CONSIDERING THE CASE STUDY

Ask a volunteer to read aloud the Case Study that begins on text page 264. Suggest that students close their eyes as the scenario is read to help them visualize the events described in it. You can use the following questions as a starting point for teaching the chapter—a sort of chapter preview in a functional setting.

When the chapter is completed, you may wish to return to the Case Study and encourage further discussion aimed at answering the questions.

CASE STUDY DISCUSSION QUESTIONS (AND ANSWERS)

1. What are the providers' first clues that their patient is receiving home care?
   (They notice oxygen bottles on the floor and see that the patient is using a nasal cannula for oxygen delivery.)
2. Do these clues suggest that the called-in chief complaint may be related to the reason for home care or that it is a distinct problem?
   (The call stated "short of breath," so it is reasonable for the paramedics to assume that the current condition may be related to the patient's chronic condition.)
3. What two pieces of historical information would be especially valuable to the paramedics as they recognize that the chief complaint may represent an exacerbation or complication of the patient's chronic condition?
   (They need to know the patient's diagnosis or diagnoses and what medications he is on, as well as when he last took them.)
4. Once the paramedics have learned the patient's major diagnoses (emphysema, bronchitis, and hypertension) and realize his age (74 years), what additional piece of information should they seek as they finish assessment and plan to initiate treatment?
   (They need to know the home care plan and, specifically, whether the patient has a Do Not Resuscitate [DNR] order in effect or another stipulation on limitations of treatment.)

TEACHING STRATEGIES

People learn in a variety of ways. Some do better with the spoken word, while others prefer the written. Some prefer to work alone, whereas others profit from working in groups. Recognizing these different ways of acquiring knowledge, the authors of this *Instructor's Resource Manual* have provided a variety of teaching strategies for the different types of learners. These strategies are intended to foster higher-level cognitive skills and encourage creative learning and problem solving.

For greatest effectiveness, incorporate these strategies into your class lecture. Marginal notes in the Teaching Outline indicate the points at which various exercises might be most appropriate. Other strategies can be used to preview the lesson or to summarize it.

The following strategies are keyed to specific sections of the lesson:

1. A Day with a Home Health Care Provider. Arrange for students to spend a day of clinical time with a home health care provider. It could be enlightening for students to witness the depth and scope of home health care. Additionally, students should gain an appreciation for the challenges of caring for terminal and chronic care patients. Often the conditions of one's home are far more difficult to work within than those of the hospital. Home health providers are excellent creative problem solvers and can teach students a great deal about their role, chronic care patients, and the advanced care devices in homes today.

2. Home Health Care Device In-Service. Provide in-service training to students on the advanced technology of home care devices so they are more likely to know how to use this equipment when they encounter it in the field. Have a representative from the manufacturer, a medical equipment representative, or home care nurse bring the equipment and manuals to class. Also, emphasize to students that patients and family members are often good resources for use of the equipment. Be sure the representative provides students with a contact number to call should they encounter an equipment problem in the field.

3. Hospital Clinical Time with Wounds and Ostomies. Consider clinical time for students on a hospital floor that deals with wounds and ostomies or with a wound care clinic. The paramedic's knowledge of wound care is often limited to direct pressure and elevation. Intensive time spent learning to recognize the early signs of local and systemic infection will be helpful in their careers. Additionally, caring for wounds, managing dressing changes, and cleaning ostomies will likely be part of the expected practice of the paramedic in the near future.

4. Simulating Bodily Functions. Students are often taken aback by the products of bodily functions encountered on calls because classroom simulations lack this type of realism. When appropriate, simulate an incontinent patient by using Depends and chocolate cake frosting, fill an ostomy bag with mushroom soup, or attach (tape) a seemingly full Foley to the patient. These additions in classroom situations seem small, but a lack of familiarity with the products of bodily functions can derail an assessment and treatment plan when encountered on an actual call.

5. Questioning Techniques. Emphasize to students how to respect a person's intelligence by directing questions first to the patient. It is appropriate to interview the family or caregiver in lieu of the patient only after the patient has been determined by you to be incapable of providing an accurate history. Too many providers insult and alienate patients by assuming they are incompetent to answer questions.

6. *Practicing Ostomy Care on Ostomy and Stoma Manikins.* Ostomy and stoma manikins are available from all of the major manikin manufacturers. If your budget does not allow a purchase, consider borrowing one from your nursing education department or home health care company. Create skills sheets for ostomy care much the way you would for other emergency procedures such as intubation or patient assessment. By practicing and testing these procedures and skills in class, you place importance on these competencies. This is an important message for students about caring for all patients equally well, regardless of level of acuity of the call.

The following strategy relates to Special Features in the student textbook and can be used to enhance the student's understanding:

Legal Notes: Legal Considerations and the Home Care Patient. Facilitate a class discussion on living wills, durable power of attorney for health care, Do Not Resuscitate orders, and the Uniform Anatomical Gift Act, and how they affect patient care. Cases related to "difficulties" involving these documents could also be discussed with the students, asking how they would handle the situation.

The following strategy can be used at various points throughout the lesson or to help summarize and demonstrate what students have learned:

The Nature of EMS Calls for Chronic Care Patients. Have students break into groups to discuss the patients listed for each category in the exercise for Framing the Lesson. This time, have your students think of possible reasons for EMS calls to these patients. Encourage them to think about the kinds of chief complaints these patients might have, as well as any kind of equipment or procedural difficulty that might result in an EMS call.

TEACHING OUTLINE

Chapter 6 is the sixth lesson in Volume 5, *Special Considerations/Operations.* Distribute Handout 6-1 so that students can familiarize themselves with the learning goals for this chapter. If students have any questions about the objectives, answer them at this time.

Then present the chapter. One possible lecture outline follows. In the outline, the parenthetical references in regular type are references to text pages; those in bold type are to figures, tables, or procedures.

I. Introduction. The movement in the United States toward early hospital discharge (or no hospital admission) and establishment of home care has resulted in large numbers of people cared for at home. Note that this number will probably increase with time. The primary driving force in home health care is cost containment. (p. 266)

II. Epidemiology of home care. (pp. 266–275)

A. Factors that promoted the growth of home health care in recent years (p. 266)

  1. Enactment of Medicare in 1965

  2. Advent of health maintenance organizations (HMOs)

  3. Improved medical technology

  4. Changes in attitudes of doctors and patients toward hospital care

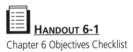

HANDOUT 6-1
Chapter 6 Objectives Checklist

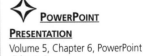

POWERPOINT PRESENTATION
Volume 5, Chapter 6, PowerPoint slides 1–3

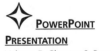

POWERPOINT PRESENTATION
Volume 5, Chapter 6, PowerPoint slides 4–6

READING/REFERENCE
Brown, L., et al. "Field Implementation of ADs," *JEMS*, Apr. 1999.

SLIDES/VIDEOS
"Chronic Disorders." Pulse: *Emergency Medical Update*, June 1997.

TEACHING STRATEGY 1
A Day with a Home Health Care Provider

TEACHING STRATEGY 2
Home Health Care Device In-Service

LEGAL NOTES
Legal Considerations and the Home Care Patient, p. 267

TEACHING STRATEGY 3
Hospital Clinical Time with Wounds and Ostomies

POINT TO EMPHASIZE
Remember that cardiac decompensation is a true medical emergency that can lead to life-threatening shock.

B. Arguments in favor of home health care (p. 266)
  1. Recovery often faster in familiar environment
  2. Speeds dismissal from hospitals and nursing homes
  3. Costs less
C. Patients receiving home care (pp. 266–267)
  1. In 1992, almost 75 percent of patients were 65 years or older.
  2. In 1992, of elderly home care patients, almost two-thirds (66 percent) were women.
  3. Today some 8 million patients—with both acute and chronic conditions—receive formal health care treatment from paid providers.
  4. Patients require home care for various reasons.
D. ALS response to home care patients (pp. 267–275) (**Fig. 6-1**)
  1. Common reasons for ALS intervention
    a. Equipment failure
    b. Unexpected complications
    c. Absence of a caregiver
    d. Need for transport
    e. Inability to operate a device
  2. The primary role of the paramedic is to identify and treat any life-threatening problems.
E. Typical responses (pp. 268–272)
  1. Chief complaints are similar to those in other populations, but the home care patient is fragile and more likely to decompensate and go into crisis more quickly than the general population.
  2. Airway complications
  3. Respiratory failure
    a. Emphysema
    b. Bronchitis
    c. Asthma
    d. Cystic fibrosis
    e. Congestive heart failure
    f. Pulmonary embolus
    g. Sleep apnea
    h. Guillain-Barré syndrome
    i. Myasthenia gravis
  4. Cardiac decompensation
    a. Congestive heart failure
    b. Acute MI
      i. Home care patients are at higher risk
    c. Cardiac hypertrophy
    d. Calcification or degeneration of the heart's conductive system
    e. Heart transplant
    f. Sepsis
  5. Alterations in peripheral circulation
  6. Altered mental status
    a. Common reason for EMS calls
    b. Causes
      i. Hypoxia
      ii. Hypotension
      iii. Sepsis
      iv. Altered electrolytes or blood chemistries
      v. Hypoglycemia
      vi. Alzheimer's disease
      vii. Cancerous tumor or brain lesions
      viii. Overdose
      ix. Stroke (brain attack)
  7. GI/GU crises (gastrointestinal/genitourinary)

8. Infections and septic complications
   a. Be alert to infections in the home care patient with any of the following:
      i. Indwelling devices
         • Gastrostomy tubes
         • PICC lines
         • Foley catheters
         • Colostomies
      ii. Limited lung function and tracheotomies
      iii. Decreased sensorium
      iv. Surgically implanted drains
      v. Decubitus wounds (bedsores) (**Fig. 6-2**)
   b. Signs of infection
      i. Redness and/or swelling, especially at insertion site of indwelling device
      ii. Purulent discharge at the insertion site
      iii. Warm skin at the insertion site
      iv. Fever
   c. Signs and symptoms of sepsis
      i. Redness at an insertion site
      ii. Fever
      iii. Altered mental status
      iv. Poor skin color and turgor
      v. Signs of shock
      vi. Vomiting
      vii. Diarrhea
9. Equipment malfunction
   a. Home ventilators
   b. Oxygen delivery systems
   c. Apnea monitors
   d. Home dialysis machines
10. Other medical disorders and home care patients
   a. Brain or spinal trauma
   b. Arthritis
   c. Psychological disorders
   d. Cancer
   e. Hepatitis
   f. AIDS
   g. Transplants (including patients awaiting transplantation)
F. Commonly found medical devices (pp. 272–273) (**Fig. 6-3**)
   1. Glucometers
   2. IV infusions and indwelling IV sites
   3. Nebulized and aerosolized medication administrators
   4. Shunts, fistulas, and venous grafts
   5. Oxygen concentrators, oxygen tanks, and liquid oxygen systems
   6. Oxygen masks and nebulizers
   7. Tracheotomies and home ventilators
   8. G-tubes, colostomies, and urostomies
   9. Surgical drains
   10. Apnea monitors, cardiac monitors, and pulse oximeters
   11. Wheelchairs, canes, and walkers
G. Intervention by a home health care practitioner or physician (p. 273)
   1. Most cases require acute intervention.
   2. In some cases the paramedic's role is supportive.
      a. Chemotherapy
      b. Pain management
      c. Hospice care

POINT TO EMPHASIZE

You will be foolish and endanger the patient if you pretend to understand a device but don't.

POINT TO EMPHASIZE

On any call involving a home care patient, be sure to ask whether another health care professional has been called.

H. Injury control and prevention (pp. 274–275) **(Table 6-1; Table 6-2)**
1. Prevent the creation of the hazard to begin with.
2. Reduce the amount of the hazard brought into existence.
3. Prevent the release of the hazard that already exists.
4. Modify the rate of distribution of the hazard from the source.
5. Separate the hazard and that which is to be protected in both time and space.
6. Separate the hazard and that which is to be protected by a barrier.
7. Modify the basic qualities of the hazard.
8. Make that which is to be protected more resistant to the hazard.
9. Counter the damage already done by the hazard.
10. Stabilize, repair, and rehabilitate the object of the damage.

III. General system pathophysiology, assessment, and management. (pp. 275–280)

A. Assessment (pp. 276–279)
1. Scene size-up: safety
   a. Any patient with limited movement may be contaminated with urine, feces, or emesis.
   b. Any bed-bound patient may have weeping wounds, bleeding, or decubitus ulcers.
   c. Sharps may be present.
   d. Collection bags for urine or feces sometimes leak.
   e. Tracheostomy patients clear mucus by coughing, which can spray.
   f. Any electrical machine has the potential for electric shock.
   g. A hospital bed, wheelchair, or walker could be contaminated with body fluid.
   h. Contaminated medical devices, such as a nebulizer, may be left unprotected.
   i. Oxygen in the presence of flame has the potential for fire or explosion.
   j. Equipment may be in the way and cause you to fall, or it may be unstable and fall on you.
   k. Medical wastes may not be properly contained or discarded.
2. Scene size-up: Patient milieu
   a. Evaluate the patient's environment.
   b. Assess the quality of home care received by the patient.
   c. Note any signs of abuse or neglect.
   d. Note the condition of medical devices.
   e. Remember: The paramedic not only has a responsibility to treat the patient, but also to act as an advocate.

B. Initial assessment, focused history, physical exam (pp. 277–279)
1. Initial assessment
   a. Try to establish a baseline presentation for patient.
   b. Assess for changes from the norm.
   c. If unable to stabilize a patient, complete the rapid assessment and transport immediately.
   d. In noncritical patients, compare vital signs to bedside records if they are kept.
   e. Focus your exam on the chief complaint and how it might relate to the patient's chronic condition.
   f. Be sure to check for decubiti, because they pose a significant danger to the patient through infection.
   g. Be meticulous.

POWERPOINT
PRESENTATION
Volume 5, Chapter 6, PowerPoint slides 7–79

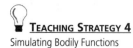

TEACHING STRATEGY 4
Simulating Bodily Functions

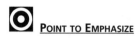

POINT TO EMPHASIZE
Be sure to remove any medical waste you generate so that the patient does not return to an unsafe environment.

2. Mental status (**Fig. 6-4**)
  a. If patient has preexisting altered mental status, have a good understanding of patient's normal mentation before transport.
  b. Follow same general procedures as with other patients.
  c. If patient unable to answer questions, rely on family members or caregivers.
  d. Remember that home care patients, particularly older or terminal patients, fear being moved from the home.
3. Other considerations
  a. Take into account the condition that led to home care and the events that led to the current crisis.
  b. Talk to the health care provider and the patient.
  c. Before beginning any life-saving measures, ascertain whether or not the patient has DNR or DNAR orders.
C. Transport and management treatment plan (pp. 279–280)
  1. Paramedic may have to replace home treatment modalities with ALS modalities.
  2. Paramedic may have to transport patient's home devices.

IV. **Specific acute home health situations.** (pp. 280–302)
A. Respiratory disorders (pp. 280–291)
  1. Common home respiratory equipment
    a. Oxygen equipment
    b. Portable suctioning machines
    c. Aerosol equipment and nebulizers
    d. Incentive spirometers
    e. Home ventilators
    f. Tracheostomy tubes and collars
  2. Chronic diseases requiring home respiratory support
    a. COPD (**Fig. 6-5**)
      i. Bronchitis
      ii. Emphysema
      iii. Asthma
    b. Congestive heart failure (CHF)
    c. Cystic fibrosis (CF)
    d. Bronchopulmonary dysplasia (BPD)
    e. Neuromuscular degenerative diseases
      i. Muscular dystrophy
      ii. Poliomyelitis
      iii. Guillain-Barré syndrome
      iv. Myasthenia gravis
    f. Sleep apnea
    g. Patients awaiting lung transplants
  3. Medical therapy found in the home setting
    a. Home oxygen therapy (**Table 6-3**)
    b. Artificial airways/tracheostomies
      i. Common complications
      ii. Management (**Fig. 6-6**)
    c. Home ventilation
      i. Positive pressure ventilators
      ii. Negative pressure ventilators
      iii. PEEP, CPAP, and BIPAP (**Fig. 6-7**)
    d. General assessment considerations
    e. General management considerations

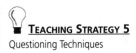
TEACHING STRATEGY 5
Questioning Techniques

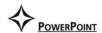
POWERPOINT
PRESENTATION
Volume 5, Chapter 6, PowerPoint slides 80–84

POINT TO EMPHASIZE
Home care patients often have a high dosing regimen, which may make them less responsive to medications.

TEACHING STRATEGY 6
Practicing Ostomy Care on Ostomy and Stoma Manikins

B. Vascular access devices (pp. 291–293)
    1. Types of VADs
        a. Hickman, Broviac, and Groshong catheters (**Fig. 6-8**)
        b. Peripherally inserted central catheters (PICCs) (**Fig. 6-9**)
        c. Surgically implanted medication delivery systems
        d. Dialysis shunts (**Fig. 6-10**)
    2. Anticoagulant therapy
    3. VAD complications
        a. Various types of obstructions cause most common complications.
            i. Thrombus at catheter site
            ii. Air embolus at catheter site
            iii. Catheter kinking
            iv. Catheter tip embolus
        b. Signs and symptoms of an air embolus
            i. Headache
            ii. Shortness of breath with clear lungs
            iii. Hypoxia
            iv. Chest pain
            v. Other indications of myocardial ischemia
            vi. Altered mental status
C. Cardiac conditions (p. 294)
    1. Post-MI recovery
    2. Post-cardiac surgery
    3. Heart transplant
    4. CHF
    5. Hypertension
    6. Implanted pacemaker
    7. Atherosclerosis
    8. Congenital malformation (pediatric)
D. GI/GU crisis (pp. 294–298)
    1. Urinary tract devices (**Fig. 6-11**)
    2. Urinary device complications (**Fig. 6-12**)
    3. Gastrointestinal tract devices (**Fig. 6-13; Fig. 6-14; Fig. 6-15**)
    4. Gastrointestinal tract complications
    5. Psychosocial implications
E. Acute infections (p. 298)
F. Maternal and newborn care (pp. 298–300)
    1. Common maternal complications
        a. Massage of uterus, if not already contracted
        b. Administration of fluids to correct hypotension
        c. Administration of certain medications, such as Pitocin, if ordered
        d. Rapid transport to hospital, if necessary
    2. Common infant/child complications
        a. Cyanosis
        b. Bradycardia (<100 beats/min)
        c. Crackles
        d. Respiratory distress
G. Hospice and comfort care (pp. 300–302) (**Table 6-4**)
    1. ALS intervention
    2. Common diseases at hospice
        a. Congestive heart failure
        b. Cystic fibrosis
        c. COPD
        d. AIDS
        e. Alzheimer's (**Fig. 6-16**)
        f. Cancer

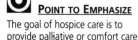

POINT TO EMPHASIZE

The goal of hospice care is to provide palliative or comfort care rather than curative care.

3. Stages of death and grief
    a. Denial
    b. Anger
    c. Depression
    d. Bargaining
    e. Acceptance

V. Summary. The shift toward home care will have an increasing impact on the ALS profession, and you can expect to see acute intervention calls for a wide range of chronic care disorders in patients of all ages and in all stages of disease progression. These calls will challenge you to develop effective management plans, and in many cases you will need to collaborate with home health care workers. (p. 302)

◆ **POWERPOINT**
PRESENTATION
Volume 5, Chapter 6, PowerPoint slide 85

YOU MAKE THE CALL

Review student responses to the You Make the Call scenario on text pages 302–303. Suggested responses to the questions that follow the scenario are given below. Point out to students that these are acceptable answers but not necessarily the only ones. Discuss with students the pros and cons of points where their responses differ from these.

  1. What does the condition of the apartment tell you?
     (A messy, dirty apartment may indicate that the patient is on her own and has little support from family or friends. It may also show that she is receiving inadequate home care. These social factors may help you understand the patient's state of mind and interact with greater compassion.)

  2. Why is it important to immediately interview the home care worker?
     (The home care worker usually knows the patient well and can tell you exactly what is different, if anything, about the patient. If you don't fully understand the patient's baseline mental status and disability, you cannot adequately assess and compare your own findings.)

  3. What are some of the causes of urinary incontinence?
     (Causes include seizures, spinal injury, abdominal trauma, and overdoses, among others.)

  4. How can you rule out spinal injury to this patient?
     (You can't. The possibility of spinal injury in a patient with a preexisting neurologic deficit cannot be ruled out without knowing the exact nature of the patient's baseline deficit. That decision is best left to the patient's own physician or the emergency department staff.)

  5. Why do you think the patient denies a history of diabetes and seizures if she takes Tegretol and glucophage?
     (Imagine how you would feel if confined to a wheelchair at age 18 for the rest of your life. Such patients can become unhappy, lonely, resentful, and bitter. They may also deny certain aspects of their disability in an attempt to feel better or to gain acceptance. In this case, because the patient exhibited no complicating factors related to diabetes or seizures, the crew decided not to argue with her. However, they had a responsibility to report all medications—and suspicions—as a part of their transfer of care.)

  6. Why is it acceptable to defer the glucose test when patient medications indicate a possible blood glucose problem?
     (The patient seems to be sensitive to her condition. Because she shows no signs of hypoglycemia, it is probably better to keep the patient calm than to argue with her about the test. If the crew had any doubts about their actions, they should, of course, consult with medical direction.)

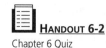
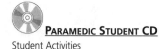
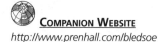

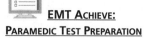
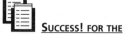
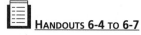
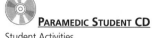
HANDOUTS 6-4 TO 6-7
Reinforcement Activities

PARAMEDIC STUDENT CD
Student Activities

POWERPOINT
PRESENTATION
Volume 5

COMPANION WEBSITE
http://www.prenhall.com/bledsoe

---

7. Was there any need for an IV?
   (*No. The patient was showing no signs of shock, nor did she need to have any medications given.*)
8. Should the patient have been placed on oxygen?
   (*Oxygen would not have hurt the patient in any way, but there was no indication for its use. The patient exhibited no shortness of breath, was in no distress, and had good skin color. She was getting enough oxygen from room air.*)

ASSIGNMENTS

Assign students to complete Chapter 6 of the Workbook. Also assign them to read Chapter 7, "Assessment-Based Management," before the next class.

EVALUATION

Chapter Quiz and Scenario   Distribute copies of the Chapter Quiz provided in Handout 6-2 to evaluate student understanding of this chapter. Make sure each student reads the scenario to reinforce critical thinking on the scene. Remind students not to use their notes or textbooks while taking the quiz.

Student CD   Quizzes for every chapter are contained on the dynamic and highly visual in-text student CD.

Companion Website   Additional quizzes for every chapter are contained on this exciting website.

TestGen   You may wish to create a custom-tailored test using *Prentice Hall TestGen for Paramedic Care: Principles & Practice*, 3rd edition, to evaluate student understanding of this chapter.

Online Test Preparation (for students and instructors)   Additional test preparation is available through Brady's new online product, EMT Achieve: Paramedic Test Preparation, at *http://www.prenhall.com/emtachieve*. Instructors can also monitor student mastery online.

Success! for the Paramedic   Keyed to *Paramedic Care: Principles & Practice* and *Essentials of Paramedic Care*, this comprehensive exam review contains hundreds of test questions and rationales.

REINFORCEMENT

Handouts   If classroom discussion or performance on the quiz indicates that some students have not fully mastered the chapter content, you may wish to assign some or all of the Reinforcement Handouts for this chapter.

Student CD (for students)   A wide variety of material on this CD-ROM will reinforce and also expand student knowledge and skills.

PowerPoint Presentation (for instructors)   The PowerPoint material developed for this chapter offers useful reinforcement of chapter content.

Companion Website (for students)   Additional review quizzes and links to EMS resources will contribute to further reinforcement of the chapter.

OneKey Online support is offered for this course on one of three platforms: CourseCompass, Blackboard, or WebCT. Includes the IRM, PowerPoints, Test Manager, and Companion Website for instruction. Ask your local sales representative for more information.

Brady Skills Series: Advanced Life Skills (Video or CD) Have your students watch the skills come to life on VHS or CD-ROM, or they can purchase the highly visual, full-color text with step-by-step procedures with rationales.

Paramedic National Standards Self-Test Another comprehensive review manual containing hundreds of review questions with page references keyed to several Brady texts.

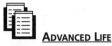
OneKey
Volume 5, Chapter 6

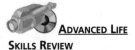
ADVANCED LIFE SUPPORT SKILLS
Larmon & Davis. *Advanced Life Support Skills*

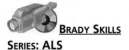
ADVANCED LIFE SKILLS REVIEW
Larmon & Davis. *Advanced Life Skills Review*

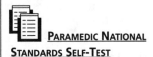
BRADY SKILLS SERIES: ALS
Larmon & Davis. *Brady Skills Series: ALS*

PARAMEDIC NATIONAL STANDARDS SELF-TEST
Miller. *Paramedic National Standards Self-Test,* 5th edition

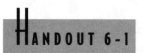

OBJECTIVES

Student's Name _____

CHAPTER 6 OBJECTIVES CHECKLIST

Knowledge Objective	Date Mastered
1. Compare and contrast the primary objectives of the paramedic and the home care provider.	
2. Identify the importance of home health care medicine as it relates to emergency medical services.	
3. Differentiate between the role of the paramedic and the role of the home care provider.	
4. Compare and contrast the primary objectives of acute care, home care, and hospice care.	
5. Discuss aspects of home care that enhance the quality of patient care and aspects that have the potential to become detrimental.	
6. List pathologies and complications in home care patients that commonly result in ALS intervention.	
7. Compare the cost, mortality, and quality of care for a given patient in the hospital vs. the home care setting.	
8. Discuss the significance of palliative care programs as related to a patient in a home health care or hospice setting.	
9. Define hospice care, comfort care, and DNR/DNAR as they relate to local practice, law, and policy.	
10. List and describe the characteristics of typical home care devices related to airway maintenance, artificial and alveolar ventilation, vascular access, drug administration, and the GI/GU tract.	
11. Discuss the complications of assessing each of the devices described in objective 10.	
12. Describe indications, contraindications, and techniques for urinary catheter insertion in the male and female patient in an out-of-hospital setting.	
13. Identify failure of GI/GU, ventilatory, vascular access, and drain devices found in the home care setting.	
14. Discuss the relationship between local home care treatment protocols/SOPs and local EMS protocols/SOPs.	
15. Discuss differences in the ability of individuals to accept and cope with their own impending death.	

©2009 Pearson Education, Inc.
Paramedic Care: Principles & Practice, Vol. 5, 3rd. Ed.

Knowledge Objective	Date Mastered
16. List the stages of the grief process and relate them to an individual in hospice care.	
17. Discuss the rights of the terminally ill patient.	
18. Summarize the types of home health care available in your area and the services provided.	

Skill Objective	Date Mastered
19. Given a series of home care scenarios, determine which patients should receive follow-up home care and which should be transported to an emergency care facility.	
20. Given a series of scenarios, demonstrate interaction and support with the family members/support persons for a patient who has died.	

OBJECTIVES

EVALUATION

CHAPTER 6 QUIZ

Write the letter of the best answer in the space provided.

_____ 1. Common reasons for ALS intervention in home care settings include all of the following
EXCEPT:
A. equipment failure.   C. unexpected complications.
B. absence of a caregiver.   D. arguments between caregiver and patient.

_____ 2. Patients with which disease are at high risk for unhealed wounds or ulcers, particularly on
the feet?
A. atherosclerosis   C. coronary heart disease
B. diabetes mellitus   D. deep vein thrombophlebitis (DVT)

_____ 3. Pressure sores are classified:
A. by the depth of tissue destruction.
B. as diabetes-related and non-diabetes-related.
C. by the location on the body.
D. as gravity-dependent or non-gravity-dependent.

_____ 4. Settings in which the scope of treatment is beyond your training include all of the following
EXCEPT:
A. chemotherapy.   C. hospice care.
B. pain management.   D. home dialysis.

_____ 5. Bronchopulmonary dysplasia (BPD) primarily affects:
A. older persons, especially heavy smokers.
B. children with cystic fibrosis.
C. infants of low birth weight.
D. older persons with hypertension.

_____ 6. Chronic dilation of a bronchus or bronchi with secondary infection is termed:
A. atelectasis.   C. chronic bronchitis.
B. bronchiectasis.   D. bronchopneumonia.

_____ 7. What form of ventilation is the recommended support for acute respiratory disorders?
A. Positive-pressure ventilation (PPV)
B. Negative-pressure ventilation (NPV)
C. Positive end-expiratory pressure (PEEP)
D. Bilevel positive airway pressure (BIPAP)

_____ 8. Types of vascular access devices used in the home setting include all of the following
EXCEPT:
A. heparin lock.   C. peripherally inserted central catheter.
B. Hickman or Broviac catheter.   D. dialysis shunt.

_____ 9. Signs and symptoms of an air embolus include all of the following EXCEPT:
A. shortness of breath with clear lung sounds.
B. chest pain.
C. back pain.
D. headache.

_____ 10. Signs of postpartum depression are found in what proportion of mothers?
A. 10 to 20 percent   C. 45 to 55 percent (roughly one-half)
B. 30 to 35 percent (roughly one-third)   D. 70 to 80 percent (roughly three-quarters)

_____ **11.** Signs and symptoms of cardiac or respiratory insufficiency in newborns include all of the following EXCEPT:

    A. hypotension.   **C.** bradycardia.

    B. cyanosis.   **D.** lung crackles.

_____ **12.** Common diseases you will see in a hospice setting include all of the following EXCEPT:

    A. congestive heart failure (CHF).

    B. chronic obstructive pulmonary disease (COPD).

    C. cerebral palsy.

    D. Alzheimer's disease.

_____ **13.** A surgical diversion of the urinary tract to a stoma, or hole, in the abdominal wall is called a:

    A. ureterostomy.   **C.** cytostomy.

    B. urostomy.   **D.** nephrostomy.

_____ **14.** Signs and symptoms of respiratory distress include all of the following EXCEPT:

    A. tachypnea.   **C.** upright posturing.

    B. use of accessory muscles.   **D.** wheezing or rales on auscultation.

_____ **15.** Common causes for calls from patients with cystic fibrosis include all of the following EXCEPT:

    A. pneumothorax.   **C.** cor pulmonale.

    B. hemoptysis.   **D.** hematemesis.

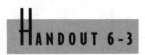

Student's Name _____

CHAPTER 6 SCENARIO

Review the following situation, and then answer the questions that follow.

The dispatcher calls you to investigate a "hysterical" call about a "man who is coughing blood." As you pull up to the house, a young woman runs down the lawn toward your unit, and you recognize her as the wife of a previous patient of yours, a man in his early 30s with advanced cystic fibrosis. He had a DNR order in place when you transported him to the hospital last month for diarrhea and dehydration.

Her husband is sitting on the floor of the living room with his back against a couch. He is breathing rapidly, shallowly, and with great effort; the muscles in his neck stand out as he leans forward. He is staring blankly at the blood that is on his hands and the front of his sweatshirt. His nasal cannula hangs loosely from his neck. As your partner goes to his side, the woman tells you that he "has had bronchitis" but had been "doing so well" on antibiotics. She says she heard coughing and came into the living room in time to see him start "coughing up all that blood" and slump from the couch to the floor.

Your partner rapidly replaces the nasal cannula, dials up the oxygen, and suctions the patient's airway. He no longer sounds as if he is choking, but he begins to cough again. He doesn't seem to be responding to your partner's presence. She shakes her head at you and reaches out to take his pulse and grab her stethoscope.

1. List two pieces of information that you need to know right away in order to provide the appropriate level and type of intervention for the patient.

She says she didn't call the cystic fibrosis clinic because "they're so negative. He needs help!" In response to your request to see current orders and plans, she reluctantly gives you information that states he has been accepted into hospice care and gives contact information for the service. The DNR order stipulates that the patient may receive oxygen and airway protection (for example, suctioning), but intubation and ventilatory assistance are precluded. You note the patient's signature on the form, as well as his doctor's.

The patient is still in a semiseated position on the floor with your partner kneeling behind him. She says he has a very rapid (about 180 beats/min), weak pulse and that she can't hear any clear areas in his lung fields. As he coughs, more blood comes out of his mouth. She suctions. The wife leans against the wall and begins to cry helplessly.

2. What is the immediate medical need? What is the immediate need in terms of coordinating your care with the established plan?

A large amount of blood comes from the man's mouth, and he falls forward so that he is lying across your partner's lap. She continues to suction, and the blood continues to come. She leans over him closely, then looks up and says "he isn't breathing and he's nonresponsive." She places her hand over his carotid and says "pulse is weakening, too."

As his wife clings to you, crying and trembling, you look over again, and your partner shakes her head once. Then she gently lays the man's body out on the floor and begins to wipe the blood off his face. Without looking, she extends her arm backward to turn off the oxygen.

3. What is your immediate medical responsibility to the patient? To his wife?

©2009 Pearson Education, Inc.
Paramedic Care: Principles & Practice, Vol. 5, 3rd. Ed.

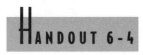

Student's Name _____

CHAPTER 6 REVIEW

Write the word or words that best complete each sentence in the space(s) provided.

1. Total health care expenditures are expected to rise by _____ percent in the first decade of the 2000s.

2. Almost _____ percent of home care patients are 65 or older.

3. The primary goal of the ALS provider in home care situations is to identify and treat any _____-_____ problems.

4. The disease that is characterized by episodic muscle weakness triggered by an autoimmune attack on the acetylcholine receptors is _____ _____.

5. A program of palliative care and support services that addresses the physical, social, economic, and spiritual needs of terminally ill patients and their families is _____.

6. The one thing home care calls have in common is their _____.

7. When making a home care call, try to ascertain from the primary care provider (if present) a(n) _____ presentation for the patient.

8. _____ habits, _____ intake, and minor _____ or _____ can have a dramatic effect on the seriously ill home-bound patient.

9. Many home care patients suffer from COPD, which is a triad of diseases including _____, _____ _____, and _____.

10. Common home treatments for respiratory illnesses include oxygen, _____ or _____ medications, and possibly a ventilator utilizing _____, _____, or _____.

11. The most common problems faced by tracheostomy patients include _____ of the airway by _____ and a dislodged _____.

12. _____ _____ _____ are used to provide any parenteral treatment on a long-term basis.

13. The most common complications seen in patients with VADs result from _____ of various types.

14. Most complications related to urinary support devices result from _____ or _____ _____.

15. For the mother who has recently given birth, the most common complications are _____ _____ and _____.

Student's Name _____

ACUTE INTERVENTIONS TRUE OR FALSE

Indicate whether each statement is true or false by writing T or F in the space provided.

_____ 1. Almost 75 percent of home care patients are age 65 or older, and about 75 percent are female.

_____ 2. A home care patient is more likely to decompensate and go into crisis more quickly than a patient in the general population.

_____ 3. Cardiac decompensation is considered a true medical emergency in patients with preexisting cardiac or pulmonary compromise.

_____ 4. A high risk of infection is not seen in all patients with decreased immune response.

_____ 5. A stage 2 pressure sore involves the epidermis, whereas a stage 3 sore involves the full thickness of the skin, exposing subcutaneous tissue.

_____ 6. On any call involving a home care patient, ask whether another health care professional, in addition to EMS, has been called.

_____ 7. Many home care patients have a baseline lung capacity that only minimally meets their normal requirements.

_____ 8. Home care patients usually have a high dosing regimen, which may make them more responsive to additional medication.

_____ 9. When treating a patient with cystic fibrosis, always inquire about the stage of the disease and about any standing orders.

_____ 10. Pulmonary congestion or frank pulmonary edema may develop in infants with bronchopulmonary dysplasia when excessive amounts of fluid have been given.

_____ 11. Tracheostomy patients who have had a laryngectomy do not have any remaining air connection with the nasopharynx, so it is not necessary to block nose and mouth when ventilating the patient.

_____ 12. Tracheostomy stomas close slowly when the tube is not replaced.

_____ 13. Some common reasons patients use a home ventilator include decreased respiratory drive, weakness of respiratory muscles, obstructive pulmonary disorders, and sleep apnea.

_____ 14. Do not obtain vascular access or blood pressure readings in an extremity with a shunt.

_____ 15. Have a high index of suspicion for infection in the wounds of home care patients

©2009 Pearson Education, Inc.
Paramedic Care: Principles & Practice, Vol. 5, 3rd. Ed.

Student's Name _____

ACUTE INTERVENTIONS ABBREVIATIONS

Interpret the following Chapter 6 abbreviations by writing out their meanings in the spaces provided.

1. DNR _____

2. DNAR _____

3. GI/GU _____

4. PEG _____

5. G-tube _____

6. COPD _____

7. VAD _____

8. PEEP _____

9. CPAP _____

10. BIPAP _____

11. CNS _____

12. CHF _____

13. CF _____

14. BPD _____

15. IMV _____

16. TPN _____

17. ARDS _____

18. PPV _____

19. NPV _____

20. PICC _____

Student's Name _____

HOME CARE SAFETY GUIDELINES

In responding to any home care situation, keep in mind the following guidelines about scene safety.

1. Any patient with limited movement may be contaminated with feces, urine, or emesis.
2. Any bed-bound patient may have weeping wounds, bleeding, or decubitus ulcers (bedsores).
3. Sharps may be present.
4. Collection bags for urine or feces sometimes leak.
5. Tracheostomy patients clear mucus by coughing, which can spray.
6. Any electrical machine has the potential for electric shock.
7. A hospital bed, wheelchair, or walker could be contaminated with body fluid.
8. Contaminated medical devices, such as a nebulizer, may be left unprotected.
9. Oxygen in the presence of flame has the potential for fire or explosion.
10. Equipment may be in the way and cause you to fall, or it may be unstable and fall on you.
11. Medical wastes may not be properly contained or discarded.

Be sure that the following safety tips on home use of oxygen are followed.

1. Alert the local fire department to the presence of oxygen in the home.
2. Keep a fire extinguisher on hand.
3. If a fire does start, turn off the oxygen immediately and leave the house.
4. Don't smoke—and do not allow others to smoke—near the oxygen system. (No open flames or smoking within 10 feet of oxygen.)
5. Do not use electrical equipment near oxygen administration.
6. Store the oxygen tank in an approved, upright position.
7. Keep a tank or reservoir away from direct sunlight or heat.
8. Ground all oxygen cylinders.

Additional guidelines on oxygen use that you should know include the following.

1. Ensure the ability of the patient/home care provider to administer oxygen.
2. Make sure the patient knows what to do in case of a power failure.
3. Evaluate sterile conditions, especially disinfection of reusable equipment.
4. As with any patient with chronic respiratory problems, remain alert to signs and symptoms of hypoxemia.

Chapter 6 Answer Key

Handout 6-2: Chapter 6 Quiz

1. D	**5.** C	**9.** C	**13.** B
2. B	**6.** B	**10.** D	**14.** C
3. A	**7.** A	**11.** A	**15.** D
4. D	**8.** A	**12.** C	

Handout 6-3: Chapter 6 Scenario

1. You need to ask the wife whether she called the patient's physician or other telephone contact and, if so, what instructions were given. Secondly, exactly what DNR or other orders are currently in place?
2. Medically, you and your partner need to support airway, breathing, and circulation to the extent you can do so within the DNR order. You need to ask the wife once again whether she has called anyone—doctor at the clinic, hospice service, or other family—and what, if anything, she was told.
3. You and your partner need to confirm lack of heartbeat and respiration and notify medical direction of the patient's death. After an initial cleanup of the patient's body, one of you needs to assist his wife in sitting with and grieving him. The other needs to call hospice to see what support they will get in place for his wife before you leave. Finally, you need to attend to whatever responsibilities are yours in the situation of a home death from natural causes.

Handout 6-4: Chapter 6 Review

1. 7.5
2. 75
3. life-threatening
4. myasthenia gravis
5. hospice
6. diversity
7. baseline

8. Eating, fluid, illnesses, injuries
9. emphysema, chronic bronchitis, asthma
10. nebulized, aerosol, PEEP, CPAP, BIPAP
11. blockage, mucus, cannula
12. Vascular access devices
13. obstructions
14. infection, device malfunctions
15. postpartum bleeding, embolus

Handout 6-5: Acute Interventions True or False

1. F	**5.** T	**9.** T	**13.** T
2. T	**6.** T	**10.** T	**14.** T
3. F	**7.** T	**11.** F	**15.** T
4. F	**8.** F	**12.** F	

Handout 6-6: Acute Interventions Abbreviations

1. Do Not Resuscitate
2. Do Not Attempt Resuscitation
3. Gastrointestinal/genitourinary
4. Percutaneous endoscopic gastrostomy (tube)
5. Gastrostomy tube
6. Chronic obstructive pulmonary disease
7. Vascular access device
8. Positive end-expiratory pressure
9. Continuous positive airway pressure
10. Bilevel positive airway pressure
11. Central nervous system
12. Congestive heart failure
13. Cystic fibrosis
14. Bronchopulmonary dysplasia
15. Intermittent mandatory ventilation
16. Total parenteral nutrition
17. Acute respiratory distress syndrome
18. Positive-pressure ventilation
19. Negative-pressure ventilation
20. Peripherally inserted central catheter

7

Assessment-Based Management

INTRODUCTION

You need to think before you act as a paramedic, in a manner similar to that for many other roles in life. This chapter addresses the focal role of thoughtful assessment in decision making regarding patient care and in ongoing evaluation and reassessment of the patient's condition. The chapter opens with presentation of the core concept of inverted pyramid thinking, clinical decision making. Then it addresses the components of effective assessment and presentation of patient information, as well as factors that may hinder either or both elements of patient care. After working through this chapter, students should be able to synthesize a large amount of material they have already encountered into a working model of a paramedic in action.

 TOTAL TEACHING TIME: 14.40 HOURS

The total teaching time is only a guideline based on the didactic and practical lab averages in the National Standard Curriculum. Instructors should take into consideration such factors as: the pace at which students learn, the size of the class, and breaks. The actual time devoted to teaching objectives is the responsibility of the instructor.

CHAPTER OBJECTIVES

Knowledge Objectives

1. Explain how effective assessment is critical to clinical decision making. (pp. 311–312)
2. Explain how the paramedic's attitude and uncooperative patients affect assessment and decision making. (pp. 312–313)
3. Explain strategies to prevent labeling and tunnel vision and decrease environmental distractions. (pp. 310–312)
4. Describe how personnel considerations and staffing configurations affect assessment and decision making. (p. 314)
5. Synthesize and apply concepts of scene management and choreography to simulated emergency calls. (pp. 314–315)
6. Explain the roles of the team leader and the patient care person. (pp. 314–315)
7. List and explain the rationale for bringing the essential care items to the patient. (pp. 315–316)
8. When given a simulated call, list the appropriate equipment to be taken to the patient. (pp. 315–316)
9. Explain the general approach to the emergency patient. (pp. 316–320)
10. Explain the general approach, patient assessment differentials, and management priorities for patients with various types of emergencies that may be experienced in prehospital care. (pp. 319–320, 322, 323–333)

11. Describe how to effectively communicate patient information face to face, over the telephone, by radio, and in writing. (pp. 320–322)

Skill Objective

12. Given various preprogrammed and moulaged patients, provide the appropriate scene size-up, initial assessment, focused assessment, and detailed assessment; then provide the appropriate care, ongoing assessments, and patient transport. (pp. 309–333)

FRAMING THE LESSON

You might begin the lesson by demonstrating use of the inverted pyramid of clinical thinking to your students through interaction with a paramedic on an actual case. Ask a paramedic to bring in blinded records of a medical or injury case that he feels is a good example of the importance of critical thinking/clinical decision making skills. Have the paramedic read the dispatcher's comments and then have the class (or the group working with him) brainstorm about questions that occur to them. Have them work through the case to the point at which the patient is transferred to the receiving team. Have one student write down the major time points (dispatcher call, arrival on-scene, scene size-up, initial assessment, focused history and physical exam, ongoing assessment, and detailed physical exam) and the questions/thoughts that are on the paramedic's mind.

After the exercise is complete, review the questions to demonstrate the inverted pyramid of broad/multiple questions narrowing toward more focused and fewer questions as patient care progresses. As a last step, ask students to name factors that helped or hindered their thinking. (If you have a radio playing softly in the background, someone may think of background noise or other environmental factors. If you have a large group of students rather than a small group, someone may think that too many providers present makes proceeding more difficult. Use the list of factors given in the chapter for other suggestions.)

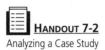
HANDOUT 7-2
Analyzing a Case Study

You also might distribute Handout 7-2 to help students analyze the Case Study in the text. Have students work through it as a group. Afterward, have them compare their responses with those given in the text presentation of the case. See "Considering the Case Study" for sample questions to get them to demonstrate understanding of the inverted pyramid and the importance of environmental and other factors in helping or hindering their thinking.

Make sure students understand—before you proceed with the chapter—that this chapter should help them synthesize a lot of material they have already encountered, from differential diagnoses for various organ systems to the basic steps of an encounter. It is a capstone to previous work, not simply a repetition of earlier material.

CONSIDERING THE CASE STUDY

Ask a volunteer to read aloud the Case Study that begins on text page 307. Suggest that students close their eyes as the scenario is read to help them mentally visualize the events described in it. You can use the following questions about the Case Study as a starting point for teaching the lesson—a sort of chapter preview in a functional setting.

When the chapter is completed, you may wish to return to the Case Study and encourage further discussion aimed at answering the questions. Some questions—for example, those on provider roles on-scene—will make far more sense to students after they read the chapter.

CASE STUDY DISCUSSION QUESTIONS (AND ANSWERS)

1. What roles do the narrator and his partner take in handling this emergency? How do the additional EMTs who arrive on-scene function in management of this case?

   (The narrator acts as the information-taker and impression-maker, while the partner attends to patient care. The narrator decides how to delegate work to the additional EMT-Basics who arrive on-scene and accepts their suggestion to have an EMT-Basic drive the ambulance so that both ALS-qualified providers can attend to the patient.)

2. Look through the narrator's thoughts, questions, and impressions at each point in time. For each comment that you did not anticipate, consider what it represents in the context of your current level of clinical thinking.

   - For example, do any of the narrator's thoughts seem too basic or too obvious?
   - Are any of his impressions ones that were more sophisticated than you were able to form at this stage in your education?
   - Are there any of the narrator's ideas with which you simply disagree?

   (The comment about the agreement between the narrator and his partner on not having tunnel vision may strike some students as contrived because this statement is so elementary. Others may feel it is something that needs to be discussed openly with a partner, especially if it is someone with whom you do not have a lot of team experience.

   The narrator's early thought about the possible correlation of intact telephone poles and absence of electrocution threats is one that many students might not have formed for themselves because of their lack of field experience in settings with potential hazards such as live electrical lines.

   The analysis synthesizes a number of physical findings into the field diagnosis of shock [presumably hypovolemic secondary to hemorrhage] and the implication for transport prioritization and need to wrap up on-scene care. Did students reach the same conclusions before the narrator stated them or not?

   Did students expect the narrator's thoughts about the absence of an identifiable medical medallion and possible underlying medical conditions? Did any feel it was unnecessary to think consciously about stroke or heart attack in an apparently healthy man in his mid-twenties? Did any feel there should have been a search for the man's wallet or other items of personal documentation? If so, did the students feel that locating a wallet was necessary for historical information/past medical history information or for another reason? Did any student feel that personal field experience might have changed his conclusion that a search for a medallion was sufficient or not?)

TEACHING STRATEGIES

People learn in a variety of ways. Some do better with the spoken word, while others prefer the written. Some prefer to work alone, whereas others profit from working in groups. Recognizing these different ways of acquiring knowledge, the authors of this *Instructor's Resource Manual* have provided a variety of teaching strategies for the different types of learners. These strategies are intended to foster higher-level cognitive skills and encourage creative learning and problem solving.

For greatest effectiveness, incorporate these strategies into your class lecture. Marginal notes in the Teaching Outline indicate the points at which various exercises might be most appropriate. Other strategies can be used to preview the lesson or to summarize it.

The following strategies are keyed to specific sections of the lesson:

1. 20 Questions. Use a variation of "20 questions" to get students to see how they start with broad questions and work down to more focused ones. Place students in small groups. Have one student in each group think of an illness or injury he has had. Then have the others ask questions about the chief complaint, history, or expected findings and guess the diagnosis or diagnoses that would need further testing to confirm.

2. Making a Diagnosis. Assign common chief complaints to small groups of students. Have them create a list of differential diagnoses as a group, then complete the narrowing process with the class, finally arriving at a field diagnosis by asking for additional information as needed. This cooperative learning exercise prevents tunnel vision while working toward a field diagnosis. Additionally, it builds oral presentation skills.

3. Thinking about Diagnoses. Get in the habit of asking students to present a list of differentials and a field diagnosis during simulations and patient assessment labs. This encourages the inverted pyramid format of critical thinking and will help you identify the students who are unsure of their assessment skills. This early identification of students needing patient assessment or pathophysiology remediation will save you and the students much anxiety later in the field internship.

4. Stressing Patient History. Be sure to share with students the fact that diagnoses are made with as much as 80 percent of the decision coming from the history. This fact adds justification to the reason paramedics should ask so many questions in the field. Too often paramedics feel that a comprehensive history is the job of the hospital staff or doctor and take shortcuts with patients. This is inappropriate and could lead to a mistake or oversight. Encourage students to obtain a full history on every patient.

5. Thinking about Biases. To help students identify the biases they may harbor, ask students to describe different types of patients that they encounter. Give them categories according to dispatch information such as "drunk," "homeless person," "domestic violence," or "nursing home patient." Allow them to free-form ideas without regard for being polite or politically correct. Then, help them work through the negative connotations and stereotypes with facts and information that clearly debunk their "theories." This activity helps students to identify biases and replace opinions based on feelings with those based in reality.

The following strategy relate to Special Features in the student textbook and can be used to enhance the student's understanding:

Patho Pearls: Your Education Begins with Graduation. Make arrangements to visit a local college cadaver lab. While the professor shows anatomy and discusses the physiology and pathophysiology, discuss with the students the various assessment and management points. Discuss the various programs and activities in your area to help fulfill the continuing education requirements and improve knowledge and skills.

The following strategies can be used at various points throughout the lesson or to help summarize and demonstrate what students have learned:

Clipping File. Gather newspaper clippings and case law rulings about EMS providers who have failed to treat legitimate medical conditions because the

©2009 Pearson Education, Inc.
Paramedic Care: Principles & Practice, Vol. 5, 3rd. Ed.

provider assumed the patient to be faking or not worthy of care. Many of these cases have harsh consequences for the providers, including fines, loss of income, suspensions, and job loss. This lends reality to the discussion of why we always treat every patient with the same level of respect and professionalism. Often, those not motivated by morals can be motivated to do the right thing by fear of the consequences.

Role-Play. If you don't do the group exercise as a start for the lesson, use group role-play to teach and reinforce the main points of the lesson. Have one group of students write a scenario, including dispatch call, scene size-up, initial assessment, pertinent history, physical exam, vitals, and so on. Then give the scenario to one student in a second group. He plays the role of patient with the information given to him while the others act as EMS providers. Get everyone's perspective—those who wrote the scenario and watch the role-play, the patient, and the providers. Show students how much "thinking" really goes on during a provider–patient interaction.

TEACHING OUTLINE

Chapter 7 is the seventh lesson in Volume 5, *Special Considerations/Operations.* Distribute Handout 7-1 so that students can familiarize themselves with the learning goals for this chapter. If students have any questions about the objectives, answer them at this time.

Then present the chapter. One possible lecture outline follows. In the outline, the parenthetical references in regular type are references to text pages; those in bold type are to figures, tables, or procedures.

I. Introduction. Much of patient assessment is based on concepts of inverted pyramid reasoning (called clinical decision making or critical thinking) and differential diagnosis. (pp. 309–310) **(Fig. 7-1)**

II. Effective assessment. Proper assessment is the foundation for patient care. (pp. 310–315)

A. Importance of accurate information (pp. 311–312)
    1. Decisions are only as good as the information collected. (p. 311)
    2. The history **(Fig. 7-2)**
    3. The physical exam
    4. Pattern recognition
    5. Assessment/field diagnosis
    6. BLS/ALS protocols
B. Factors affecting assessment and decision making (pp. 312–314)
    1. Personal attitudes
    2. Uncooperative patients **(Fig. 7-3)**
    3. Patient compliance
    4. Distracting injuries
    5. Environmental and personnel considerations
C. Assessment/management choreography (pp. 314–315) **(Fig. 7-4)**
    1. Role of the team leader
    2. Role of the patient care provider

III. The right equipment. The paramedic should learn to think of equipment as essential items carried in a backpack. (pp. 315–316)

A. Infection control supplies (p. 315)
B. Airway control items (p. 315)
    1. Airways (oral and nasal)

HANDOUT 7-1
Chapter 7 Objectives Checklist

POWERPOINT PRESENTATION
Volume 5, Chapter 7, PowerPoint slides 1–4

PATHO PEARLS
Your Education Begins with Graduation, p. 310

POWERPOINT PRESENTATION
Volume 5, Chapter 7, PowerPoint slides 5–16

TEACHING STRATEGY 1
20 Questions

TEACHING STRATEGY 2
Making a Diagnosis

TEACHING STRATEGY 3
Thinking about Diagnoses

TEACHING STRATEGY 4
Stressing Patient History

TEACHING STRATEGY 5
Thinking about Biases

POINT TO EMPHASIZE
The decisions you make as a paramedic will be only as good as the information you gather.

POINT TO EMPHASIZE
A large number of rescuers moving around can be as distracting as a large number of bystanders.

READING/REFERENCE
Werfel, P. "20 Tips to Perfect Your Assessment Skills," *JEMS,* Jan. 2000.
Augustine, J., "Enhancing Assessment Senses," *JEMS,* March 2004.

2. Suction
    3. Catheters
    4. Laryngoscopes and blades
    5. ET tubes and equipment
C. Breathing (pp. 315–316)
    1. Pocket mask
    2. Bag-valve mask (BVM)
    3. Variously sized masks
    4. Oxygen tank and regulator
    5. Oxygen masks and cannulas
    6. Occlusive dressings
    7. IV catheter for decompression
D. Circulation (p. 316)
    1. Dressings
    2. Bandages
    3. Tape
    4. Sphygmomanometer
    5. Stethoscope
    6. Notebook and pen/pencil
E. Disability (p. 316)
    1. Rigid collars
    2. Flashlight
F. Dysrhythmia (p. 316)
    1. Cardiac monitor/defibrillator
G. Exposure and protection (p. 316)
    1. Scissors
    2. Space blankets

IV. General approach to the patient. Use an ordered approach when confronting a patient. Use the basic elements of the assessment process. (pp. 316–320)

A. Scene size-up (p. 317)
B. Initial assessment (pp. 317–318)
    1. Resuscitative approach
    2. Contemplative approach
    3. Immediate evacuation (**Fig. 7-5**)
C. Focused history and physical exam: four categories of patients (pp. 318–319)
    1. Trauma patient with a significant mechanism of injury or altered mental status
    2. Trauma patient with an isolated injury
    3. Medical patient who is responsive
    4. Medical patient who is unresponsive
D. Ongoing assessment and the detailed physical exam (p. 319)
E. Identification of life-threatening problems (pp. 319–320)

V. Presenting the patient. Learning to communicate effectively is key to transferring patient information. (pp. 320–322)

A. Establishing trust and credibility: best done through use of the SOAP (Subjective findings, Objective findings, Assessment, Plan) format (p. 320) (**Fig. 7-6**)
B. Developing effective presentation skills (pp. 320–322)
    1. Guidelines for effective presentation
        a. Lasts less than 1 minute
        b. Is very concise and clear
        c. Avoids extensive use of medical jargon
        d. Follows a basic format, usually the SOAP format or variation

  e. Includes both pertinent findings and pertinent negatives (findings that might be expected, given the patient's complaint or condition, but are absent or denied by the patient)

  f. Concludes with specific actions, requests, or questions related to the plan

 2. Information in ideal presentation

  a. Patient identification

  b. Chief complaint

  c. Present illness/injury

  d. Past medical history

  e. Physical signs

  f. Assessment

  g. Plan

VI. Review of common complaints. (p. 322)

A. Practice sessions (p. 322)

B. Laboratory-based simulations (p. 322)

C. Self-motivation (p. 322)

VII. Summary. (p. 323)

A. Assessment is the basis of patient care because you must gather information and then evaluate and synthesize it in order to make correct decisions.

B. Factors affecting decision making include paramedic attitude, uncooperative patients, obvious but distracting injuries, narrow or tunnel vision, the environment, patient compliance, and personnel considerations.

C. Also important in assessment are availability of right equipment and effective communication and transfer of patient information.

SKILLS DEMONSTRATION AND PRACTICE

Assessment Practice. You can distribute Handouts 7-8 through 7-22 to students at any point during the lesson. The handouts are set up using the same format as in the scenarios accompanying You Make the Call in this chapter of the text. Use the handouts in the same manner that the ones in the text were used. Encourage students to put themselves one step ahead of the paramedics in the scenarios. If the paramedics in the scenarios take action, see if the students arrive at reasons for the actions similar to those given in the handout. What would they have done differently? Or for different reasons? Have class discussions about each of the scenarios.

YOU MAKE THE CALL

Work through each of the three scenarios given in the textbook. Encourage students to share their thoughts at each stage, even when they disagree with each other or the reasoning given in the book. Get them to see that in many cases there is no "one right way" to work through a clinical problem. Many factors go into a paramedic's thinking, including medical knowledge, familiarity with local protocols, and past experience.

ASSIGNMENTS

Assign students to complete Chapter 7 of the Workbook. Also assign them to read Chapter 8, "Ambulance Operations," before the next class.

POWERPOINT PRESENTATION
Volume 5, Chapter 7, PowerPoint slides 25–26

POWERPOINT PRESENTATION
Volume 5, Chapter 7, PowerPoint slide 27

WORKBOOK
Chapter 7 Activities

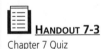
READING/REFERENCE
Textbook Chapter 8, pp. 335–359

HANDOUT 7-3
Chapter 7 Quiz

HANDOUT 7-4
Chapter 7 Scenario

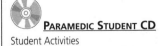
PARAMEDIC STUDENT CD
Student Activities

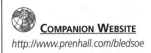
COMPANION WEBSITE
http://www.prenhall.com/bledsoe

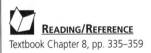

TestGen
Volume 5, Chapter 7

EMT Achieve:
Paramedic Test Preparation
Mistovich & Beasley. *EMT Achieve: Paramedic Test Preparation,* *http://www.prenhall.com/emtachieve.*

Success! for the
Paramedic
Cherry. *SUCCESS! for the Paramedic,* 4th edition

Handouts 7-5 to 7-7
Reinforcement Activities

Paramedic Student CD
Student Activities

PowerPoint
Presentation
Volume 5

Companion Website
http://www.prenhall.com/bledsoe

OneKey
Volume 5, Chapter 7

Advanced Life
Support Skills
Larmon & Davis. *Advanced Life Support Skills.*

Advanced Life
Skills Review
Larmon & Davis. *Advanced Life Support Skills.*

Brady Skills
Series: ALS
Larmon & Davis. *Brady Skills Series: ALS.*

Paramedic National
Standards Self-Test
Miller. *Paramedic National Standards Self-Test,* 5th edition.

EVALUATION

Chapter Quiz and Scenario   Distribute copies of the Chapter Quiz provided in Handout 7-3 to evaluate student understanding of this chapter. Make sure each student reads the scenario to reinforce critical thinking on the scene. Remind students not to use their notes or textbooks while taking the quiz.

Student CD   Quizzes for every chapter are contained on the dynamic and highly visual in-text student CD.

Companion Website   Additional quizzes for every chapter are contained on this exciting website.

TestGen   You may wish to create a custom-tailored test using *Prentice Hall TestGen for Paramedic Care: Principles & Practice,* 3rd edition, to evaluate student understanding of this chapter.

Online Test Preparation (for students and instructors)   Additional test preparation is available through Brady's new online product, EMT Achieve: Paramedic Test Preparation, at *http://www.prenhall.com/emtachieve.* Instructors can also monitor student mastery online.

Success! for the Paramedic   Keyed to *Paramedic Care: Principles & Practice* and *Essentials of Paramedic Care,* this comprehensive exam review contains hundreds of test questions and rationales.

REINFORCEMENT

Handouts   If classroom discussion or performance on the quiz indicates that some students have not fully mastered the chapter content, you may wish to assign some or all of the Reinforcement Handouts for this chapter.

Student CD (for students)   A wide variety of material on this CD-ROM will reinforce and also expand student knowledge and skills.

PowerPoint Presentation (for instructors)   The PowerPoint material developed for this chapter offers useful reinforcement of chapter content.

Companion Website (for students)   Additional review quizzes and links to EMS resources will contribute to further reinforcement of the chapter.

OneKey   Online support is offered for this course on one of three platforms: CourseCompass, Blackboard, or WebCT. Includes the IRM, PowerPoints, Test Manager, and Companion Website for instruction. Ask your local sales representative for more information.

Brady Skills Series: Advanced Life Skills (Video or CD)   Have your students watch the skills come to life on VHS or CD-ROM, or they can purchase the highly visual, full-color text with step-by-step procedures with rationales.

Paramedic National Standards Self-Test   Another comprehensive review manual containing hundreds of review questions with page references keyed to several Brady texts.

CHAPTER 7 OBJECTIVES CHECKLIST

Knowledge Objective	Date Mastered
1. Explain how effective assessment is critical to clinical decision making.	
2. Explain how the paramedic's attitude and uncooperative patients affect assessment and decision making.	
3. Explain strategies to prevent labeling and tunnel vision and decrease environmental distractions.	
4. Describe how personnel considerations and staffing configurations affect assessment and decision making.	
5. Synthesize and apply concepts of scene management and choreography to simulated emergency calls.	
6. Explain the roles of the team leader and the patient care person.	
7. List and explain the rationale for bringing the essential care items to the patient.	
8. When given a simulated call, list the appropriate equipment to be taken to the patient.	
9. Explain the general approach to the emergency patient.	
10. Explain the general approach, patient assessment differentials, and management priorities for patients with various types of emergencies that may be experienced in prehospital care.	
11. Describe how to effectively communicate patient information face to face, over the telephone, by radio, and in writing.	

Skill Objective	Date Mastered
12. Given various preprogrammed and moulaged patients, provide the appropriate scene size-up, initial assessment, focused assessment, and detailed assessment; then provide the appropriate care, ongoing assessments, and patient transport.	

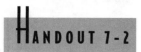
ANALYZING A CASE STUDY

*As you read through this case study, consider what questions or conclusions occur to you at each point marked in boldface type as "**I'm thinking.**" Write notes for yourself as you walk through the exercise. When you have finished, read the case study with thoughts included as it is printed at the opening of Chapter 7 in the textbook. Where are your thoughts the same as the narrator's? Where do they differ?*

It's after midnight. In fact, a glance at the clock on the station wall tells me it's 3:05 on Sunday morning. I sigh with relief, thinking the worst is probably over for the weekend. Just then, the bell rings, signaling another call. Dispatch reports a single-vehicle crash on Moonglow Road, just outside of town. The caller has given no additional information.

I'm thinking:

My partner and I agree that we have to keep an open mind. No tunnel vision. We need to be prepared for anything. While my partner drives to the scene, I'm making a mental list of all the possible medical conditions and injuries that could be involved, and I'm mentally reviewing equipment that we'll need, including airway and ventilation devices, scissors to cut away clothing, dressings and bandages, immobilization equipment, and ECG monitor/defibrillator.

As we near the scene, I pull on gloves. Anticipating blood spatter, I have mask and eye protection ready, too. I look around carefully to determine scene safety. All the nearby telephone poles appear undamaged. . . .

I'm thinking:

. . . and the police already have traffic under control. I spot the vehicle and surmise from the damage that it has rolled several times. Out in the field, about 50 yards from where the vehicle finally landed, I observe a crowd of people surrounding someone lying on the ground. A police officer tells us this is the driver. There were no passengers and nobody else has been hurt, they say. However, the person who called in the accident seems to have left the scene, so there are no witnesses to interview.

I'm thinking:

As we approach the patient, I notice that he is in the supine position with his right leg flexed under him at an unnatural angle. He appears unresponsive to the crowd and the glare of flashlights. Any blood would be soaking into the ground, so it's hard to estimate how much he's lost. But the only blood I see on his clothing is a spreading stain on the pants legs where one leg is bent under the other.

● **I'm thinking:**

When we reach the patient, my partner immediately stabilizes his head and neck. I call out to the patient but get no response. I squeeze his shoulder, and he makes a slight pushing-away gesture. I open the airway, using a jaw thrust. The patient is breathing, but shallowly and only about eight times a minute. My partner has already grabbed a BVM out of the jump kit and is ready to assist the patient's ventilations with supplemental oxygen.

Checking pulses, I find that the patient has no radial pulses but does have a carotid pulse, indicating that his systolic blood pressure is probably somewhere between 60 and 80 mmHg. His skin is pale, cool, and clammy. As I noted earlier, a considerable amount of blood is coming from an injury to his right leg where it is bent under him. Two EMT-Basics have just arrived on the scene, and I assign one of them to quickly get the bleeding under control with direct pressure while I continue my assessment.

I'm thinking:

I perform a head-to-toe rapid trauma assessment in less than 60 seconds, finding a reddened area over the right upper abdominal quadrant. When I palpate the area, the patient flinches.

● **I'm thinking:**

As I expose and assess the extremities, I confirm an open right tibial fracture. I direct one of the EMTs to assess vital signs while the other EMT and I apply gentle traction to straighten the right leg. I quickly place a pressure dressing over the open wound. Then, the EMTs, my partner, and I log-roll the patient and immobilize him to a long backboard.

I have found no medical ID medallion. The pulse is weak and rapid but steady. The patient has responded to painful stimulus with no indication of weakness or paralysis. There is a strong odor of alcohol on the patient's breath, and one of the policemen says they found an open container of bourbon in the car.

I'm thinking:

Further assessment and emergency care will have to be done en route to the emergency department. We have been on the scene for approximately 8 minutes.

One of the EMTs offers to drive the ambulance to the hospital so my partner and I can both attend to the patient. En route, I complete an ongoing assessment. The patient is stable, and I have time to perform a detailed physical exam but make no further findings. Meanwhile, my partner has started two IVs of lactated Ringer's. I complete another ongoing assessment. By the time we arrive at the emergency department, the patient has begun to respond when we call to him.

●

Student's Name _____

CHAPTER 7 QUIZ

Write the letter of the best answer in the space provided.

_____ 1. When the patient has a medical (nontrauma) complaint, as much as _____ of the diagnosis will be made upon the history.
   A. 30 percent   C. 66 percent
   B. 50 percent   D. 80 percent

_____ 2. Your ability to recognize patterns in the history and physical findings depends on your knowledge base and:
   A. the patient's ability to provide a full history.
   B. your experience.
   C. the quality of your medical direction.
   D. the quality of your local protocols.

_____ 3. Medical causes of patient restlessness and lack of cooperation with the paramedic include all of the following EXCEPT:
   A. emotional response to poor previous EMS experiences.
   B. hypoxia.
   C. intoxication with alcohol or other drugs.
   D. hypoglycemia.

_____ 4. Factors that can affect assessment and decision making negatively include all of the following EXCEPT:
   A. patients who are not compliant.
   B. environmental considerations such as scene chaos and dangerous situations.
   C. having only one paramedic for assessment.
   D. presence of distracting injuries.

_____ 5. In multiple-casualty situations, who acts as the triage group leader?
   A. most experienced provider present
   B. patient care provider
   C. team leader
   D. equipment manager

_____ 6. The list of essential equipment for all calls includes all of the following EXCEPT:
   A. a long spine board.   C. oral and nasal airways.
   B. cardiac monitor/defibrillator. D. oxygen tank and regulator.

_____ 7. If you may need additional equipment or support, call for it during the:
   A. initial assessment.   C. scene size-up.
   B. focused history and physical exam. D. detailed physical exam.

_____ 8. Whenever you suspect a life-threatening problem, use the:
   A. contemplative approach.   C. ABC approach.
   B. immediate evacuation approach. D. resuscitative approach.

_____ 9. A patient who hit a tree while sledding and appears to have broken an ankle but seems fine otherwise without positive finding would probably fit into what category after the focused history and physical exam is done?
   A. trauma patient with a significant mechanism of injury or altered mental status
   B. trauma patient with an isolated injury
   C. medical patient who is responsive
   D. medical patient who is unresponsive

_____ **10.** A patient in great distress who is complaining of angina-like pain that hasn't subsided with nitroglycerin would probably fit into what category after the focused history and physical exam is done?
   A. trauma patient with a significant mechanism of injury or altered mental status
   B. trauma patient with an isolated injury
   C. medical patient who is responsive
   D. medical patient who is unresponsive

_____ **11.** Ongoing assessments should be done at which interval if the patient is stable and at which interval if unstable?
   A. 10 minutes, 2 minutes
   B. 10 minutes, 5 minutes
   C. 15 minutes, 2 minutes
   D. 15 minutes, 5 minutes

_____ **12.** For trauma patients, if time and patient condition permit, you should perform a:
   A. focused physical exam.
   B. detailed physical exam.
   C. rapid trauma assessment.
   D. thorough trauma assessment.

_____ **13.** The resuscitative approach would be taken with all of the following conditions, EXCEPT:
   A. respiratory distress or failure.
   B. altered mental status.
   C. all spinal injuries.
   D. status epilepticus.

_____ **14.** The ongoing assessment includes all of the following, EXCEPT the:
   A. transport priority consideration.
   B. rapid head-to-toe exam.
   C. mental status.
   D. vital signs.

_____ **15.** The most effective oral presentations of patients include all of the following characteristics, EXCEPT:
   A. avoiding extensive use of medical jargon.
   B. following a basic format, usually SOAP or a variation.
   C. lasting less than 5 minutes.
   D. concluding with actions, requests, or questions related to the plan.

HANDOUT 7-4

CHAPTER 7 SCENARIO

Review the following real-life situation. Then answer the questions that follow.

Dispatch sends you to a local park for "a child hurt while sledding." While your partner drives, you wish you knew the approximate age of the child and what kind of trauma is suggested by the word "hurt."

1. What other thoughts might go through your head while en route to the scene?

On arrival at the park, you and your partner head toward a large group of people near a stand of tall pine trees. As you approach, you see a child of perhaps age 7 or 8 years lying still on the ground. You don't see any blood on the snow.

2. What thoughts run through your head now?

You are told that the little girl was playing happily. Then she took "one last" afternoon ride down the hill, went straight into a tree, and fell off the sled. She seemed to be dazed, then complained of a headache and laid down. She hasn't spoken since, but moans intermittently.

Your partner notes that the child is lying on her back with limbs in seemingly proper alignment, no bleeding, and abrasions on one side of her face. The child focuses on your partner's face as he kneels by her side, but she doesn't move.

3. What thoughts are probably running through the partner's head as he gets an immediate impression of the patient?

As your partner talks to the little girl, he learns her name is Emily, she is 7 years old, and she feels sick. When asked for specifics, she says her head hurts and she feels very dizzy if she moves at all. She is not sure what happened, but does know she is at the park near her grandmother's house and that she had gone sledding with friends. She can feel all four extremities but doesn't want to move because that makes her feel as if she might vomit.

The only additional historical information is that the child might have been unconscious briefly after the accident, but mostly she "just seemed out of it." No adults or children have any impression of whether her level of consciousness or mental status has changed since the accident.

4. What are your thoughts on the nature of injury and how to proceed?

Your partner places a cervical collar on the little girl. As you position the spine board to move her onto it, she sits up suddenly and leans against your partner. Head examination reveals a large swelling on the patient's forehead, mostly behind the hairline. There is only slight oozing from surface abrasions. The child's pupils are equal and reactive to light. There is no evidence of any foreign matter in either eye. The rest of the rapid exam is notable only for tachycardia. There is no tenderness or swelling around the collarbones or on any of her extremities. She has no chest or abdominal discomfort.

At this point, the child becomes increasingly aware of the people staring at her and she begins to cry. An adult tells you that someone has gone to her grandmother's house and her parents are on the way and should be here within 5 minutes.

5. What do you do next? Is your next action affected by the fact that the patient is a child and not an adult?

The patient is moved to the ambulance. Medical direction suggests immediate transport, with the parents to meet the ambulance at the hospital, which is about 15 minutes away by car.

6. What elements should be emphasized during the ongoing assessment of this child?

The parents arrive at the hospital shortly after Emily is transferred to the care of the emergency department staff. Her vitals remained stable during transport and her mental status improved somewhat, with greater ability to show orientation to day, place, nature of her situation ("I'm riding in the ambulance with you"), and the names of her paramedics.

She is eventually diagnosed with a concussion, from which she recovers without sequelae.

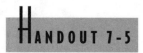
Student's Name _____

CHAPTER 7 REVIEW

Write the word or words that best complete each sentence in the space(s) provided.

1. The three elements of the inverted pyramid are _____ _____,
   _____ _____, and _____ _____.

2. _____ forms the foundation for patient care.

3. You must be as nonjudgmental as possible to avoid "short circuiting" data collection and pattern recognition by _____ conclusions before _____ a thorough assessment.

4. The roles of the team leader include the following:

   _____

   _____

   _____

   _____

   _____

   _____

5. The roles of the patient care provider include the following:

   _____

   _____

   _____

   _____

   _____

6. Be aware of your _____ _____ and the messages it sends, either intentionally or unintentionally.

7. The scene size-up has four components, which are:

   _____

   _____

   _____

   _____

8. The initial assessment has six components, which are:

   _____

   _____

   _____

   _____

   _____

   _____

   _____

©2009 Pearson Education, Inc.
Paramedic Care: Principles & Practice, Vol. 5, 3rd. Ed.

9. After the focused history and physical exam are complete, patients can be classified into one of four groups:

_____

_____

_____

_____

10. The seven components of the ongoing assessment are:

_____

_____

_____

_____

_____

_____

_____

11. At all stages of the assessment, you must actively and continuously look for and manage any
_____ - _____ _____.

12. The underlying principle of assessment-based management is to rapidly and accurately assess the patient and then to treat for the _____ - _____ _____.

13. SOAP stands for S _____ _____, O _____
_____, A _____, P _____.

14. The ability to _____ _____ is the key to transferring patient information.

15. The most effective oral presentations usually last less than _____ _____.

Student's Name _____

CHECKLIST OF ESSENTIAL EQUIPMENT

- Infection Control

  ___infection control supplies, namely gloves and eye shields

- Airway Control

  ___oral airways

  ___nasal airways

  ___suction (electric or manual)

  ___rigid tonsil-tip and flexible suction catheters

  ___laryngoscope and blades

  ___endotracheal tubes, stylettes, syringes, tape

- Breathing

  ___pocket mask

  ___manual ventilation bag-valve mask

  ___spare masks in various sizes

  ___oxygen tank and regulator

  ___oxygen masks, cannulas, and extension tubing

  ___occlusive dressings

  ___large-bore IV catheter for thoracic decompression

- Circulation

  ___dressings

  ___bandages and tape

  ___sphygmomanometer, stethoscope

  ___note pad and pen or pencil

- Disability

  ___rigid collars

  ___flashlight

- Dysrhythmia

  ___cardiac monitor/defibrillator

- Exposure and Protection

  ___scissors

  ___space blankets or something to cover the patient

©2009 Pearson Education, Inc.
Paramedic Care: Principles & Practice, Vol. 5, 3rd. Ed.

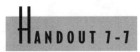

Student's Name _____

CHECKLIST FOR ELEMENTS IN PATIENT PRESENTATION

✔ Patient identification, age, sex, and degree of distress

✔ Chief complaint (why EMS call was made)

✔ Present illness/injury

   __Pertinent details about present problem

   __Pertinent negatives

✔ Past medical history

   __Allergies

   __Medications

   __Pertinent medical history

✔ Physical signs

   __Vital signs

   __Pertinent positive findings

   __Pertinent negative findings

✔ Assessment

   __Paramedic impression

✔ Plan

   __What has been done

   __Orders requested

Student's Name _____

CHEST PAIN SCENARIO

Actions	Reasoning
Dispatch	
I am working overtime at Medic 3 when we get dispatched to a 63-year-old male with chest pain. My partner, John, and I head to the ambulance and sign on en route to the call 2 minutes later.	I recognize the street that we are going to and realize I have 4 to 5 minutes to think about the situation on the way to the call. Chest pain in a 63-year-old male can be any one of several things, from a heart attack to an aneurysm to musculoskeletal chest pain. I have to be prepared for anything, so when we arrive on-scene, I grab the O_2 and the monitor while John grabs the drug bag. We throw it all onto the stretcher and head into the house.
Scene Size-Up	
We arrive on-scene and find a one-story ranch house with only two steps up to the front door. I am grateful that I don't have to carry my stretcher up a flight of stairs. The house looks clean and well kept.	I have always been concerned about a back injury working this job. Easy access to the patient decreases my chances of that happening. The walk-way to the house is clear of any obstacles, and the porch appears to be in good repair.
Initial Assessment	
We get into the living room to find a gentleman sitting straight up in his recliner. He is pale, short of breath, and holding his chest. I notice a walker beside the chair. John places our pulse oximeter on the patient's finger for a room air reading as he prepares to place the patient on high-flow O_2. He will place the patient on the monitor after the oxygen.	I am concerned because the patient is pale and appears to be in significant pain. I immediately wonder if he is having an MI because of his chest pain. Although he is pale, he does not appear diaphoretic, so I can't rule out several other possibilities as well. His pulse ox reads 88 percent on room air, which has me wondering why he is not oxygenating well. Does he have a history of COPD? I would like to see what his ECG strip shows, to help me narrow what is going on.
History	
Our patient introduces himself as Steven Willis. He tells us that he was sitting in the recliner, and as he sat up to get himself something to drink he had a sudden onset of sharp left-sided chest pain that took his breath away. He has been feeling short of breath ever since. He tried to rest for several minutes, hoping it was just a pulled muscle, but the pain hasn't gotten any better so he called 911.	As Mr. Willis is telling us that he is short of breath, I notice that his breathing is slightly labored, although he can speak in complete sentences. I have approached him, and as he is talking I check a radial pulse and find a rapid, regular pulse rate. I count the rate in the 120s, which rules out SVT as the cause of his chest pain. The oxygen that he has been getting seems to be helping a little, and his breathing is starting to slow down.

©2009 Pearson Education, Inc.
Paramedic Care: Principles & Practice, Vol. 5, 3rd. Ed.

History *(continued)*	
John now has Mr. Willis on the monitor, and Mr. Willis appears to be in a sinus tachycardia.	I am relieved to see that he is not in V-tach or having any other rhythm disturbances, such as PVCs. His rate could be fast due to the fact that he is having pain, or it could also be related to his chest pain.
John has rechecked Mr. Willis' pulse ox, and it is now at 94 percent. He takes a blood pressure reading and reports 132/88.	I am happy to see that he is oxygenating better, but I am concerned about what caused the decreased oxygen saturation to begin with. The fact that Mr. Willis is able to sit up without complaining of lightheadedness or diaphoresis, plus the fact that he has a strong radial pulse, leads me to believe that he has a good blood pressure. Mr. Willis described his pain as "sharp" and not as "ripping" or "tearing." This, along with the fact that he is normotensive, leads me to rule out a dissecting thoracic aneurysm.
When asked, Mr. Willis describes the pain as sharp. His shortness of breath is somewhat relieved with the oxygen. He denies nausea, vomiting, and diaphoresis. The pain started as soon as he sat up, and until then he had been pain-free at rest.	I know from experience that patients having an MI describe their pain as "pressure" or "tightness in the chest," not usually as sharp, so I am thinking that this is probably not an MI. The fact that the pain started with movement and not at rest also leads me to think that this is not unstable angina, although I would like to know what his medical history is.
Mr. Willis tells us that he has a history of non-insulin-dependent diabetes and hypertension and has recently been discharged from a rehabilitation unit for a hip fracture he suffered 3 weeks ago. He had surgery on the hip 2 1/2 weeks ago.	With this last piece of medical history, I think I can narrow Mr. Willis' chest pain and shortness of breath to a pulmonary embolism (PE). He is post-op from a recent hip fracture and has been sedentary for 3 weeks. A PE would explain his decreased oxygenation level, as a result of an occluded vessel in his lung. I would like to finish a physical exam, though, before I make a final decision.
Physical Exam	
I ask Mr. Willis to lean forward so I can listen to his lung sounds. He has decreased breath sounds with scattered wheezes bilaterally. At this point he admits to being a two-pack-a-day smoker.	My last thought was that perhaps Mr. Willis had a spontaneous pneumothorax, but since I can hear breath sounds in all lung fields, I can rule this out as a cause of his chest pain and shortness of breath.
We place Mr. Willis on the stretcher carefully, because of his recent fractured hip. I take this opportunity to palpate femoral pulses bilaterally, which he indeed does have.	If Mr. Willis had a dissecting aneurysm, I would not be able to palpate femoral pulses because of the aorta leaking blood into the retroperitoneal cavity. This helps to confirm my thought that Mr. Willis is suffering from a PE.

Interventions

We move Mr. Willis to the ambulance, where we place him on onboard oxygen, which continues through a nonrebreather mask at 15 L/min. I start an IV as John starts to drive to the hospital with lights and sirens. Unfortunately, there isn't much more for me to do for Mr. Willis besides supportive care and frequent vital sign checks.	I would like to get Mr. Willis to the hospital quickly so they can get him to V/Q scan or CT for a final diagnosis. If he is having a PE, they need to start him on heparin as soon as possible.

Ongoing Assessment

During the short trip to the hospital, Mr. Willis states he is starting to feel increased relief from his shortness of breath with the oxygen, but the sharp chest pain remains.	I note his pulse ox is up to 95 percent, so I know he is oxygenating better, but this just doesn't seem to be helping his pain.

Communications and Written Report

I called ahead to the ED to let them know we were coming. As it turned out, they were having a quiet shift and had already called ahead for the V/Q scan. We settle him on an ED stretcher and give a final report with a final set of vital signs.	I had started filling out my run sheet in the back of the ambulance, so I just need to finish the narrative section. I grab a cup of coffee and head to the EMS room to finish my chart so I can leave it with his nurse before I go.

Follow-Up

I called the ED the next day to see what happened with Mr. Willis. The V/Q scan did indeed show a PE, and they heparinized him pretty quickly.	Well, at least I got that one right! I just wish there was more we could do for these patients in the field.

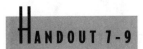

ANDOUT 7-9

Student's Name _____

CARDIAC ARREST—PULSELESS ELECTRICAL ACTIVITY SCENARIO

SCENARIOS

Actions	Reasoning
Dispatch	
My partner, Sue, and I are hanging out in the dispatch center after dropping off a box of donuts when a 911 call comes in for a woman down on the street about three blocks away. Because we aren't doing anything, we volunteer to take the call. We are already in the ambulance and heading to the call when we are officially dispatched.	"Woman down on the street." I'm thinking, in this city, this could be anything. Is she awake, dead, drunk? I tell Sue that I'll grab the monitor and the drug box if she grabs the airway kit and the O_2. We arrive on the scene in about 2 minutes.
Scene Size-Up	
By the time we get there, a large crowd has gathered around our patient, so we really can't see her. There is a police officer there trying to clear an area with easy access to the patient for us to park. I can see that there are a couple of people, one of whom is another police officer, kneeling on the ground near the patient. When the crowd sees us get out of our ambulance they clear an area for us.	I am relieved to see the scene is safe. It adds to my comfort level on this job to see the police arrive ahead of me. A job outside like this attracts a crowd, and you never know when the scene can get hostile. The crowd seems concerned about the woman and allows us through easily.
Initial Assessment	
We find the woman in the supine position, with a man doing chest compressions and the police officer holding a nonrebreather mask over the patient's face. She is cyanotic. I get down next to her and ask the man to hold compressions while I check for a carotid pulse. There isn't one. I ask him to continue compressions.	"Oh great!" Sue says to me as she looks at the patient's oxygen mask. She goes to the woman's head and proceeds to take out the airway equipment. I am trying to figure out what is going on here. Was this woman walking down the street when she suddenly collapsed? Could this have been a traumatic event? I start to look around for any evidence of trauma.
History	
"Can anyone around here tell me what happened?" I yell to the crowd as I start to get out the ECG monitor. A man tells me that he saw the woman walking down the street when two men gave her a shove, grabbed her bag, and then ran down the street. She staggered a bit after being pushed, started to run after them while yelling, and then fell to the ground.	This is interesting. While trying to figure out the cause of the cardiac arrest, several things go through my head. How hard did they shove her? Could they have caused some kind of blunt trauma, like a tension pneumothorax or a cardiac tamponade? Does she have a cardiac history, and the exertion of what has happened to her put too much strain on her heart?

History (continued)

I ask the man doing compressions if he is doing OK and if he needs relief. He says he is fine, that he took a CPR class at the gym, and he doesn't mind continuing. I take advantage of this and prepare to attach the monitor. As I start to take out the monitor, a woman comes running through the crowd. She is crying and tells us that the woman is her mother and she had just left her apartment down the street. Her elevator is broken, and she had just run down six flights of stairs after a neighbor told her what had happened to her mother. Just then our supervisor shows up as well. He puts the patient on the monitor for me.

When asked, she tells us her mother has a history of heart disease and has recently been told she needed to have a cardiac catheterization and possible angioplasty. She has high blood pressure and her cholesterol level has been high.

I am glad we have someone here who could tell us something about our patient. We still don't know what has caused this woman to go into cardiac arrest.

This may help narrow things, but I don't want to rule out trauma as the cause of this event yet. After all, who knows how hard she got pushed and if that could have caused any problems.

Physical Exam

Sue gets the ET tube in, and I watch for equal rise and fall of her chest. I listen for breath sounds over the epigastrium, which I don't hear, and then I listen for breath sounds bilaterally.

Sue dumps around two times the normal dose of epi down the tube, followed by 20 mL of saline.

She has clear and equal breath sounds bilaterally, with equal rise and fall of her chest. Sue ventilates her, and I do not note any tracheal deviation. I can now rule out a tension pneumothorax as a cause for this cardiac arrest.

Looking around, I don't see any other cause for blunt trauma. There is nothing she could have been pushed into to cause electrocution. It is pretty warm out, so I can safely say she wasn't hypothermic, and she obviously didn't drown.

Interventions

I ask the man to hold compressions so I can see if there is any activity on the monitor. I note a coarse V-fib and get ready to shock her. I make sure everyone is clear and shock at 360 joules. Immediately following defibrillation, I instruct the man to resume CPR.

We continue compressions as I get the IV started. I run normal saline wide open as I secure the IV. Sue has been ventilating the patient after the epi. Just then I hear someone in the crowd telling the patient's daughter what happened. I hear him say that right before she fell, he saw her clutch her chest and take a few deep breaths; then she fell.

I know she's got a cardiac history, so I'm thinking that she just had too much stress put on her heart as she was mugged and then tried to run down the street. I know that taking the time to check for a pulse after defibrillating will interrupt compressions for an unacceptable length of time. I'll check for a pulse when I reevaluate the rhythm in two minutes, after five cycles of CPR.

Why couldn't he have told me this? I'm thinking. It appears as if she might have suffered an MI from the activity. I begin thinking about the PEA and what I can do next to convert her to a perfusing rhythm. If the PEA is being caused by hypoxia, then the hyperventilation should have helped. The atropine hasn't increased her rate.

Interventions (continued)

I give the patient another epi via the IV. Now that 2 minutes have passed since defibrillation, I ask the man to pause compressions while I reevaluate the rhythm and check for a pulse. The monitor is showing a sinus bradycardia, but the patient does not have a pulse. I tell the man to resume CPR. It is time to get her loaded into the ambulance. As we load her up, I profusely thank the man for doing compressions.	Still no pulse. Maybe she is acidotic. If she doesn't convert soon, I'll consider giving her some bicarb.

Ongoing Assessment

We head to the hospital with lights and sirens. Our supervisor is driving, so we can work on the patient in the back. Sue continues to bag the patient as I do compressions. We continue to give epi and atropine IV, but her rhythm never changes. I give her sodium bicarbonate 1 mEq/kg via IV. We hold compressions and check again for a pulse. There is still no pulse, so we continue CPR.	Once again I consider pericardial tamponade, but it appears that this event occurred before the woman fell to the ground, so I have ruled out trauma as the cause for the arrest. If she is in PEA from hypokalemia, a round of sodium bicarb may help now. I know this can work if the patient is hypokalemic or acidotic, two more causes of PEA. I hope something works.

Communications and Written Report

My supervisor called ahead, so the hospital knew we were coming. They had the code room ready for us. I give a report as someone takes over compressions for me. We hang back and watch as they continue working on her. She soon goes from PEA to asystole, and they call the code.	The only thing left that they could have done was a pericardiocentesis, but the ED staff decided that they didn't want to do this once she converted to asystole.

Follow-Up

It turns out that the cops grabbed the kids that did this just a few blocks away. They had stolen a few bags that day but didn't think anything like this would happen.	I love being a paramedic, but sometimes the job is a little distressing. I can't help but feel bad for this woman and her daughter.

SCENARIOS

Student's Name _____

ACUTE ABDOMINAL PAIN SCENARIO

Actions	Reasoning
Dispatch	
It's 2:00 in the afternoon, and Chris and I have had a pretty slow day when we get dispatched for a 78-year-old female with abdominal pain. It's my turn to work up the patient, so Chris hops in the driver's seat as I jump in the front seat next to him. I know the address, and I know that we have about a 5-minute response time.	I've been doing this job for a long time, so I realize that although this is probably just a routine call, it could turn out to be more than that. The patient could have a long-standing history of abdominal problems, such as colitis or diverticulitis, but there is also a chance that this could be an acute problem, such as an aortic aneurysm. That's what I like about this job; you just never know.
Scene Size-Up	
We arrive on-scene to find two cars in the driveway, so we park on the road in front of the house. This makes it difficult for us to get our stretcher to the door, because we now have to take it up to the front door. Then I notice five steps leading up to the front door. This does not make me happy.	I am always concerned about a back injury working this job. We try to minimize the amount of lifting we need to do. Hopefully there will be someone in the house who can move the car blocking the driveway. If we have to, we can call for lifting assistance.
Initial Assessment	
We've made it into the house with the stretcher, our jump kit, oxygen, and the monitor. There is a middle-aged woman, who is not our patient, waiting at the door, telling us that her mother is in the bedroom on the first floor (thank goodness for the small things!). I get to the bedroom and find the patient lying in bed in her nightclothes, pale and dry, sitting up in the bed. There is a bedside commode at the side of the bed and several pill bottles on the bedside table.	For several reasons, I am guessing that my patient has chronic medical problems. The bedside commode makes me wonder if she is bedridden, and the number of pill bottles leads me to think that she has a significant medical history. I need to start asking her some questions to find out what is going on.
History	
I introduce myself and my partner, and the patient tells me her name is Nancy. She hasn't been feeling well for several days, and over the last 2 days she has been having abdominal pain, which is getting worse. She says she also has been short of breath, which is getting worse as well.	Well so far this doesn't really help me narrow down what is going on. I need to find out where exactly the pain is. If she is having pain that she describes as indigestion and shortness of breath, this may not be an abdominal problem but could be an MI. I ask her to show me exactly where her pain is.

©2009 Pearson Education, Inc.
Paramedic Care: Principles & Practice, Vol. 5, 3rd. Ed.

History *(continued)*	
Nancy uses her hands to cover her entire abdomen and says she cannot pinpoint exactly where the pain is. When asked, she denies feeling indigestion and heartburn.	Well, at least this rules out a cardiac problem. And if she were having renal colic, she would be complaining more of back pain and not generalized abdominal pain, so I don't think that is what is going on either. I still need more information. This could still be something quite serious, like a dissecting abdominal aortic aneurysm (AAA).
She tells me she has been having small, frequent episodes of diarrhea for about 2 days and started vomiting this morning. She points to a bowl sitting on her bedside table.	Although patients may experience vomiting from a dissecting AAA, they usually don't have several days of diarrhea before it. This could still be appendicitis, but I think that by now her pain would have localized to the right lower quadrant. I also don't think that this is cholecystitis, because she doesn't have epigastric pain that is radiating to her back between her shoulder blades.
I ask Nancy what her medical history is as Chris starts getting a set of vital signs. Nancy's daughter starts handing me the pill bottles. I see that she is on blood pressure medication, an antidepressant, an anti-inflammatory, and a narcotic. I am told that Nancy has recently been having pain in her left knee after a fall and that she has been taking the narcotic on a regular basis. She denies any heart disease. She tells me her last normal bowel movement was 3 days ago.	Well, now we are getting somewhere. The fact that she has recently been placed on narcotics helps me. I know that narcotics can cause constipation, especially if the patient is not mobile, which Nancy apparently isn't due to knee pain. In a patient Nancy's age, constipation can easily lead to a bowel obstruction.

Physical Exam	
Chris tells me that Nancy's blood pressure is 92/70 and her heart rate is 102. On physical exam, I find Nancy's abdomen to be firm and distended. I try not to press too hard, but even with slight palpation she complains of pain. I have her lean forward so I can listen to her breath sounds, which are clear and equal throughout all lung fields. Her skin is cool and dry. I look over to the bowl at the side of her bed and find a small amount of dark brown emesis.	
I am pretty certain that Nancy is suffering from a bowel obstruction. Her abdomen is distended and she has pain with palpation. She hasn't had a normal bowel movement for 3 days. I am also concerned, because of her vital signs, that she is bordering on shock. This could be caused by necrosis within an organ, in this case her intestines.	

Interventions	
She is not experiencing all of the signs of hypovolemic shock, and she is tolerating her vital signs well. I am not going to aggressively treat her for shock but will just give her supportive care. I do want to see if a 500-mL fluid bolus will help her.	Nancy needs an IV so we can give her a fluid bolus. Chris takes out the oxygen and puts her on a nonrebreather at 15 lpm as I start her IV. We assist her to the stretcher, and, although her blood pressure is a little low, she tells me she is more comfortable sitting at a 45-degree angle. We move her down the hall, and together are able to carry her down the stairs and into the ambulance.

Ongoing Assessment	
Since I just started the fluid bolus I don't really expect to see any immediate changes. I will check again in a few minutes.	En route to the hospital, I place Nancy on the monitor and notice a sinus tach of 104. Her pulse ox is 100 percent on the nonrebreather mask. Her blood pressure hasn't changed. Nancy continues to complain of nausea, so I've given her an emesis basin.
I give her another blanket to help warm her up. We are almost at the hospital now.	Five minutes later, I notice her heart rate is now in the 90s and her BP is 100/72. It seems that the fluid bolus is doing her some good. She still feels cool and remains pale.

Communications and Written Report	
Since it is a quick trip to the hospital, I haven't got much charting done. I can get that finished after I've given my patient report.	I call ahead to let the ED know that they are receiving a 78-year-old female with probable bowel obstruction. They say they will give me a room assignment upon arrival.

Follow-Up	
Chris and I say goodbye to Nancy as we head out. I hope she does well, because she apparently has a long road ahead of her.	Before we leave the ED, I check on Nancy one last time. Her vital signs have stabilized, although she isn't feeling any better. They are doing blood work and X-rays and have already consulted with a surgeon. It looks like she does, indeed, have a bowel obstruction.

©2009 Pearson Education, Inc.
Paramedic Care: Principles & Practice, Vol. 5, 3rd. Ed.

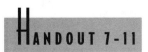

Student's Name _____

GI BLEEDING SCENARIO

Actions	Reasoning
Dispatch	
"Medic 210, respond to 5891 Cedar Lane, Apartment 3, for a 56-year-old male vomiting blood." Robin and I had just sat down to eat lunch when our radio sounded. "Great, another day without a meal," Robin says as we head to the ambulance.	Vomiting blood—this is not going to be pleasant, I'm thinking as we head to the call. Especially on an empty stomach.
Scene Size-Up	
The apartment complex is large, and we are having a little trouble finding the right apartment. This isn't in a great part of town, so the police respond to calls here with us, and the officer in front of us has finally found the right one. Lucky for us, this is a first-floor apartment. The officer gets to the door first and finds it unlocked, so he heads in the door in front of us. We find our patient on the floor of the bathroom, sitting up against the wall near the toilet.	It eases my mind to have the police on the scene with us. We don't always get this lucky, but when I am concerned about my safety on a call, it is a relief to have them there. After looking around the apartment, I don't see any reason to feel unsafe here.
Initial Assessment	
The patient is pale and sitting straight up against the wall. When we come in, he tries to get up, but winces as if in pain, so he goes right back to the same position he was in. We introduce ourselves, and I go over to the patient, whose name is John.	John is probably pale because of blood loss from his vomiting. I don't have any information from him yet, but I am guessing he may have lost a significant amount of blood. He also seems hesitant to move, probably from extreme abdominal pain. I quickly try to find out what is going on.
History	
John tells us that he hasn't been able to work the last couple of days because of abdominal pain. At first, he thought it was indigestion, so he went out and bought some antacids, hoping they would help, which they did for a few hours. Yesterday the pain got worse, and he just lay in his bed. This morning he woke up nauseous and had several episodes of vomiting blood along with one episode of soft stool. He tells us he was barely able to get up and call 911 when he had to come back into the bathroom to vomit again.	I'm wondering if John has any history of peptic ulcer disease. I'm guessing that he doesn't because he didn't recognize the signs of it and tried medicating himself. I know this is common for patients complaining of upper GI bleeds. Bleeding in the GI tract can be very irritating to the stomach and intestines. I ask him to describe the bleeding for me before I jump to any conclusions about what is going on.

History *(continued)*	
John says that he has been vomiting bright red blood, but he noted that his stool was black and tarry.	John is having an upper GI bleed. This has been going on long enough for older blood to pass through his lower GI tract. If this were a lower GI bleed, the blood in his stool would be a brighter color and he would probably be vomiting blood that looked like coffee grounds, if he were vomiting at all.

Physical Exam	
We need to get a quick set of vital signs and then get some treatment started. Robin gets out the BP cuff as I get ready to do a physical assessment. I would like to do this quickly so we can get him comfortable on the stretcher.	His blood pressure is 104/72, and his heart rate is 98. He is still hemodynamically stable, but I know this can change quickly so I still want to get two large-bore IVs started.
On physical exam, John is very tender on palpation of the right upper quadrant. I also note bulging in the RUQ.	We assist John onto the stretcher and place him supine on it. I would like to perform a tilt test to see if there are any changes in his blood pressure or his pulse. When we stand him up, I am going to get another set of vital signs.
Robin and I help John to his feet. He complains of severe pain with movement, but I explain why I am getting another set of vital signs before he sits on the stretcher. He agrees to let us do this, so Robin helps hold him up while I check his blood pressure and pulse.	His blood pressure is now 88/52, and his pulse rate has gone to 118. This means that he has failed his tilt test and will need aggressive fluid resuscitation.

Interventions	
Once John is on the stretcher, I start one of the two IVs that he will need. I figure I can get a fluid bolus going while we load him into the ambulance and then start another IV en route to the hospital. We also put him on oxygen. I am concerned about his positioning on the stretcher. I know that if he continues to vomit and, because he has a decreasing level of consciousness, there is risk for aspiration. However, with his vital signs, I don't want to sit him up straight on the stretcher. I place John in the left lateral recumbent position, which should help avoid aspiration.	John needs the fluid resuscitation because he is beginning to go into hypovolemic shock. I don't want him to decompensate any more than he already has. Although he has been awake, alert, and oriented times 3 up until this point, I still want to make sure I do everything for him I can to prevent aspiration.

Ongoing Assessment	
I've got two IVs started, and I've drawn some blood off the second IV. His bolus continues, and he hasn't vomited since we've been in the ambulance. I continue to check his vital signs every 5 minutes until we get to the hospital.	I need to continue to monitor John for signs of worsening shock. His vitals remain stable, and he has maintained his level of consciousness. He reports no change in his pain.

Communications and Written Report	
I alert the ED that we are en route with an active upper GI bleed. They tell us to report to their trauma room, where they can easily do fluid resuscitation and give blood if necessary.	Once in the ED, I report to the waiting nurse. I've labeled my bloods, and they get sent to the lab quickly for a CBC and type and crossmatch in case John needs a blood transfusion.
Follow-Up	
I follow up with the nursing staff later in the day. John's first set of blood work came back within normal limits, but the second set, done a couple of hours later, showed a significant blood loss, and he wound up needing to get a couple of units of blood.	I'm glad John called when he did. If he had continued to decompensate while alone in his apartment, his outcome could have been a lot worse.

ALTERED MENTAL STATUS SCENARIO

SCENARIOS

Actions	Reasoning
Dispatch	
What a day! Matt and I are both on overtime at Medic 3, which is usually a quiet station, but we haven't stopped all day. We just sit down to put our feet up for 5 minutes when we get dispatched. "Medic 3, respond to 176 West 59th Street, Apartment 5J, for an unconscious male." When we sign on that we are responding, dispatch tells us that we have an unconscious male in his early-to-mid-30s, and the caller has no idea what is going on.	Matt hops in the driver's seat and hits the lights and sirens as I get in the passenger's seat. We start discussing what is going on here, and he starts testing me. "OK," he says, "let's review our AEIOU-TIPS," as he tests my memory. "I'll buy lunch if you can remember them all." This time I can outsmart him, and I know I'll be saving $5 on lunch today. AEIOU-TIPS is a mnemonic that helps us remember some of the common causes for altered mental status. I tell him I know them all. A is acidosis; E is epilepsy; I is infection; O is an overdose; U is uremia (or kidney failure); T can be trauma, tumor, or a toxin; I is for insulin (or diabetic emergency); P is for psychosis or poisoning; and S is for stroke or seizure. "I'm in the mood for Italian today," I tell him as we arrive on-scene.
Scene Size-Up	
We pull up to a pretty old apartment building with a several-step walk up to the front door. There is a doorway to get into the building, which I am assuming is locked, then a vestibule and then another doorway. I only hope this building has a working elevator. There is no one around this afternoon, and this is usually a pretty safe neighborhood, but I always look around to see who is hanging around and who can mess with the ambulance while we're inside. Matt locks up the front as I grab the stretcher from the back. We grab all of our equipment and he finishes locking up.	We have to stay on our toes with regard to our safety, as far as lifting and moving and environmental factors as well. We both know how to lift and move stretchers and patients up and down stairs without getting hurt, but you can never be too cautious. And scene safety is important no matter where you work, whether it's in the heart of the city or in the quietest suburb.
Initial Assessment	
The elevator is working and we head up to 5J. We get off the elevator to find a man waiting at the door of one of the apartments. He yells down to us when he sees us. We get inside to find a male, mid 30s, in the bed, profusely sweaty, pale, bordering on unconscious. He is in gym clothes, and there is a gym bag at the side of the bed. His friend tells us he doesn't know anything about the patient's medical history; he came to pick him up for lunch and found him like this.	Matt starts getting out the monitor and IV equipment while I start assessing the patient. He is cool to the touch and very sweaty. I start getting a blood pressure. I look around to see if there are any pill bottles or alcohol around; perhaps this was an overdose, or maybe he had a seizure. I am glad we reviewed the mnemonic on the way here, because I am now going through them all again in my head.

History

Our patient's friend, John, tells us that he called Larry, our patient, this morning to see if he wanted to go to lunch. Larry was off from work today, so they made plans for John to pick Larry up at 12:00. John didn't show up until 12:45, and Larry didn't answer the buzzer downstairs. Someone let him into the building, and luckily Larry didn't lock his door, so John let himself in and found Larry like this. There is also vomitus in the bathroom.	I ask John to start looking around the apartment for any medications his friend may take or to find anything that may give us a clue as to what's going on. I don't see any alcohol bottles nearby, and I don't smell it on Larry's breath, and with the story that John has told us, I don't think Larry is drunk. His breath doesn't smell fruity, so I don't think this acidosis. He could have had a seizure, and if he takes seizure meds, hopefully John will find them. I think I can also rule out an infectious process, because he was willing to go to lunch up to the last minute, so he must have been feeling well. I guess this could be a drug overdose, but again, if there are any bottles, hopefully John will find them. I get to "T" for trauma, and I think, maybe this is a head injury—he could have suffered a head injury, didn't feel well afterward, and decided to lie down, and that's how he got to the bed. So far, I'm not really getting anywhere here. Now I'm at "I" for insulin. There is a good chance that Larry could be hypoglycemic, because he hadn't eaten lunch yet. When Matt gets the IV started, we'll have to check his dex stick. I guess Larry could have a psych history or could have been poisoned in some way. We'll find out about the psych history if John can find any meds. I think it is unlikely that Larry had a stroke, based on his initial presentation of diaphoresis and vomiting.

Physical Exam

Matt keeps calling Larry's name, and Larry is looking at him but isn't speaking. Matt has him on the monitor, which shows a sinus tach. Matt reports a weak, rapid pulse. Larry can move all extremities and even tries to fight Matt as Matt takes his arm to start the IV. Matt is having trouble with the IV because Larry is really fighting now. He has strong movements of his extremities, so I go to hold him down.	I yell out to John, who is searching Larry's medicine cabinet, to see if he has found anything yet. When he says he hasn't, I tell him to look in the kitchen and to make sure he checks the refrigerator. If Larry is diabetic, there should be insulin in there. I tell Matt that I don't think Larry had a stroke, because of the strong, equal movements of his extremities. It appears that he just came back from the gym, so I don't think this is an intentional overdose or alcohol-related, but we can't rule that out just yet.

Physical Exam (continued)

We get the IV started, and Matt draws blood and gets a dex stick, which I throw in the glucometer. Just then John comes into the room with two bottles of insulin, NPH and regular, and a box of syringes.	Larry's glucose reading is 23. He is diabetic and is hypoglycemic.

Interventions

I grab the drug kit and throw Matt an ampule of 50 percent dextrose. He is pushing it as fast as he can, but the dextrose is thick and it takes some time.	While we are waiting for Larry to become more alert, we are trying to piece together what happened. We are guessing that Larry had been exercising before lunch. Regular exercise can actually lead to a decrease in the amount of insulin a patient needs to take. He may have then taken his regular insulin, expecting to eat lunch at a certain time, but then John was late and Larry probably didn't eat. All this could have led to Larry becoming severely hypoglycemic.

Ongoing Assessment

A few minutes later Larry starts to wake up and looks around. He manages to sit up in the bed, and his skin is becoming dry. He begins to regain color in his face.	The D_{50} is working and Larry's blood glucose is coming up. He is alert and oriented and can tell us what is going on. Basically, we got the story right. He tells us he usually wears a medical ID bracelet, but one of the links broke and he hadn't replaced it yet.
This episode has scared Larry because this is the first time that this has happened to him. He agrees to go the hospital with us, and transport is uneventful. His heart rate is coming down, and his skin is warm and dry.	Many diabetics, once they wake up, refuse transport to the hospital. To avoid medical liability for not transporting a patient for whom we have begun treatment, we call a supervisor who reviews with the patient the procedure for refusal of medical transport and then has the patient sign a refusal form. In this case, Larry realizes that his insulin needs to be adjusted because he has been working out regularly and wants to be seen in the ED.

Communications and Written Report

We call ahead to the ED and let them know we are coming. They give us a room assignment as we head in without an emergency.	This is a nonemergent transport because Larry has regained his normal mental status and he is no longer hypoglycemic. I write my report en route to the hospital.

Follow-Up

The ED runs Larry's preglucose blood for a glucose level, which shows 23. His dextrose stick is now 69, so they give him some orange juice and lunch to eat, because they would like to see it a little higher.	We say goodbye and head to lunch ourselves. After all, it's time for Matt to pay off his bet.

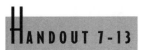
DYSPNEA SCENARIO

Actions	Reasoning
Dispatch	
It is 4:30 in the afternoon, and we've just had one of the slowest days I can remember for a long time. I'm telling my partner, Maria, that I am almost bored when we are dispatched for a 26-year-old male in a local park complaining of shortness of breath. I am actually relieved to have some work to do.	The park that we are dispatched to has several different areas. We are directed to go to the basketball courts when we get there. The park is very busy this time of year, with lots of ball players coming around in the afternoon for pickup games, but there is also a crowd that is into the drug scene, and you can usually find one or two drug dealers there. The occasional crack overdose or drug bust is never a surprise here. So we don't know what we are getting into when we head to the park.
Scene Size-Up	
We pull into the parking lot at the basketball courts to find a crowd of people standing around in a circle. There are two cop cars already there, and I can see at least three police officers in the crowd. One car has its trunk open, and I see an officer heading toward the crowd with an oxygen tank.	The fact that there are several police officers there is not surprising. The city is pretty good about making sure that EMS is not alone in areas that have a reputation for drugs and crime, even in the middle of the day. Maria and I grab our monitor, airway kit, and stretcher and head toward the basketball courts.
Initial Assessment	
A young man is sitting up against a basketball pole with labored respirations, sternal retractions, and diaphoresis. He is complaining of chest pain.	En route to the scene, I had been thinking that this could be drug-related because of the location. Perhaps the patient had been smoking crack or inhaling fumes as some kids have become fond of doing, but it appears that the patient had been playing ball. He is working hard to breathe, but I don't hear any stridor, so I can rule out a foreign body obstruction. Although it is hard to say right now, the fact that he was playing ball leads me to think he is in good health, so I don't think there is anything infectious like pneumonia. He may be a smoker, but he is too young to have any chronic breathing problems from it, like emphysema or acute bronchitis. He is tall and thin, so I can't rule out a spontaneous pneumothorax or even a pneumothorax from trauma, if he was hit in the chest by another player. He is breathing fast and his respirations are obviously labored, so he is clearly not hyperventilating. I need to get a little medical history and do a respiratory assessment to rule out heart failure, MI, and pulmonary embolism.

History

Our patient, Jason, cannot speak in complete sentences because of his shortness of breath. Another player tells us that they had been playing ball for about an hour when Jason started to slow down and walk toward the bench. Then he couldn't walk anymore. He sat down against the pole because he was able to breathe a little better sitting straight up, but he didn't have the strength to hold himself up.	Jason cannot speak, so I ask him only to answer yes or no to my questions. When asked, he denies any cardiac history. He does tell me that he has a history of asthma. I ask him if he uses medicine for his asthma every day, and he shakes his head no and points to his bag. I give it to him and he pulls out an albuterol inhaler. He manages to get out that he only uses it when he becomes short of breath with exercise. I shake it, and it feels empty. He tells me he can't remember when he used it last.

Physical Exam

As we are getting Jason's medical history, Maria puts the pulse ox on Jason's finger. He is already on 15 lpm of oxygen via a nonrebreather mask that one of the police officers put on him. His pulse ox reading is 90 percent.	He isn't oxygenating well, which means he must be pretty tight, meaning that his bronchioles are pretty closed up.
I ask Jason to lean forward so I can listen to his lungs. He has high-pitched inspiratory and expiratory wheezing throughout all lung fields.	He doesn't have unilateral wheezing, so I can rule out an aspirated foreign body and a pneumothorax. The wheezing is clearly related to his asthma, so I am no longer concerned that his shortness of breath and chest pain are from a pulmonary embolism.

Interventions

Maria puts Jason on the albuterol treatment and assists him to our stretcher. I place him on the monitor and note sinus tachycardia in the 110s. His respiratory rate is 36.	Shortness of breath can lead to tachypnea and tachycardia. I want to monitor his vital signs regularly to watch for any changes.

Ongoing Assessment

En route to the ED, I start an IV in case the physician wants to give steroids when Jason gets to the ER. When the first albuterol treatment is over, I start a second. I note that his heart rate is now in the 120s, but his respiratory rate is now 28. I reassess his breath sounds, and the wheezing is becoming a little coarser.	Steroids are important to relieve the inflammation in the bronchioles. Albuterol is a beta agonist, and one of its side effects is tachycardia. As Jason's airway starts to open, the wheezing should become less high-pitched, like whistling, and become coarser. This means that he is having more air movement. He is still breathing fast, although it is good to see his respiratory rate come down a little.

Communications and Written Report

We call ahead to the ED to let them know we are coming. It is a quick trip, so I don't have time to get my chart written in the back of the ambulance.	I give the report and sit down in the EMS room to get my chart done while Maria restocks the respiratory equipment.

©2009 Pearson Education, Inc.
Paramedic Care: Principles & Practice, Vol. 5, 3rd. Ed.

Follow-Up	
Jason has finished his third treatment by the time I am done with my chart. He is still on oxygen, but they've put him on a nasal cannula and his pulse ox is now 95 percent. He is speaking in complete sentences and thanks us for our help.	I remind him that he needs to keep a new inhaler in his bag if he is going to play ball. Even if he had gotten to the one he had with him, it wouldn't have done him any good.

Student's Name _____

SYNCOPE SCENARIO

Actions	Reasoning
Dispatch	
Miguel and I have just spent the day cleaning the ambulance. It is 4:30 P.M., and we are looking forward to resting for the rest of the shift when we get dispatched for a 59-year-old female with a syncopal episode. We clear the buckets and mop out of the way so we can get the ambulance out and sign on en route to the scene.	Well, so much for getting some rest this afternoon. I ask the dispatcher if they have any more information for us, because syncope is kind of vague—at least let us know if the patient is conscious. We find out that the caller is the patient's daughter, who was a bit hysterical on the phone and didn't give much information. We do know that the patient is now awake. That's a start.
Scene Size-Up	
We arrive on-scene 6 minutes later. We are in a typical suburban neighborhood and there are bikes and toys in the driveway, so we park in the street. We usually don't have police on the scene with us, unless there is reason to believe the scene is unsafe, so we are the only ones to arrive. A young woman comes running out of the house, telling us to hurry up.	We look at each other and move a little quicker. Perhaps something has changed and her mother is no longer awake.
Initial Assessment	
We are shown to the living room, where a middle-aged woman is lying on the couch with her feet up on some pillows. She looks pale and clammy. She is awake, alert, and oriented times 3. Her respirations are easy and nonlabored. When she sees us, she begins to sit up, but we encourage her to lie back down.	At least someone knew to lie her down and elevate her feet to help the blood flow back to her head. I wonder if she was here in the living room when she experienced the syncope or if she was helped here after she woke up.
History	
Mrs. Dunn, our patient, tells us that she was standing at the sink, washing dishes, when she felt lightheaded and became sweaty. As she was reaching the table to sit down, she fell to the floor, and that is where her daughter found her. Her daughter, Lynn, tells us through her tears that her mother "was out" for a long time but woke up and was able to walk to the couch.	I can see we are going to have trouble getting information from the daughter, but Mrs. Dunn seems to be doing pretty well. She was standing at the sink when she became lightheaded. I wonder if she became orthostatic because of a fluid volume problem or if she had a vasovagal episode. Her respirations are easy and nonlabored, so her syncope does not appear to be caused by hyperventilation. She may have a glucose problem or a cardiac problem that we don't know about yet. I saw her move all extremities equally when she sat up, so I don't think she had a stroke, although she may have had a TIA. Her daughter did not describe any seizure activity, so I am ruling that out as a cause for her syncope.

©2009 Pearson Education, Inc. *Paramedic Care: Principles & Practice, Vol. 5, 3rd. Ed.*

History (continued)

When asked, Mrs. Dunn denies any chest pain or shortness of breath before her syncopal episode, nor is she experiencing either one now.	This can still be cardiac-related, such as an arrhythmia. She denies chest pain, so I don't think this is an MI.

Physical Exam

Miguel gets out the monitor as I start my physical assessment. Mrs. Dunn is cool and clammy to the touch. She has clear lung sounds bilaterally and no pedal edema. I've checked her pulse and it feels pretty slow. I'd like to see what her rhythm looks like.	With a quick pulse check, I can rule out SVT and V-tach as a cause for the syncope. Her rate is pretty slow, so I am thinking that her bradycardia could be the problem. I'd like to know more about that.
Miguel reports a sinus bradycardia on the monitor with no ectopy. Mrs. Dunn's blood pressure is 180/110. Her daughter reminds her to tell us about her blood pressure problem.	I wonder what this blood pressure problem is all about? She may have been hypotensive due to a fluid volume problem, although with a BP of 180/110 now, I doubt that is what happened.
Mrs. Dunn has recently been diagnosed with hypertension. Her daughter comes back with the pill bottle and I see that Mrs. Dunn is taking atenolol. She just started the medication this past week.	Atenolol is a beta-blocker that is used for hypertension. It can also cause bradycardia. Mrs. Dunn just couldn't compensate for her low heart rate while standing up washing dishes, and that is what caused her syncopal episode.

Interventions

Miguel starts an IV and draws blood. He starts a line of normal saline at a KVO rate.	If Mrs. Dunn remains symptomatic from the bradycardia, we may need to give her atropine or possibly even use our pacer. We need to have an IV started to be prepared for either.

Ongoing Assessment

We get Mrs. Dunn loaded into the ambulance, and I recheck her vital signs. Her blood pressure is 176/112, and her heart rate is 42.	Mrs. Dunn is tolerating her vital signs well, but I realize that this could easily change. I've taken out an amp of atropine just to be on the safe side. I also have my pacer pads ready, in case I need to take them out quickly. If she were still feeling lightheaded, I may even consider putting the pads on her in case I needed to use the pacer quickly, but I don't think it is necessary at this time.

Communications and Written Report

I let the ED know that we need a monitored bed for a syncopal episode related to bradycardia. They give me a room assignment as I finish my report. We now have about a 10-minute transport, so Mrs. Dunn and I talk in the back of the ambulance as I finish my run sheet.	The trip to the ED was uneventful. Mrs. Dunn remained asymptomatic, with no change in her vital signs. I give the report to the ED nurse and hand her my run sheet. Now maybe we can head back to the station to put our feet up.

Follow-Up

Mrs. Dunn was admitted to the hospital for monitoring. She shouldn't be there for more than a day or two. Her physician will also be changing her blood pressure medication.	There are many other drugs available that will keep Mrs. Dunn's blood pressure under control but will not cause the bradycardia and syncope that she experienced today.

SEIZURE SCENARIO

Actions	Reasoning
Dispatch	
The call comes in the middle of the night. "Medic 206, respond to 218 Treebrooke Road for a seizure." Kayla and I throw our boots on and head out the door. I knew it was too much to expect to be able to sleep through the night on a Friday. Things were just going too well.	Kayla is driving as I am looking up the street on the map. Treebrooke is in one of the little subdivisions in our district—it is just a matter of finding the right one.
Scene Size-Up	
We arrive in a quiet little neighborhood to find the house well lit. This is always a relief in the middle of the night. There is one step up to the front door. We head up the driveway with our stretcher and equipment.	I am always concerned about going out to someone's house in the middle of the night. If they don't turn lights on, we never know what we may find the hard way. I have tripped over children's toys and fallen off porches. Thankfully, none of this ever led to an injury.
Initial Assessment	
We get into the house, and a woman named Pat meets us at the door and quickly directs us upstairs. We carry up our equipment and leave the stretcher downstairs. We are led into the bathroom of the master bedroom to find a man in his mid-40s on the bathroom floor, with jerking motions noted in his arms and legs. He has vomited on the floor.	The patient appears to still be seizing. I grab suction equipment as Kayla grabs the oxygen and a bag-valve mask. While I start to suction, Pat tells us the seizure is getting better and that he isn't jerking as much. Kayla passes me the BVM, and I start to bag our patient, Bobby, as Kayla gets out the IV kit and prepares to start an IV.
History	
As I am bagging Bobby, his jerking continues. I yell out a bunch of questions to Pat. Does Bobby have any medical problems we need to know about? Does he have a history of seizures? Can she tell us what happened prior to Bobby having the seizure?	Bobby does not have a history of seizures. Pat now starts getting upset, so I have to start asking more specific questions. I want to know exactly what is causing this seizure, but Pat is becoming less helpful as she gets more upset.
I ask specifically about medical history. Has he been complaining of not feeling well recently? Specifically, has he been complaining of a headache? She tells me that Bobby does not have any medical problems at all.	By asking about any recent headaches, I can rule out more than one cause of the seizure. I am concerned that he may have an infectious process going on, such as meningitis. Pat denies any recent headaches. The fact that she denies any medical history doesn't mean that this isn't caused by something like a brain tumor or a neurovascular disease. He may have either one, and this could be the initial presentation.

History *(continued)*	
Has Bobby recently experienced any trauma or head injury?	A head injury, even several days ago, could have led to a cerebral bleed or contusion, which could result in a seizure several days later. Pat is unaware of any head injury.
I tell her I have to ask some sensitive questions. I ask if Bobby takes drugs or drinks alcohol on a regular basis. She starts to cry and tells me that he usually drinks at least 2 six-packs over the course of the day, but lately they have been arguing about it. Two days ago he told her he could prove that he wasn't an alcoholic by going "cold turkey" and not drinking anymore. Tonight he was shaking and sweating and complaining of nausea before going to bed.	It appears that Bobby is going through alcohol withdrawal. Pat describes the symptoms of detoxification, and patients going through withdrawal frequently have seizures.

Physical Exam	
Bobby continues to have jerking motions in his arms and his legs. He has urinated in his pajama pants. I take the bag-valve mask off his face to look in his mouth to see if he has bitten his tongue.	Incontinence and a bitten tongue are both signs of a generalized tonic-clonic, or grand mal, seizure.

Interventions	
Because Bobby hasn't stopped jerking yet, we are concerned that he may have another seizure. Kayla calls medical direction for an order for Valium so we can get this seizure activity stopped.	Due to local protocols, we need to call the hospital for medical direction before we give any narcotics. We get an order for 10 mg of Valium, which I give via slow IV push through the normal saline IV that Kayla started. We start a normal saline IV on seizure patients because of the fact that if the physician wants to give the patient IV Dilantin, it is compatible only with normal saline.
As we are waiting for the fire department to show up, we have time to put Bobby on the monitor. He is now breathing on his own, so I switch him to a nonrebreather mask.	I also call for lifting assistance, because I am concerned that Kayla and I will not be able to safely carry this patient down the stairs by ourselves, especially if he starts to seize again.

Ongoing Assessment	
We get Bobby loaded into the ambulance. His seizure activity has stopped, and he is postictal. He is taking slow deep breaths, so I check his respiratory rate, which is 12. His pulse ox is 99 percent on the nonrebreather mask. His blood pressure is 132/78, and his heart rate is 92.	I need to closely monitor his vital signs. Valium is a CNS depressant, which means he could stop breathing as a result of the medication. It can also lower his blood pressure, so I need to make sure that his BP stays within normal limits.

SCENARIOS

Communications and Written Report	
We notify the ED that we are coming, and we are told that we will get a room assignment on arrival.	I wait until I get to the ED to write my report. I want to monitor Bobby closely in case he seizes again or has any change in his vital signs.
Follow-Up	
Bobby is starting to come around as we are getting ready to leave the ED. Pat has arrived at the hospital and thanks us for helping her husband.	If there were any doubts that Bobby has an alcohol problem, this incident should settle it. Bobby has a long road ahead of him.

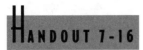

Student's Name _____

HYPOTHERMIA SCENARIO

Actions	Reasoning
Dispatch	
"Medic 112, respond to 357 South East Drive for an elderly male, unresponsive." Our radio alerts us of a call, and Lucas and I head out to the rig.	While en route, I call dispatch to see if there is any other information I can get. I know the address—it's one of the many nursing homes in our district. Many times they call us and the chief complaint isn't even close to what's going on when we get there, so we like to have a little more information before our arrival. We find out that the patient had been missing for several hours and was found outside in nightclothes.
Scene Size-Up	
We arrive on-scene to find several police cars and fire trucks already on location. We are directed to the ambulance entrance by a police officer, who escorts us into the building and fills us in on what is going on. The police had been called several hours ago because one of the Alzheimer's patients was missing. The police and fire department searched for 3 hours and found the patient in the woods behind the nursing home. It is close to winter and the temperatures dropped into the low 40s last night. They wrapped the patient in some blankets, carried him back to the nursing home on a Reeves stretcher, and called us.	I do not have any concerns regarding my safety or the safety of my partner on this call. However, I wonder how this patient was able to just leave during the night without anybody noticing. But this is not my problem. I just need to make sure I do the best I can for this patient.
Initial Assessment	
We arrive in the patient's room to find him wrapped in several blankets. He is unresponsive and lying very still, and his muscles are stiff and rigid. He has shallow respirations and a weak pulse. He is not on any oxygen or monitoring equipment. I ask what the patient's temperature is and no one seems to know.	This patient is exhibiting signs of severe hypothermia. He is not shivering, which means his body temperature must be pretty low. I am concerned about his shallow respirations, because this may indicate an impending respiratory or cardiac arrest.

History

The head nurse comes in to give us a report, but doesn't add much more to what we already know. The patient has been a resident for several months and has a history of wandering the halls, but has never tried to leave the building before. He has a medical history of hypertension and coronary artery disease. She also tells us that he has a Do Not Resuscitate order on his chart and that his daughter is on her way.	This medical history doesn't really change anything that we are going to do for the patient right now. However, I am concerned about cardiac and respiratory arrest, and the fact that he has a DNR can completely change the way we care for this patient.

Physical Exam

Lucas starts to get out the monitor and IV equipment as I start a physical assessment. I unwrap the blankets the patient is in and find that he is still in the wet nightclothes that he was found in. A nursing assistant takes a quick rectal temperature and reports 30°C (86°F). We place the patient on the monitor and find he is in atrial fibrillation. I ask the head nurse if he has a history of A-fib, which she denies. I attempt to get a blood pressure, but I cannot hear one.	I immediately take out my shears and start cutting off the wet clothes. I ask for some new blankets and a nursing assistant runs to get some. His body temperature indicates that he is in need of active internal rewarming, which should not be attempted in the field unless we have more than a 15-minute response time to the hospital. A-fib is the most common presenting dysrhythmia seen in hypothermia and can be seen in those patients with a body temperature of less than 30°C. This concerns me, because if he gets any cooler, the patient can easily go into ventricular fibrillation.

Interventions

The patient is still lying in the Reeves stretcher, and I would like to get it out from under him because it is also cold and a little damp. I ask for some moving assistance from the firefighters who are still there. The nursing assistant hands me some heat packs, which she wants me to place under his arms and in his groin. I say thanks but no thanks and continue doing what I am doing.	I know it is important to limit handling of the patient and to move him carefully, because rough handling can lead to ventricular fibrillation. However, I want to do everything I can to get whatever is cold and wet away from the patient. We can move him to our stretcher on a sheet when the time comes. Applying external heat to this patient can result in rewarming shock by causing reflex peripheral vasodilation. This causes the return of cool blood and acids from the extremities to the core. This may cause a paradoxical "afterdrop" core temperature decrease and further worsen core hypothermia.

©2009 Pearson Education, Inc.
Paramedic Care: Principles & Practice, Vol. 5, 3rd. Ed.

Interventions (continued)

I want to get this patient to the hospital quickly, because there is nothing more that I can do for him here. I quickly get him covered up in dry blankets after we start an IV. We slowly and carefully move him over to our stretcher and load him carefully into the back of the ambulance. We keep warm IV fluids in an IV warmer in the ambulance, so I grab a bag and hang it on the patient en route to the hospital.	Active internal rewarming requires warm IV fluids, warm, humidified oxygen, peritoneal lavage, and extracorporeal rewarming. I know that the warmed IV fluids that I have will contribute little to the rewarming effort, but their use may prevent further heat loss and can prevent the onset of rewarming shock. We have less than a 15-minute response time to the hospital, so even if I had the means of further active rewarming, I wouldn't attempt it in the field.

Ongoing Assessment

We transport the patient to the hospital slightly inclined with his head down. Although Lucas is using his lights and sirens, he is driving slowly to avoid any rough handling of the patient. The patient remains in A-fib.	I am still concerned about the possibility of V-fib, so we do our best to keep the patient still. Although we have the heat blasting in the back of the truck and we are hanging warm IV fluids, nothing is going to help this patient until we get him to the hospital.

Communications and Written Report

I call the ED and let them know we have a 7-minute ETA with a severely hypothermic patient. They tell me to report to the trauma room, where they keep all of their equipment for active rewarming.	We head to the trauma room and I quickly give the report and hand them the patient's DNR order, along with the rest of the copies of his chart. The DNR order will become very important, should the patient convert to V-fib. This is going to be a long report to write, so I grab a cup of coffee and head to the EMS room.

Follow-Up

We head out about 25 minutes later. The ED staff has started the active rewarming process and his core temperature is now 32°C. His daughter has arrived and would like to know what happened, so we take a few minutes to fill her in a little on what we know took place before our arrival.	It's a shame that this patient was able to get out of the nursing home as easily as he did. They need to review how they care for Alzheimer's patients, because it is all too common for them to wander off as this man did.

Student's Name _____

HAZARDOUS MATERIALS/TOXICOLOGY SCENARIO

Actions	Reasoning
Dispatch	
I am working an overtime night shift at Station 3 with Mary. It's the middle of the night, and we get toned out for a 36-year-old male in respiratory arrest. Lucky for him, the call is right down the street.	I throw my boots on and head out the door. I offer to drive, but because Mary is used to working nights and I'm not, she says she would prefer to drive. It's fine with me because it gives me a minute or two to shake the sleep out of my head. I tell her that I'll grab the oxygen, monitor, and airway kit if she takes the jump box. We'll just throw it all on the stretcher as we head inside.
Scene Size-Up	
We arrive on the scene to find a dark, run-down apartment building. I can't believe anyone even lives here. The neighborhood is known for the drug dealers and addicts who hang around, and it is protocol to dispatch police along with the ambulance on any calls here. Just as I am getting ready to ask if the police are on the way, I hear their siren in the background. We follow protocol and wait in the ambulance until the cops arrive.	This is a frustrating part of the job. I remember learning the very first day of EMT class that I always have to make sure the scene is safe for me and my crew. This scene is definitely not safe, and, although I am told that the patient is in respiratory arrest, I am not going to take any chances with my own safety.
Initial Assessment	
We are escorted up the stairs and find ourselves in an abandoned apartment. Several people run out the door when they see the police arrive. A woman stands in the doorway to another room and motions for us to come in there. We find a man in his mid 30s leaning up against a wall, breathing at about four times a minute. I look around him before I get down next to him to make sure I don't get stuck with any needles. As I kneel down, I feel for a pulse, which is slow.	I am assuming that this is a heroin overdose, based on what I know about the area and the fact that this patient is experiencing severe respiratory depression and bradycardia.
History	
We ask the woman what happened, but she looks at the cops and says she doesn't know; she just found him like this.	She obviously isn't going to tell us the truth, especially with the cops around.
I ask if she knows if he has any medical problems, and she says she has no idea and that she hasn't known him for very long.	Although I am assuming that this is a heroin overdose, I cannot rule out the possibility of a medical problem. However, as my husband always says, "When you hear hoof beats, think horses and not zebras," so we are going to treat the obvious first.

Physical Exam	
We lay him down and Mary gets out the oxygen and bag-valve mask. I do a quick pupil check with my flashlight while she is doing this and find constricted pupils.	Constricted pupils are another sign of a heroin overdose.

Interventions	
I then start bagging the patient with 100 percent oxygen.	The patient is basically in a coma and isn't fighting the BVM at all. Mary puts the pulse ox on his finger, and his oxygen saturation goes from 79 percent to 98 percent after a short time. This gives Mary a little more time to get an IV started, as I am not having any difficulty managing his airway.
Because I am not having any problems managing the patient's airway with a bag-valve mask, Mary attempts an IV rather than intubation. We both know that this patient needs naloxone as soon as possible.	I don't want to bag him for too long, because of increased gastric distention and the risk of aspiration from vomiting. However, we both know that the opiate antagonist naloxone can reverse a heroin overdose quickly, thereby reversing the respiratory depression quickly. Many times these patients wake up intubated and proceed to pull out their tubes, which can cause trauma to the airway.
Mary gets lucky and finds a good vein in the patient's thumb and is able to start an IV on the second attempt.	Frequently, IV drug abusers are very difficult IV sticks. They have been abusing their veins for a long time and therefore don't have any usable veins left. If this were to happen, we would give the naloxone as an intramuscular injection. Although it takes longer to work this way, the advantage of IM naloxone is that it lasts longer as well.
Mary gives the patient naloxone 2 mg slow IV push.	We have both had the experience of giving this drug too rapidly, causing vomiting.
The patient starts to breathe on his own and starts to become combative, pushing the BVM off his face. Mary had just finished securing the IV.	Many times these patients wake up combative. I have also had the experience of the patient getting very angry because we have taken away his high. Such patients don't realize that we have saved their lives, because they weren't breathing and would have died.
The police jump in and secure him until he has had a chance to calm down. He becomes quiet and cooperative once he realizes what is going on. We convince him to go to the hospital with us and load him up on the stretcher.	Naloxone reverses the symptoms of a narcotic overdose, but has a shorter half-life than the drug that the patient overdosed on. It is important to get the patient to the hospital in case the drug wears off before the heroin does.

Ongoing Assessment	
En route to the hospital, I get a full set of vital signs, which are now all within normal limits. He is breathing 20 times a minute, and he is in a normal sinus rhythm at 88. His blood pressure is 118/62. I recheck his vital signs every 5 minutes.	I want to do frequent vital sign checks, in case the naloxone wears off and he starts to experience signs of overdose again.

Communications and Written Report	
Mary calls in a report from the front of the ambulance as I ride in the back with the patient. We have a short trip to the hospital, and transport is uneventful.	I give the report to the nurse in charge and sit at the desk to finish the run sheet while Mary restocks the equipment we used.

Follow-Up	
While in the ER, the patient starts to exhibit signs of the overdose again, so they give him another dose of naloxone. Although he wants to leave, he isn't going anywhere for a while.	The patient won't be discharged until the physician is convinced that the patient won't go into respiratory arrest when he leaves. We head back to the station to hopefully finish out our shift quietly.

SCENARIOS

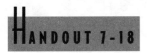

Student's Name _____

BLUNT TRAUMA SCENARIO

Actions	Reasoning
Dispatch	
My partner, Antonio, and I are just cleaning up at the hospital after bringing in a bad MI when dispatch calls us on the radio to see if we are available to take a call. The last thing we want to do is run another call right now, but we have just finished cleaning up so we agree to do it. The call is for a pedestrian struck at the corner of Howard and Mills, which is just a few blocks from the hospital.	Great, we go from taking care of a huge MI to a trauma. I call dispatch to find out if this is a child or an adult, because this type of trauma affects these types of patients differently. I am told that this is a male patient in his mid-to-late-20s.
Scene Size-Up	
We reach Howard pretty quickly, but traffic is backed up, presumably because of the accident. Antonio maneuvers around the cars that are trying to get out of our way. We get to the intersection to find a car in the middle of it, with a man lying in the road about 12 feet away. There are a few people around the man, including a police officer. I get out of the ambulance and note that the engine of the car is turned off. I don't see any fluids leaking from the car.	I want to make sure the scene is safe. The car is safely turned off, and I don't need to worry about any leaking fluids causing a problem.
Initial Assessment	
We approach the patient and find him lying on his stomach. He appears to be unconscious and is not moving. There is a moderate amount of blood by his head, but I can't see where it is coming from. I can see that he is breathing, but I am not certain about airway compromise.	Right away I am concerned about a head injury, because of the mechanisms of injury and the bleeding from his head. We also need to protect his C-spine, in case he has a cervical spine injury.
History	
The driver of the car is clearly upset, stating that he didn't see the patient walk in front of the car. Witnesses say that the patient was trying to run across the street against the light when he got hit. They saw him roll onto the hood of the car and slide into the windshield, then get thrown to the ground as the car stopped suddenly. Another witness says that she didn't think the car was going very fast when it hit the victim.	From this story I am figuring that he got hit on the side, possibly causing a lower leg injury on the side that was hit. Hitting the hood could have caused a femur or chest injury. Hitting the windshield could have caused head, neck, or shoulder trauma. He could have suffered additional trauma from being thrown to the ground.

Physical Exam and Interventions	
Antonio immediately measures the patient for a cervical immobilization collar, while at the same he assesses the patient's airway, breathing, and circulation. The patient is breathing on his own but has blood coming from his mouth. He has a radial pulse, which means he has a blood pressure of at least 60 systolic. I help Antonio put the C-collar on, and, with the assistance of the police officer, we gently log-roll the patient onto his back.	The blood in the patient's mouth concerns me. If the patient cannot protect his airway, then he can aspirate on the blood or any teeth that may have been loosened.
I use the portable suction to suction his mouth and find out where the bleeding is coming from. This starts to wake the patient up. I don't see any loose teeth or other objects, and I see that he has a cut on his tongue, probably from biting it. Once I finish suctioning, I see the cut isn't bleeding anymore. I start the patient on 100 percent oxygen via a nonrebreather mask.	Suctioning is important to clear the airway and to visualize the mouth for trauma even though the patient has a patent airway.
Now that he is on his back and his airway is clear, I can evaluate for a flail chest or other chest injury such as pneumothorax or hemothorax. I note equal expansion of the chest cavity, and as I listen to his breath sounds I note clear and equal breath sounds bilaterally.	The type of blunt trauma that this patient suffered can lead to internal chest injuries. If he were having any compromise in his breathing, this could lead to respiratory arrest.
The patient starts to moan and starts moving his arms to grab at his C-collar. He opens his eyes after I ask him to several times. He is trying to speak, but I don't understand what he is saying, and he is withdrawing from pain. I figure his Glasgow coma score at 10.	The Glasgow coma score is a moderately good predictor of head injury severity. A score between 9 and 12 indicates moderate injury. I had been considering intubating him to protect his airway, especially with the blood in his mouth, but I think I can hold off on that for now.
I instruct the patient to lie still and not to move his head or neck and stop grabbing at his collar. I explain that, if he has a neck injury, all the movement can make the injury worse. I do a quick neuro assessment and ask him to squeeze my hands and to push down and then pull up with his feet. I find he moves all extremities equally.	The fact that he is moving his arms and legs is a good sign that he hasn't suffered an obvious C-spine injury. This certainly is not a guarantee, however, and, if he has any broken bones in his neck, I want to keep him from moving them to prevent further injury.
I already know that the patient has a strong radial pulse. I check capillary refill, and it is less than 2 seconds. I do a quick look to see if there is evident bleeding from additional injuries, and right now I don't see any.	A capillary refill of more than 3 seconds can be caused by hypovolemia, although I also realized that if he were a smoker or taking certain meds, those things could also cause a delayed capillary refill. It is important to detect any signs of early shock.

Physical Exam and Interventions *(continued)*	
Due to the mechanism of injury, I decide that this patient needs a rapid trauma assessment. I have already done a quick evaluation of the patient's head, neck, and chest during my initial assessment. I need to now evaluate his abdomen, pelvis, and extremities.	I focus on these areas first because they are where serious life threats are most likely to occur.
Because we are concerned about hypothermia, we don't want to leave him lying on the ground, especially since we'll have to cut off his clothes to perform our exam, further lowering his body temperature. The ambulance is right here, so we decide to quickly get him loaded in the back before going any further. We know he has a decent blood pressure and pulse from our initial assessment, so we take a few minutes to put him in the ambulance now.	We want to keep the patient as warm as possible to prevent hypothermia.
We are now in the back of the ambulance. The patient has become more alert and is starting to ask questions. As a matter of fact, he has asked the same questions several times. I do a quick pupil check and find his pupils are equal and reactive.	The repetitive questioning convinces me that the patient has a concussion, as exhibited by the memory loss. He is not suffering any herniation in his brain from swelling or bleeding, at least not yet, which I note since his pupils are equal and reactive.
Antonio checks the patient's vital signs and gets the following: blood pressure 102/68, pulse 104, with sinus tachycardia on the monitor, and respirations 22.	His vital signs are good but bordering on possible shock. We need to check them frequently and do what we can to prevent the patient from going into shock. If he is bleeding, I need to find out from where.
I try to get the patient to tell me if he is having any pain anywhere, but he isn't answering my questions. I try to get him to pay attention, but I'm not getting anywhere. Antonio gets ready to start his IVs as I go on with my assessment. I start cutting his clothes off so I can do a visual inspection, but I cover him up with blankets so I can keep him warm.	My physical evaluation of the patient is going to be very important, because he is not answering my questions because of his head injury.
I inspect his abdomen for any asymmetry or apparent pulsing masses. I palpate each quadrant to see if this elicits any pain response from the patient, which it does not.	I carefully palpate all four quadrants of his abdomen, and I watch his face for any evidence of pain, but this does not seem to bother him. He denies pain on palpation when I ask him.
Next, I evaluate his pelvis. I place firm pressure on the iliac crests directed medially and on the pubic bone directed downward. Everything feels fine, and again the patient denies pain in the area.	I am checking for crepitus and/or any instability of the pelvis. A patient can bleed heavily from a pelvic fracture.

Physical Exam and Interventions (continued)	
I carefully examine each extremity for muscle tone, distal pulse, temperature, color, and capillary refill time. I also check for motor response, sensory response, and limb strength. I do not see any evidence of injury.	When a patient has a major area of injury, such as a head injury, he may not complain about pain from a broken bone in an extremity because he is focused on the major injury.
Antonio and I now need to log-roll the patient to check his back for injury. I examine the total surface of the back and palpate the spinal column from top to bottom. Again, the patient has no complaints of pain, although I still find his answers unreliable.	Careful examination for slight deformities, minor reddening, and very subtle pain or tenderness may reveal the only signs or symptoms of a spinal cord injury.
Antonio takes one more set of vitals before heading up front to drive. The patient's blood pressure remains stable at 108/70 and pulse rate is 107, he is still in sinus tach, and his respirations are still 22.	His vital signs are stable, and there really isn't much more to do for this patient except transport him to the hospital.

Ongoing Assessment	
I recheck vital signs every 5 minutes en route to the hospital. I also do a repeat neuro exam and check the patient's pupils for any changes. He is responding to my questions better, although he is still asking repetitive questions. I'm glad it's a short ride to the hospital!	With any major trauma, a patient can compensate for a while and then decompensate quickly. This is why I am checking vital signs and neuro status frequently.

Communications and Written Report	
Our dispatcher has called the ED for us to let them know they are getting a trauma. The trauma team is waiting for us in the trauma bay. The leader of the trauma team takes my report and takes over from here.	A trauma chart is a hard one to write. I have to make sure I have documented every assessment that I have done. This chart is going to take a while to complete.

Follow-Up	
By the time we clean up the ambulance and finish charting, the patient is back from a CT scan. Miraculously for the patient, it is negative. So far, all X-rays have been negative as well. It seems that he is going to walk away from this with just a bad concussion.	I realize that not everyone is this lucky, and I'm glad he is going to have a good outcome.

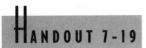

Student's Name _____

ALLERGIC REACTION SCENARIO

SCENARIOS

Actions	Reasoning
Dispatch	
It's a warm Sunday afternoon, and I'm sitting around the station feeling sorry for myself. It's too nice to be working today! My partner, Luz, is taking a nap and I'm watching the Yankees game when the tones go off. We are dispatched for an allergic reaction. Why are we getting this call? The closer unit must already be out.	En route to the call we are told that our patient is a 42-year-old male who was stung by several bees while mowing the lawn. The caller's wife states that the patient is in the backyard, too weak to go into the house.
Scene Size-Up	
We arrive in 9 minutes and pull up to the house. I am concerned about the fact that if the patient is still in the back, then the bees are, too. The patient's son meets us at the ambulance and tells us that his father is "passed out." We ask about the bees, and he says that his father was able to move away from the hive before he got sick.	We don't normally think of insects when we think of scene safety, but I was concerned about what we would find when we got there. The last thing I would want to do is have to approach a patient who is still surrounded by angry bees.
Initial Assessment	
We get to the yard to find our patient, Mr. Mann, sitting in a deck chair, with his upper body lying across the picnic table. His skin is red, and I can see hives on his exposed skin. His breathing is labored. He sees us coming and weakly lifts up his head.	Without even talking to the patient I can see he is in anaphylaxis, a severe allergic reaction. Although his condition appears to be bad, we want to make sure he isn't in shock and then prevent that from happening.
History	
His wife tells us that he was mowing the lawn, and suddenly she heard him screaming. She ran outside and found him running from the bees after being stung several times. When asked, she says that he has been stung by a bee twice before. The first time he was fine; the second time the area where he was stung became red and swollen, but he never got this bad.	Before a patient has an allergic reaction, he needs to have an initial exposure to the antigen, known as sensitization. A subsequent exposure induces a much stronger secondary response, such as the localized reaction that Mr. Mann had with the second bee sting. Hypersensitivity is an unexpected and exaggerated reaction to a particular antigen, such as the multiple bee stings that Mr. Mann experienced.
Physical Exam	
We get a quick set of vital signs and find the following: BP 90/60, pulse 110, respirations 28. Mr. Mann has wheezing throughout all lung fields. He is complaining of dizziness and abdominal pain.	Mr. Mann is experiencing many of the symptoms of anaphylactic shock. We need to get him treated immediately.

Interventions	
Luz gets out a nonrebreather mask and starts Mr. Mann on high-flow oxygen.	Oxygen is the first drug to administer in anaphylactic shock.
Mr. Mann needs an IV, but first I am going to give him epinephrine 1:10,000 subcutaneously.	Epinephrine is a sympathetic agonist, the primary drug used in anaphylaxis. It causes increased cardiac contractility and peripheral vasodilation and can also reverse some of the bronchospasm that Mr. Mann is having.
Luz starts Mr. Mann on an albuterol treatment as I start his IV.	As a beta agonist, albuterol will help reverse some of the bronchospasm and laryngeal edema associated with anaphylaxis. Mr. Mann needs an IV so that we can administer additional medication and for a fluid bolus.
Mr. Mann's IV is started, and I give him 50 mg of IV diphenhydramine. I also start a 500-mL fluid bolus.	Antihistamines are the second-line drugs used in anaphylaxis. Antihistamines block the effects of histamine, which is the principal chemical mediator in allergic reactions. I give him a fluid bolus to correct the hypotension.

Ongoing Assessment	
Treating Mr. Mann takes several minutes. Once we have completed the initial round of drugs and fluid, I recheck his vital signs. His BP is 100/62, pulse is 122, and respirations are 24.	We are starting to see some improvement. His blood pressure is coming up, and he is breathing a little slower. I am not surprised that his pulse rate is higher, because the epinephrine and the albuterol can both raise a patient's heart rate.
I reassess Mr. Mann's breath sounds, and the wheezing is getting coarser.	His airway is opening, so he is getting more airflow through his bronchioles.
Mr. Mann is still in the deck chair, but we have brought the stretcher over to him and assist him onto it. He says his dizziness is getting better and he wants to sit up a little bit.	Since his blood pressure is coming up, I assist Mr. Mann in sitting up to a semi-Fowler position. This helps with his breathing, but he is still wheezing.
En route to the ED, I take another set of vital signs, which remain stable.	I could have given another dose of epinephrine 3 to 5 minutes after the first dose, but Mr. Mann didn't need it.

Communications and Written Report	
We load Mr. Mann into the ambulance and head to the ED. We call to let them know we are coming. They will give additional medication, such as corticosteroids.	Corticosteroids do not help in the initial stages of anaphylaxis, but they help suppress the inflammatory response later on.

SCENARIOS

Communications and Written Report *(continued)*

We arrive at the hospital and give a report. The first albuterol treatment is done, but Mr. Mann is still wheezing, so the ED staff starts another one as soon as he is transferred to the stretcher.	I sit down to write up the run report. This call went very quickly, so this shouldn't take me very long.

Follow-Up

I stick my head in Mr. Mann's room to see how he is doing before I go. I ask him if anyone has told him that he could give himself epinephrine if he should get stung again, and he laughs and tells me that three different people have already told him this. He won't be leaving without a prescription.	Patients who experience severe allergic reactions can give self-administered epinephrine. Hopefully, this will help Mr. Mann avoid any more incidents like this in the future.

Handout 7-20

Student's Name _____

BEHAVIORAL—DEPRESSION SCENARIO

Actions	Reasoning
Dispatch	
It's 3:34 in the morning, and Brandon and I get dispatched for a patient requesting transport because of suicidal thoughts. We have just gotten back from another call, and I am tired. Hopefully, this won't take very long, I think as I am getting in the ambulance.	This could turn out to be a simple transport to the hospital, or it could be much more difficult than that, especially if the patient has already made an attempt to end his life. If that's the case, he may not want to go willingly with us. We'll have to see when we get there.
Scene Size-Up	
We arrive on-scene and find we are the first ones here. It is departmental policy that we do not enter the scene of the call until we have a police escort, so we wait a few minutes until they show up.	Although I know that most patients experiencing behavioral emergencies are not violent, if this patient is in crisis, his behavior is unpredictable. We approach these patients cautiously, to protect ourselves from potential injury.
Initial Assessment	
The police officer goes in the house and comes to get us after a couple of minutes. We go into the house and find the patient sitting at the kitchen with three pill bottles in front of him. He is fully dressed and speaks quietly. His affect is flat, and he doesn't look at me.	As soon as I see the bottles I am concerned that he may have taken an overdose of the medication. We need to find out what is going on as quickly as possible, but I don't want to proceed too fast and cause the patient any extra anxiety.
History	
I approach the patient, who is named Sam, quietly and sit down next to him. Brandon keeps his distance, along with the police officer. I ask him if he has taken any of the pills in the bottles, and he says he hasn't. I look at them and note two antidepressants and an anti-anxiety medication. I see they were just filled the day before. I ask him if Brandon can count them, and he tells us to go ahead.	Brandon takes the bottles to count the pills and make sure that they are all accounted for. Unfortunately, we cannot believe a patient when he says he hasn't taken an overdose. By counting out the pills, Brandon can confirm that he hasn't. All of the pills, except for his daily dose, are accounted for.
I ask Sam what is going on. He tells me that over the last couple of weeks he has been feeling worthless and depressed and that he went to see his doctor for it yesterday. He can barely get himself up in the morning to go to work, and he didn't make it in at all the last 2 days. He hasn't been able to sleep and hasn't been eating much. Tonight he sat up thinking that everything would be much better if he just took all of his pills and "got it over with." That scared him, so he called us.	Sam is experiencing five of the symptoms that must be present in a 2-week period in order to be diagnosed with major depressive disorder.

History (continued)

He denies any recent events that could have caused him to feel this way, such as a recent death of a family member. He also denies drug and alcohol abuse. When asked, he states he doesn't have any medical history.	Before a patient can be diagnosed with depression, other causes of these symptoms need to be ruled out. Bereavement can cause symptoms similar to depression, as can drug and alcohol abuse. A medical condition, such as hypothyroidism, also can cause such symptoms.

Physical Exam

I take a quick set of vital signs and find them to be within normal limits. We then walk him out to the ambulance and seat him in the captain's chair in the back with his seat belt on.	We need to remove the patient from the crisis area, so we decide to head to the hospital. I can get the rest of the information I need en route to the ED.

Interventions

I talk to Sam in a quiet, nonthreatening tone. I start to ask some open-ended questions about what has been going on over the last 2 weeks. I do not interrupt him while he is speaking.	There isn't much I can do for Sam except to make him feel nonthreatened and cared for. By listening and paying attention, I show that I am not ignoring his problems.

Ongoing Assessment

Sam starts to open up and tells me that he has a history of depression, but this is the first time he has seen a doctor for it or has taken medication. He also tells me that he has never attempted suicide, although he has thought about it before. It scared him, because he has never come this close to actually trying to kill himself.	Since he has opened up and started talking to me, I don't want to interrupt him by taking another set of vital signs, although I normally would get a set en route to the hospital.

Communications and Written Report

Brandon is driving to the hospital and notifies them that we are en route with a quiet and cooperative patient who is feeling suicidal. He is instructed to take the patient to one of the three behavioral emergency rooms when we get there.	Many hospitals have BE rooms for psych patients. If a patient becomes violent or cannot be controlled, there isn't anything in the room that can cause harm to the patient or a staff member.
Upon arrival we walk Sam to BE 3 and give a report to the nurse and the social worker.	The social worker will talk with Sam and will determine the safest plan for him, whether that is admission to a psychiatric hospital or sending him home.

Follow-Up

I follow up the next day and find out that Sam was admitted to the psychiatric hospital for depression and suicidal thoughts.	I hope they get his medication under control and he starts to feel better. He is a nice man, and I hope everything works out well for him.

Student's Name _____

VAGINAL BLEEDING SCENARIO

Actions	Reasoning
Dispatch	
"Medic 12, respond to 5234 North Main Street, 5th floor, for an obstetrical emergency." It's 2:00 in the afternoon, and we just finished watching our daily soap when Trevor and I got dispatched to one of the office buildings downtown.	We sign on that we are en route to the scene, and dispatch tells us that we are responding to a 27-year-old who is having vaginal bleeding in her first trimester. This is good to know. We know we don't have an impending delivery, which, although it can be exciting, also can be very dangerous for the mother and the baby.
Scene Size-Up	
We pull up to the door and security is waiting for us, keeping the elevator clear. We get to the 5th floor and we are directed to the ladies' restroom, where several women are standing in the doorway. They clear out of the way, and we find the patient sitting on the bathroom counter, crying softly.	The scene is safe and well controlled. We have no difficulty getting upstairs or finding the patient.
Initial Assessment	
I approach the patient and introduce Trevor and myself. I do a quick pulse check and find it to be within normal limits. Her skin is warm and dry, and her color is good.	If she were having heavy vaginal bleeding, she would be in danger of going into hypovolemic shock. So far, she does not display any symptoms of shock.
History	
As Trevor takes her blood pressure, I try to find out more about what is going on. She tells me she is 6 weeks pregnant after trying to get pregnant for a year. She woke up with mild cramping this morning, which has gotten worse throughout the day. She came into the bathroom this afternoon and noted "a lot" of bleeding. The cramping has been continuing to get worse, and now she is starting to have a backache.	What our patient is describing are all signs and symptoms of spontaneous abortion, or miscarriage. If she has passed the fetus and placenta, this would be considered a complete abortion.
I ask her if she has noticed any clots or tissue, and she said she was too upset to notice.	If she hasn't passed tissue or only partially passed tissue, then this may be considered a threatened abortion; in some cases like this, the fetus can actually be saved. Or it could be an incomplete abortion, which may need surgery. Vaginal bleeding and cramping can also be signs of an ectopic pregnancy, in which the fertilized egg is implanted in the fallopian tube instead of the uterus. This is an obstetrical emergency and may require emergency surgery if the patient suffers a ruptured tube and is bleeding excessively.

©2009 Pearson Education, Inc.
Paramedic Care: Principles & Practice, Vol. 5, 3rd. Ed.

Physical Exam	
We assist the patient to the stretcher and place her in a position of comfort. I ask her if her pain feels like it is more on one side than the other, which she denies. I palpate her abdomen to see if I can localize the pain, but again she denies any sharp pain in the right or left lower quadrant.	Ectopic pregnancies most often present as abdominal pain, which then localizes in the affected lower quadrant of the abdomen. Syncope, vaginal bleeding, and shock can accompany the pain. Although she would need an ultrasound to rule it out, I am willing to bet that this is not an ectopic pregnancy.
We do a set of orthostatic vital signs to note changes in order to determine impending shock.	Her orthostatic vital signs remain within normal limits.

Interventions	
We head downstairs and place the patient in the ambulance. Trevor jumps up front to drive, and I get in the back. En route to the hospital I start an IV of normal saline at a KVO rate after drawing a set of blood samples.	The ED staff is going to run a set of basic blood work, and, because I started an IV, I drew the blood in order to avoid a second needle stick for the patient. I prefer to have the IV line in case the patient starts to bleed heavily and goes into shock.

Ongoing Assessment	
I repeat a set of vital signs every few minutes to monitor for blood loss. The patient does not report any changes in pain or bleeding.	Everything remains within normal limits en route to the ED. Transport remains uneventful.
The patient continues to cry softly and tells me how excited she was to be having a baby.	A miscarriage is a very sad occurrence for a patient to go through and requires emotional support during transport.

Communications and Written Report	
We alert the ER that we are coming and are told that Room 8, the pelvic room, is empty. We give a report to the nurse taking the patient and head to the EMS room to write the report.	This was a quick run and shouldn't require much time to write the report.

Follow-Up	
The ER doctor hasn't even seen the patient yet by the time we leave. She thanks us for our help, and we say goodbye.	I think about our patient later in the day and hope everything turned out all right for her.

SCENARIOS

SCENARIOS

Student's Name _____

PEDIATRIC SCENARIO

Actions	Reasoning
Dispatch	
At 1:13 A.M., my partner, Jim, and I are sleeping when our radio tones go off. "Medic 206, respond to Tree Top Trailer Park, Lot #3, for a pediatric respiratory arrest." I don't think either of us has ever moved any quicker to the ambulance as we sign on en route. I know this trailer park, which is right up the street.	A pediatric patient always gets my blood flowing, but a pediatric respiratory arrest is even worse. We ask the dispatcher if they have any more information for us, but we are told that the caller doesn't have a telephone and had gone to the end of the road to use a pay phone to call us.
Scene Size-Up	
We pull into the trailer park and find #3 in the front. There is a gentleman waiting for us, waving his arms up and down so we can see him. As we get out, we hear him telling us to hurry up, his baby isn't breathing. I grab our pediatric emergency bag as Jim grabs the oxygen and monitor. We leave the stretcher in the back for now.	The father is obviously frantic but does not appear to be any danger to us. The scene is not well lit, and we have to carefully watch where we are going so we don't fall.
Initial Assessment	
We get inside to find an approximately 10-month-old baby in his mother's arms, pinking and breathing on his own. Mom is crying and rocking the baby.	Immediately I can see that the baby is no longer in respiratory arrest. He has spontaneous respirations and good color.
History	
I try to calm the parents down so we can get some information. I ask what happened, and Dad tells me that they heard a funny noise coming from the crib and went in and found the baby blue, with his arms and legs jerking. He was making a "funny, gagging sound" and wasn't breathing.	It sounds like the parents are describing a seizure. When a patient has a seizure, he is unable to breathe, and babies tend to become cyanotic quickly. The "funny, gagging sound" could have been the baby's tongue causing an airway obstruction during the seizure.
Physical Exam	
I ask Mom to unwrap the baby so I can do a patient assessment. She tells me that she would prefer to keep him wrapped up because he feels very warm and is afraid he has a fever.	This is making more sense now. Febrile seizures are those seizures that occur as a result of a sudden increase in body temperature. They occur most commonly between the ages of 6 months and 6 years.

Physical Exam (continued)

I explain to the mother that it is really important that I take a good look at the baby. She unwraps him, and this wakes him up. He starts to cry a little and sounds irritable. I do a quick head-to-toe assessment. He has rhonchi throughout all lung fields.	I ask Mom if the baby has been sick, and she says he has had a cold for about 2 days. He started coughing before bedtime tonight. The irritable cry could be because he is postictal, or it could mean that he has a CNS infection.

Interventions

I explain to the parents that even though the baby is breathing now and appears to have had a febrile seizure, it is important to take him to the hospital to make sure there isn't anything else going on.	The parents agree that the baby needs to be seen. Mom asks to come with us, and Dad says he'll follow us in the car.
Before we leave for the ED, I ask Jim to give me a hand in the back starting an IV.	I need to have IV access in case the patient has another seizure and needs medication. I would also like to check a glucose level to make sure we aren't missing hypoglycemia.
I call medical direction and ask for an order to give Valium in case the patient has another seizure. I am told I can give 0.2 mg/kg every 2 to 5 minutes if the patient should seize again.	I don't want to have to take the time to call should the baby start to have another seizure.
I start some blow-by oxygen, as the patient still appears postictal.	
I take a set of vital signs on the patient and get a pulse rate of 180 and a respiratory rate of 66. We do not have a thermometer on the ambulance, but he is hot to the touch and his vital signs plus his medical history indicate that he has a fever.	I convince Mom to unwrap the baby, because keeping him wrapped up in the blanket does not allow him to cool off.

Ongoing Assessment

I monitor the patient's airway and color, which remain good.	The airway obstruction that his parents described may have been from his tongue during the seizure, but he also could have had a lot of mucus in his airway, because his lungs sound infected. I want to make sure he doesn't choke again.

Communications and Written Report

I had already notified the ED that we were coming when I called medical direction. They are waiting for us when we get there. We give a report and Mom walks toward an exam room with the nurse.	We sit down at the desk, and I start to write up the run sheet.

Follow-Up

It turns out the baby had a fever of 104.2°. He was doing much better after a little ibuprofen and was actually playful by the time we left the ED.	His fever got very high, quickly, which is what caused the seizure. He was like a new child after the fever reducer.

Chapter 7 Answer Key

Handout 7-3: Chapter 7 Quiz

1. D	5. B	9. B	13. C
2. B	6. A	10. C	14. B
3. A	7. C	11. D	15. C
4. C	8. D	12. B	

Handout 7-4: Chapter 7 Scenario

1. The questions should be broad and without preconception. Possible questions include the following:

   - Parents/guardians there or not?
   - Trauma to head, chest, abdomen, limbs?
   - Neurologic deficits, need for spinal immobilization?
   - Fractured ribs or extremity(ies)?
   - Internal bleeding?
   - Abrasions or other surface injuries?
   - Any significant underlying medical problems?

2. These impressions may overlap with those already given, but many will be more specific to the case of possibly severe trauma in a child:

   - Is airway open, and is patient breathing?
   - Has patient had loss of consciousness or altered mental status?
   - Possible head or spinal injury?
   - Possible chest or abdominal trauma?
   - Fracture or serious trauma to limbs?
   - Signs of internal or external hemorrhage?

3. There are no obvious signs of major trauma and the child is conscious and responding to his presence. Thoughts might include the following:

   - Did anyone talk to her after the accident, and has her apparent mental status changed since then?
   - Can she respond to basic questions I might ask, such as her name and whether anything hurts her?

4. Thoughts on the nature of injury and how to proceed:

   - Head injury is definitely possible. Should we immobilize her neck and possibly put her on a spine board before further examination?
   - Should we do a quick check for other signs of head injury, such as state of pupils or swelling or bruising of the head, or should we proceed with rapid assessment of the rest of her body?
   - When proper protective steps have been taken, should we position her or take other measures to protect the airway, especially if there is threat of vomiting?

5. Because of the cold environmental conditions and the child's anxiety, it is definitely time to move her to the ambulance and call medical direction to see whether she should be transported immediately or if it is acceptable to wait 5 minutes to see if the parents arrive.

6. Components of ongoing assessment should include the following:

   - Ongoing assessment of airway, breathing, and circulation. Look at least once for signs of cold injury to feet and hands.
   - Otherwise focus on vital signs and neurologic reassessment for mental status, other evidence of head injury.
   - If patient is able to talk without additional distress, ask for historical information on medications, allergies, chronic problems, or recent illness or accident.

Handout 7-5: Chapter 7 Review

1. differential diagnosis, narrowing process, field diagnosis
2. Assessment
3. reaching, completing (or synonyms)
4. obtains history, performs physical exam, presents patient, handles documentation, acts as EMS commander
5. provides scene cover, gathers scene information, talks to relatives/bystanders, obtains vital signs, performs interventions, acts as triage group leader
6. body language
7. standard precautions, scene safety, location of all patients, determination of mechanism of injury or nature of illness
8. forming a general impression, mental status assessment (AVPU), airway assessment, breathing assessment, circulation assessment, determining patient's priority for further on-scene care or immediate transport
9. trauma patient with a significant mechanism of injury or altered mental status, trauma patient with an isolated injury, medical patient who is responsive, medical patient who is unresponsive
10. mental status, airway/breathing/circulation, transport priorities, vital signs, focused assessment of any problem areas or conditions, effectiveness of interventions, management plans
11. life-threatening problems
12. worst-case scenario
13. subjective findings, objective findings, assessment, plan
14. communicate effectively
15. 1 minute

Ambulance Operations

INTRODUCTION

Most students readily identify medical knowledge and procedural skills as types of content to be mastered before they become proficient as paramedics. Far fewer think of knowledge about standards for ambulances and medical equipment or skills necessary to methodically check and restock an ambulance's equipment and supplies. Yet the ability of a paramedic to function safely and effectively in the field depends on proper ambulance operation. This chapter covers five related topics: ambulance standards, maintenance of ambulance equipment and supplies, ambulance stationing, safe ambulance operations, and utilization of air medical transport.

CHAPTER OBJECTIVES

Knowledge Objectives

1. Identify current local and state standards that influence ambulance design, equipment requirements, and staffing of ambulances. (pp. 337–339)
2. Identify the elements of a vehicle, equipment, and supply checklist. (pp. 339–341)
3. Describe the process for reporting vehicle or equipment problems/failure to the director of operations. (p. 339)
4. Identify the EMS equipment that needs routine service to ensure proper field operation. (pp. 340–341)
5. Discuss OSHA standards and other federal requirements for vehicle and equipment cleaning. (p. 340)
6. Discuss the importance of completing an ambulance equipment/supply checklist. (pp. 339–341)
7. Discuss factors used to determine ambulance stationing and staffing within a community. (pp. 341–342)
8. Describe the advantages and disadvantages of air medical transport. (p. 352)
9. Identify conditions/situations that merit air medical transport. (pp. 352, 353)
10. Discuss strategies to help ensure safe operation of ambulances when responding to or at an emergency. (pp. 342–360)

TOTAL TEACHING TIME
There is no specific time requirement for this topic in the National Standard Curriculum for Paramedic. Instructors should take into consideration such factors as: the pace at which students learn, the size of the class, and breaks. The actual time devoted to teaching objectives is the responsibility of the instructor.

FRAMING THE LESSON

You can use the following exercise to get students to recognize for themselves the critical importance of sound ambulance operation: Lay out a scenario for your students, perhaps a call for a middle-aged man with a suspected acute MI or a two-vehicle car collision. Have them brainstorm about the thought and action steps they take after they receive the call (this also reinforces the concepts they learned in the preceding lesson, Chapter 7). When someone makes initial mention of a piece of equipment (such as a cardiac monitor/defibrillator) or supplies (such as those necessary for standard precautions, or standard procedures) say, "Oh, that isn't working correctly" or "the only gloves are much too large for your hands" and view their reactions.

After students share their responses to the thought that needed equipment or supplies might be missing or nonfunctional, have them review the brief Case Study for this chapter to set the tone for the upcoming discussion.

CONSIDERING THE CASE STUDY

Ask a volunteer to read aloud the Case Study on text page 336. Suggest that students close their eyes as the scenario is read to help them mentally visualize the events described in it. You can use the following questions as a starting point for teaching the chapter—a sort of chapter preview in a functional setting.

When the chapter is completed, you may wish to return to the Case Study and encourage further discussion aimed at answering the questions or solving the problems.

CASE STUDY DISCUSSION QUESTIONS (AND ANSWERS)

1. What kinds of operations do you think should be done to check the function of your ambulance itself? Why?
   (The ambulance should have the same kinds of automotive maintenance done as is proper for any vehicle and on the schedule recommended by the manufacturer. In addition, it is important that lights, sirens, and other specialized equipment be checked and kept in good functional order. This is vital because the best medical skills possible aren't enough if the ambulance cannot safely and expediently get the paramedics to the scene and get the patient to the proper receiving facility.)
2. What kinds of procedures do you think should be done at the beginning of each shift? Why?
   (Before the first call, it is important to know that the vehicle is in sound running order, that all equipment has been checked per schedule to confirm it is functional, that all supplies are in place, and that the vehicle is clean and has been disinfected as necessary after the last call. This is done in part by personal inspection and in part by reliance on documentation of efforts taken by others in the department.)
3. What kinds of procedures do you think should be done after each call? Why?
   (It is best to restock supplies and disinfect immediately after return from a call because your memory is freshest about what needs to be done. If any equipment is reaching time for inspection, it is best to document that for the administrative staff as soon as you notice the expiration date on the equipment. In this way you are least likely to forget something that may later prove important.)

4. How heavily do you depend on the skill and integrity of other personnel in your EMS service to see that these things are done and documented properly? How heavily do others depend on you?

(You depend as heavily on others in your department, and they on you, as patients rely on you in the field. Competency and integrity in matters that are not directly related to patients are as important as field skills.)

TEACHING STRATEGIES

People learn in a variety of ways. Some do better with the spoken word, while others prefer the written. Some prefer to work alone, whereas others profit from working in groups. Recognizing these different ways of acquiring knowledge, the authors of this *Instructor's Resource Manual* have provided a variety of teaching strategies for the different types of learners. These strategies are intended to foster higher-level cognitive skills and encourage creative learning and problem solving.

For greatest effectiveness, incorporate these strategies into your class lecture. Marginal notes in the Teaching Outline indicate the points at which various exercises might be most appropriate. Other strategies can be used to preview the lesson or to summarize it.

The following strategies are keyed to specific sections of the lesson:

1. Recognizing State Codes. Since the book explains that the "State EMS Code" dictates the standards for most ambulances, obtain a copy of this code, or one provided by your county health department, for students to read. There is no better reinforcement to learning than real-world examples, especially when the text refers to one of these examples.

2. Designing an Ambulance. As a class, design a new ambulance. Include all the "wish list" items such as TV and DVD player but also help students create solutions to current vehicle problems such as inability to stand up inside the vehicle or sharps containers located in the wrong places. When you have the "ultimate" vehicle, have a draftsperson draw you one or make a model and keep it in the classroom as evidence of student creativity and ingenuity. This cooperative learning exercise builds teamwork and employs problem solving.

3. Thinking about Maintenance. To emphasize the importance of equipment maintenance and calibration, challenge students to implement a system for these activities in their service or your school. Be sure they obtain the manufacturers' recommendations for each piece of equipment to be included. This activity brings the classroom to the workplace and lends realism to your lecture.

4. Staff Planning. Arm students with the description of a community and vital call volume statistics. Have each small group create a system status and staffing plan for their community using a tabletop town or actual city map. Ask them to indicate how many ambulances should be on duty at any given time, create a shift schedule, establish acceptable response times, and post their units to accomplish this goal. This activity is kinesthetic and requires actual problem-solving skills. Additionally, it may lend some empathy for their dispatch and staffing personnel.

5. Thinking about Safety. Few things are as frightening to providers as the thought of causing an injury ourselves. To emphasize the importance of meticulous care when driving, obtain a dispatch audio of a collision involving the ambulance that caused injury to another human being. The reality of this mistake will leave a powerful impression for many years to come.

The following strategy relates to Special Features in the student textbook and can be used to enhance the student's understanding:

Patho Pearls: Rooting EMS Practice in Sound Science.   Contact your local air medical provider. Most are happy to bring their aircraft for a demonstration and discuss proper procedures for contacting, preparing the landing zone, and preparing the patient.

The following strategy can be used at various points throughout the lesson or to help summarize and demonstrate what students have learned:

Building Air Medical Awareness.   Ask any of your local air medical rescue crews to land at or near your school for a helicopter safety drill. This is a special situation that cannot be fully realized with lecture alone. Several factors make helicopter evacuations unique, including the loud noise, flying debris, danger of rotors, limited cargo space, expertise of staff, and so on. The students will remember this information much better by actually seeing the helicopter land and hearing the crew cover safety information.

TEACHING OUTLINE

Chapter 8 is the eighth lesson in Volume 5, *Special Considerations/Operations*. Distribute Handout 8-1 so that students can familiarize themselves with the learning goals for this chapter. If students have any questions about the objectives, answer them at this time.

Then present the chapter. One possible lecture outline follows. In the outline, the parenthetical references in regular type are references to text pages; those in bold type are to figures, tables, or procedures.

I. Introduction. Ambulance standards, maintenance of ambulance equipment and supplies, ambulance stationing, safe ambulance operations, and utilization of air medical transport are all core concepts for effective ambulance maintenance and operation. (p. 336)

II. Ambulance standards. (pp. 337–339)

A. Levels of oversight (p. 337)
    1. Federal (DOT)
    2. State
    3. Local
B. Ambulance design (pp. 337–338) (**Fig. 8-1**)
    1. Type I
        a. Conventional truck cab-chassis with a modular ambulance body
    2. Type II
        a. Standard van, forward control integral cab-body
    3. Type III
        a. Specialty van, forward control integral cab-body ambulance
C. Medical equipment standards (p. 338)
    1. OSHA
    2. NIOSH
    3. NFPA
D. Additional guidelines (p. 339)
    1. Commission on Accreditation of Ambulance Services (CAAS)

III. Checking ambulances: vehicle and equipment checklists. (pp. 339–341) (**Fig. 8-2**)

HANDOUT 8-1
Chapter 8 Objectives Checklist

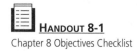
POWERPOINT
PRESENTATION
Volume 5, Chapter 8, PowerPoint slides 1–4

POWERPOINT
PRESENTATION
Volume 5, Chapter 8, PowerPoint slides 5–11

READING/REFERENCE
Dernocoeur, K., and D. M. Meade. "Patient Compartment Safety," *EMS*, Oct. 1999.

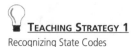
TEACHING STRATEGY 1
Recognizing State Codes

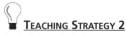
TEACHING STRATEGY 2
Designing an Ambulance

TEACHING STRATEGY 3
Thinking about Maintenance

TEACHING STRATEGY 4
Staff Planning

READING/REFERENCE
Burns, L. "So You Want to Drive an Ambulance?" *EMS*, Nov. 1999.

POWERPOINT
PRESENTATION
Volume 5, Chapter 8, PowerPoint slides 12–18

©2009 Pearson Education, Inc.
Paramedic Care: Principles & Practice, Vol. 5, 3rd. Ed.

IV. Ambulance deployment and staffing. (pp. 341–342)

A. Deployment factors (p. 341)
  1. Demographics
  2. Primary area of responsibility
B. Traffic congestion (pp. 341–342)
  1. System status management
    a. Response times of less than 4 minutes are associated with improved outcomes
  2. Tiered response system
C. Operational staffing (p. 342)

V. Safe ambulance operations. (pp. 342–350)

A. Educating providers (p. 343)
B. Reducing ambulance collisions (pp. 343–345) (**Fig. 8-3**)
C. Standard operating procedures (p. 345) (**Fig. 8-4**)
D. The due regard standard (pp. 345–346)
E. Lights and siren: A false sense of security (pp. 346–347)
F. Escorts and multivehicle responses (pp. 347–348)
G. Parking and loading the ambulance (p. 348) (**Fig. 8-5**)
H. The deadly intersection (pp. 348–350)

VI. Utilizing air medical transport. (pp. 350–357)

A. Fixed-wing aircraft (p. 351)
B. Rotorcraft (p. 351) (**Fig. 8-6**)
C. Advantages and disadvantages of air transport (p. 352)
D. Activation (p. 352)
E. Indications for helicopter transport (p. 352)
  1. Clinical criteria (**Table 8-1**)
  2. Mechanism of injury
  3. Difficult assessment situations
  4. Time/distance factors
F. Patient preparation and transfer (p. 354)
G. Scene safety and the landing zone (pp. 354–356) (**Fig. 8-7; Fig. 8-8**)
  1. Approximately 100 by 100 feet (about 30 large steps on each side)
  2. Situated on ground with less than an 8-degree slope

VII. Summary. It is important that paramedics be familiar with standards regarding ambulance operation, equipment, and staffing, as well as develop appreciation of the role of air medical transport. (p. 357)

YOU MAKE THE CALL

Review student responses to the You Make the Call scenario on text page 357. Suggested responses to the questions that follow the scenario are given below. Point out to students that these are acceptable answers but not necessarily the only ones. Discuss with students the pros and cons of points where their responses differ from these.

1. Should you drive down the open eastbound right lane with your lights and siren on? Explain.
   (No. It is strongly suggested that you do not pass other vehicles on the right with lights and siren because a motorist might hear the siren at the last minute and pull to the right, directly into your vehicle.)
2. Should you enter the oncoming traffic by going around the left side of the vehicle that is currently stopped in the left-hand, eastbound lane? Explain.
   (Yes, but be very careful. Slow down to a crawl and use lights and siren to alert all traffic as you approach.)

READING/REFERENCE
Fitch, J. "Strategic Deployment,"
JEMS, Feb. 2002.

TEACHING STRATEGY 5
Thinking about Safety

POWERPOINT
PRESENTATION
Volume 5, Chapter 8, PowerPoint
slides 19–32

POINT TO EMPHASIZE
As a general rule, do not rely solely
on lights and siren to alert other
motorists to your approach.

POWERPOINT
PRESENTATION
Volume 5, Chapter 8, PowerPoint
slides 33–44

POINT TO EMPHASIZE
Exercise extreme caution whenever
you approach an intersection.

POWERPOINT
PRESENTATION
Volume 5, Chapter 8, PowerPoint
slide 44

PATHO PEARLS
Rooting EMS Practice in Sound
Science

READING/REFERENCE
Davidoff, J. B. "Flying High: The Role
of Helicopters in EMS," *EMS*, Mar.
1999.

POINT TO EMPHASIZE
Stable patients who are accessible to
ground vehicles are best transported
by ground vehicles.

HANDOUT 8-7
Typical Unit Checklists

HANDOUT 8-8
Lights, Sirens, and Intersections

WORKBOOK
Chapter 8 Activities

READING/REFERENCE
Textbook Chapter 9, pp. 360–398

HANDOUT 8-2
Chapter 8 Quiz

HANDOUT 8-3
Chapter 8 Scenario

PARAMEDIC STUDENT CD
Student Activities

COMPANION WEBSITE
http://www.prenhall.com/bledsoe

TESTGEN
Volume 5, Chapter 8

**EMT ACHIEVE:
PARAMEDIC TEST PREPARATION**
Mistovich & Beasley. *EMT Achieve: Paramedic Test Preparation,* http://www.prenhall.com/emtachieve.

SUCCESS! FOR THE PARAMEDIC
Cherry. *SUCCESS! for the Paramedic,* 4th edition

HANDOUTS 8-4 TO 8-8
Reinforcement Activities

PARAMEDIC STUDENT CD
Student Activities

POWERPOINT PRESENTATION
Volume 5

3. How can you best deal with this very dangerous intersection? (*Avoid the intersection, if possible. If it is not possible, enter each lane slowly, making eye contact with all drivers. Use your lights and siren as suggested in this chapter. Remember—most ambulance collisions take place in intersections. So be very careful in all such situations.*)

ASSIGNMENTS

Assign students to complete Chapter 8 of the Workbook. Also assign them to read Chapter 9, "Medical Incident Management," of the textbook before the next class.

EVALUATION

Chapter Quiz and Scenario Distribute copies of the Chapter Quiz provided in Handout 8-2 to evaluate student understanding of this chapter. Make sure each student reads the scenario to reinforce critical thinking on the scene. Remind students not to use their notes or textbooks while taking the quiz.

Student CD Quizzes for every chapter are contained on the dynamic and highly visual in-text student CD.

Companion Website Additional quizzes for every chapter are contained on this exciting website.

TestGen You may wish to create a custom-tailored test using *Prentice Hall TestGen for Paramedic Care: Principles & Practice,* 3rd edition, to evaluate student understanding of this chapter.

Online Test Preparation (for students and instructors) Additional test preparation is available through Brady's new online product, EMT Achieve: Paramedic Test Preparation, at *http://www.prenhall.com/emtachieve.* Instructors can also monitor student mastery online.

Success! for the Paramedic Keyed to *Paramedic Care: Principles & Practice* and *Essentials of Paramedic Care,* this comprehensive exam review contains hundreds of test questions and rationales.

REINFORCEMENT

Handouts If classroom discussion or performance on the quiz indicates that some students have not fully mastered the chapter content, you may wish to assign some or all of the Reinforcement Handouts for this chapter.

Student CD (for students) A wide variety of material on this CD-ROM will reinforce and also expand student knowledge and skills.

PowerPoint Presentation (for instructors) The PowerPoint material developed for this chapter offers useful reinforcement of chapter content.

Companion Website (for students) Additional review quizzes and links to EMS resources will contribute to further reinforcement of the chapter.

OneKey   Online support is offered for this course on one of three platforms: CourseCompass, Blackboard, or WebCT. Includes the IRM, PowerPoints, Test Manager, and Companion Website for instruction. Ask your local sales representative for more information.

Brady Skills Series: Advanced Life Skills (Video or CD)   Have your students watch the skills come to life on VHS or CD-ROM, or they can purchase the highly visual, full-color text with step-by-step procedures with rationales.

Paramedic National Standards Self-Test   Another comprehensive review manual containing hundreds of review questions with page references keyed to several Brady texts.

COMPANION WEBSITE
http://www.prenhall.com/bledsoe

ONEKEY
Volume 5, Chapter 8

ADVANCED LIFE SUPPORT SKILLS
Larmon & Davis. *Advanced Life Support Skills*

ADVANCED LIFE SKILLS REVIEW
Larmon & Davis. *Advanced Life Skills Review*

BRADY SKILLS SERIES: ALS
Larmon & Davis. *Brady Skills Series: ALS*

PARAMEDIC NATIONAL STANDARDS SELF-TEST
Miller. *Paramedic National Standards Self-Test,* 5th edition

CHAPTER 8 OBJECTIVES CHECKLIST

Knowledge Objective	Date Mastered
1. Identify current local and state standards that influence ambulance design, equipment requirements, and staffing of ambulances.	
2. Identify the elements of a vehicle, equipment, and supply checklist.	
3. Describe the process for reporting vehicle or equipment problems/ failure to the director of operations.	
4. Identify the EMS equipment that needs routine service to ensure proper field operation.	
5. Discuss OSHA standards and other federal requirements for vehicle and equipment cleaning.	
6. Discuss the importance of completing an ambulance equipment/ supply checklist.	
7. Discuss factors used to determine ambulance stationing and staffing within a community.	
8. Describe the advantages and disadvantages of air medical transport.	
9. Identify conditions/situations that merit air medical transport.	
10. Discuss strategies to help ensure safe operation of ambulances when responding to or at an emergency.	

 ©2009 Pearson Education, Inc. *Paramedic Care: Principles & Practice, Vol. 5, 3rd. Ed.*

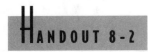

CHAPTER 8 QUIZ

Write the letter of the best answer in the space provided.

_____ 1. The plan used by an EMS agency to maneuver its ambulances and crews in an effort to reduce response times is called:
   A. use strategy.
   B. operational strategy.
   C. deployment strategy.
   D. staffing/stationing strategy.

_____ 2. Oversight for EMS services is usually handled at which level?
   A. federal government
   B. state government
   C. regional level
   D. local level

_____ 3. The agency charged with worker safety is abbreviated as:
   A. OSHA.
   B. NIOSH.
   C. NFPA.
   D. CAAS.

_____ 4. Deployment factors commonly considered by an EMS agency include all of the following, EXCEPT:
   A. location of hospitals.
   B. location of possible facilities to house ambulances.
   C. safety of neighborhood with possible housing facility.
   D. local geographic and traffic considerations.

_____ 5. Analysis of collision data indicates that almost three-quarters of ambulance collisions take place:
   A. at dusk or after dark.
   B. in inclement weather.
   C. during daylight hours.
   D. at intersections.

_____ 6. Steps to reduce ambulance collisions commonly include all of the following EXCEPT:
   A. hands-on driver training with experienced field officers.
   B. ordering paramedics to report all personal citations or accidents.
   C. use of slow-speed vehicle operations course.
   D. demonstrated knowledge of primary and backup routes to hospitals.

_____ 7. Ambulances are rarely, if ever, legally exempted from:
   A. operating during night hours with lights and siren.
   B. highway speed limits.
   C. following posted directions of travel.
   D. passing a school bus with flashing lights.

_____ 8. Common guidelines for siren use include all of the following EXCEPT:
   A. using the siren as a standard warning device during daylight hours.
   B. assuming that some motorists will hear the siren but ignore it.
   C. being prepared for erratic maneuvers from some drivers who hear the siren.
   D. never assuming all motorists will hear the siren.

_____ 9. Fixed-wing aircraft are generally employed:
   A. in areas with regional airports and landing sites.
   B. in weather conditions that make helicopter flight unsafe.
   C. whenever helicopters are unavailable.
   D. when transport distances exceed 100 miles.

_____ **10.** Indications for patient transport by helicopter include all of the following EXCEPT:
  A. certain clinical criteria relating to trauma score, crush injury, major burns, and so on.
  B. trauma team preference for the receiving facility.
  C. situations that are difficult for ground transportation.
  D. transport time to a trauma center greater than 15 minutes by a ground ambulance.

_____ **11.** When you are first to arrive at the scene of a motor vehicle collision, park the ambulance, if possible, upwind and uphill from the wreckage by:
  A. 50 feet.   **C.** 200 feet.
  B. 100 feet.   **D.** 250 feet.

_____ **12.** If the scene of a motor vehicle crash has been secured when you arrive, you should park the ambulance:
  A. next to the wreckage.   **C.** in front of the wreckage.
  B. behind the wreckage.   **D.** behind a police vehicle.

_____ **13.** An organization that allows multiple vehicles to arrive at an EMS call at different times, often providing different levels of care or transport, is:
  A. system status management.   **C.** PAR.
  B. reserve capacity.   **D.** a tiered response system.

_____ **14.** A situation likely to require patient transport by helicopter is a:
  A. multivehicle crash.   **C.** wilderness rescue.
  B. hazardous materials incident. **D.** multialarm fire.

_____ **15.** The landing zone for a helicopter should be:
  A. 25 by 25 feet.   **C.** 75 by 75 feet.
  B. 50 by 50 feet.   **D.** 100 by 100 feet.

©2009 Pearson Education, Inc.
Paramedic Care: Principles & Practice, Vol. 5, 3rd. Ed.

Student's Name _____

CHAPTER 8 SCENARIO

Review the following real-life situation. Then answer the questions that follow.

Your unit has been based for several years at a fire station in a residential section of the city. Because recent development has significantly increased the number of homes in your area and has expanded the residential neighborhood into the adjacent foothills, your area of responsibility has grown much larger. This winter has been hard, with frequent snow that has accumulated on the shoulders of roads and made some of the outlying, previously country roads very difficult to negotiate, particularly those running to a recreational area at the edge of your sector. Your unit is a type II van ambulance.

    You have an in-service meeting coming up with your city administrator, and you and the other ambulance crews that staff your unit would like to present your concerns regarding the difficulty of using your ambulance on the outlying roads and your concerns about the large geographic area you cover.

1. What, if any, suggestions might you make regarding the matching of ambulance type with the roads of your expanded area of operation?

2. You have heard that the EMS administration is considering a review of deployment over the city as a whole based on growth in city size and population over the last decade. To make your input as useful as possible, what should you consider about the peak loads in your sector and how that might affect citywide deployment plans?

Student's Name _____

CHAPTER 8 REVIEW

Write the word or words that best complete each sentence in the space(s) provided.

1. Most state regulations set _____ standards rather than a(n) _____ standard for operation.

2. _____ is an organization that makes the work environment safer by ensuring mechanical maintenance and the availability of personal protection equipment.

3. _____ _____ on medications should be checked each shift, and the older, in-date drugs marked appropriately so they are used first.

4. Ideal deployment decisions take into account two sets of data: past _____ _____ and projected _____ _____.

5. The highest volume of calls, or _____ _____, should be expressed in terms of day or week and time of day.

6. When vehicles are positioned for calls in specific high-volume areas, the crew's location is known as their _____ _____ of _____ (_____).

7. In _____ _____ management, a computerized personnel and ambulance deployment system enables the EMS service to meet service demands with fewer resources and still ensure appropriate response time and vehicle location.

8. Communities that have several levels of response, from designated first responders to backup ALS units, are said to have a(n) _____ _____ system.

9. A number of backup accidents could be avoided by use of a(n) _____.

10. The situation in which it is most likely that a police escort is appropriate for an ambulance is when the ambulance is operating in _____ _____ and needs to be guided to the scene or the hospital.

11. If your ambulance is the first vehicle on the scene of an auto collision, park _____ _____ _____ the wreckage so your warning lights alert approaching motorists.

12. Exercise _____ _____ whenever you approach an intersection.

13. For a helicopter program to be effective, the frontline first responders must consider _____ as early as possible.

14. A standard van with a forward control integral cab-body is called a(n) _____ _____ ambulance.

15. Flight crews suggest that EMS crews mark the landing zone with a single _____ in the _____ position.

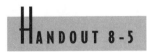

Student's Name _____

AMBULANCE OPERATIONS TRUE OR FALSE

Indicate whether the following statements are true or false by writing T or F in the space provided.

_____ 1. The days of "blowing through" intersections at high speed with lights and sirens engaged have passed.

_____ 2. Routine, detailed shift checks of ambulances are insufficient to minimize issues associated with risk management.

_____ 3. OSHA has helped to ensure there are equipment lists calling for disinfecting agents, sharps containers, red bags, HEPA masks, and personal protective equipment.

_____ 4. In general, ambulance staffing takes into account ample coverage for peak load times as well as the need for reserve capacity.

_____ 5. The New York State data on ambulance collisions included reportable collisions and crashes occurring while the ambulance was backing up.

_____ 6. The legal standard for drivers of ambulances is based on the concept of due regard.

_____ 7. As a general rule, do not rely solely on lights and siren to alert other motorists to your approach.

_____ 8. Recent data have indicated that lights/siren use shaves roughly a minute from response time, but significantly increases the possibility of injury to the responding crew.

_____ 9. The most important point in ambulance lighting is visibility: The ambulance must be clearly visible from 360 degrees to all other motorists as well as pedestrians.

_____ 10. Stable patients who are accessible to ground vehicles are best transported by ground vehicles.

_____ 11. You should consider air medical transport for any patient who has a Glasgow coma scale score of less than 12.

_____ 12. Most EMS agencies no longer suggest the use of a police escort for ambulances.

_____ 13. If your ambulance is the first vehicle on the emergency scene of a motor vehicle collision, make sure that you park in back of the wreckage.

_____ 14. Always go around cars stopped at an intersection on their left (driver's) side.

_____ 15. In general, a helicopter requires a landing zone of 75 by 75 feet.

Student's Name _____

AMBULANCE OPERATIONS ABBREVIATIONS

Fill in the words for each abbreviation used in the chapter.

1. DOT _____

2. FCC _____

3. OSHA _____

4. NIOSH _____

5. NFPA _____

6. CAAS _____

7. ACS _____

8. SOPs _____

9. AED _____

10. SSM _____

11. CAAMS _____

12. LZ _____

13. PAR _____

14. FAA _____

©2009 Pearson Education, Inc.
Paramedic Care: Principles & Practice, Vol. 5, 3rd. Ed.

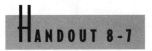

TYPICAL UNIT CHECKLISTS

The components of a typical vehicle/equipment checklist include the following:

- Patient infection control, comfort, and protection supplies
- Initial and focused assessment equipment
- Equipment for the transfer of the patient
- Equipment for airway maintenance, ventilation, and resuscitation
- Oxygen therapy and suction equipment
- Equipment for assisting with cardiac resuscitation
- Supplies and equipment for immobilization of suspected bone injuries
- Supplies for wound care and treatment of shock
- Supplies for childbirth
- Supplies, equipment, and medications for the treatment of acute poisonings, snakebite, chemical burns, and diabetic emergencies
- Advanced Life Support equipment, medications, and supplies
- Safety and miscellaneous equipment
- Information on the operation and inspection of the ambulance itself

Equipment items that should be checked regularly include the following:

- Automated external defibrillator (AED)
- Glucometer
- Cardiac monitor
- Oxygen systems
- Automated transport ventilator (ATV)
- Pulse oximeter
- Suction units
- Laryngoscope blades
- Lighted stylets
- Penlights
- Any other battery-operated equipment

Student's Name _____

REINFORCEMENT

LIGHTS, SIRENS, AND INTERSECTIONS

GUIDELINES ON USE OF LIGHTS AND SIREN

Consider the following before turning on the siren:

- Motorists are less inclined to yield to an ambulance when the siren is continually sounded.
- Many motorists feel that the right-of-way privileges given to ambulances are abused when sirens are sounded.
- Inexperienced motorists tend to increase their driving speeds by 10 to 15 miles per hour when a siren is sounded.
- The continuous sound of a siren can possibly worsen sick or injured patients by increasing their anxiety.
- Ambulance operators may also develop anxiety from sirens used on long runs, not to mention the possibility of hearing problems.

Some useful guidelines on use of sirens include the following:

- Use the siren sparingly and only when you must.
- Never assume all motorists hear your siren.
- Assume that some motorists will hear your siren, but choose to ignore it.
- Be prepared for panic and erratic maneuvers when drivers do hear your siren.
- Never use the siren to scare someone.

INTERSECTIONS

Helpful tips for negotiating an intersection include the following:

- Stop at all red lights and stop signs and then proceed with caution.
- Always proceed through an intersection slowly.
- Make eye contact with other motorists to ensure they understand your intentions.
- If you are using any of the exemptions offered to you as an emergency vehicle, such as passing through a red light or a stop sign, make sure you warn motorists by appropriately flashing your lights and sounding the siren.
- Remember that lights and siren only "ask" the public to yield the right of way. If the public does not yield, it may be because they misunderstand your intentions, cannot hear the siren because of noise in their own vehicles, or cannot see your lights. Never assume that other motorists have a clue as to what you plan on doing at the intersection.
- Always go around cars stopped at the intersection on their left (driver's) side. In some instances, this may involve passing into the oncoming lane, which should be done slowly and very cautiously. You invite trouble when you use a clear right lane to sneak past a group of cars at an intersection. If motorists are doing what they should do under motor vehicle laws, they may pull into the right lane just as you attempt to pass.

- Know how long it takes for your ambulance to cross an intersection. This will help you judge whether you have enough time to pass through safely.

- Watch pedestrians at an intersection carefully. If they all seem to be staring in another direction, rather than at your ambulance, they may well be looking at the fire truck headed your way.

- Remember that there is no such thing as a rolling stop in an ambulance weighing over 10,000 pounds or a medium-duty vehicle weighing some 24,000 pounds. Even at speeds as slow as 30 miles per hour, these vehicles will not stop on a dime. When negotiating an intersection, consider "covering the brake" to shorten the stopping distance.

©2009 Pearson Education, Inc.
Paramedic Care: Principles & Practice, Vol. 5, 3rd. Ed.

REINFORCEMENT

Chapter 8 Answer Key

Handout 8-2: Chapter 8 Quiz

1. C	**4.** C	**7.** D	**10.** B	**13.** D
2. B	**5.** D	**8.** A	**11.** B	**14.** C
3. A	**6.** B	**9.** D	**12.** C	**15.** D

Handout 8-3: Chapter 8 Scenario

1. Your unit is not built for rough roads. If a significant proportion of your current area is in the foothills and supplied by rough roads, perhaps a medium-duty ambulance or other vehicle type would be a better match for this sector.

2. Your operations area is almost entirely residential, which means you have a lower volume of people in that area during working hours on weekdays. Because people are home evenings and on weekends and your area abuts a recreational area, your peak times are weekday evenings and weekends. If deployment plans are being reviewed, that information may be helpful to the administrators. They can actually look at the records of number of calls in your area to confirm peak times and compare your peak times with those for sections of the city that are primarily business or industrial. If necessary, the administration could consider shifting your primary area of responsibility during business hours on weekdays to include some business/industrial areas. Another possibility might be to collaborate with the agency that covers the recreational area itself to see if a heavier-duty ambulance might cover the most difficult roads, at least in winter.

Handout 8-4: Chapter 8 Review

1. minimum, gold
2. OSHA (Occupational Safety and Health Administration)
3. Expiration dates
4. community responses, demographic changes
5. peak load
6. primary area of responsibility (PAR)
7. system status
8. tiered response
9. spotter
10. unfamiliar territory
11. in front of
12. extreme caution
13. Medevac
14. Type II
15. flare, upwind

Handout 8-5: Ambulance Operations True or False

1. T	**4.** T	**7.** T	**10.** T	**13.** F
2. F	**5.** F	**8.** F	**11.** F	**14.** T
3. T	**6.** T	**9.** T	**12.** T	**15.** F

Handout 8-6: Ambulance Operations Abbreviations

1. Department of Transportation
2. Federal Communications Commission
3. Occupational Safety and Health Administration
4. National Institute for Occupational Safety and Health
5. National Fire Protection Association
6. Commission on Accreditation of Ambulance Services
7. American College of Surgeons
8. standard operating procedures
9. automated external defibrillator
10. system status management
11. Commission on Accreditation of Air Medical Services
12. landing zone
13. primary area of responsibility
14. Federal Aviation Agency

©2009 Pearson Education, Inc.
Paramedic Care: Principles & Practice, Vol. 5, 3rd. Ed.

Chapter 9

Medical Incident Management

INTRODUCTION

In almost all of the material your students have read so far, the emphasis has been on the relationship between one or two EMS providers and a single patient. This chapter deals with incidents that involve multiple patients. Situations that your students may see frequently range from multiple-vehicle accidents to home fires to scenes of domestic or other violence. Less frequent incidents such as chain-reaction vehicular collisions, bus or train crashes, and natural disasters can be much more complicated and involve many more patients. Efficient responses in cases involving multiple patients depend on the skills and discipline your students will learn from this chapter and other training materials and exercises. Because EMS providers almost always interact in the larger situations with police and firefighters, and possibly even disaster officials, this chapter introduces them to the logistics of working with other types of emergency personnel.

CHAPTER OBJECTIVES

Knowledge Objectives

1. Explain the need for the Incident Management System (IMS)/Incident Command System (ICS) in managing emergency medical services (EMS) incidents. (pp. 366–369)
2. Describe the functional components (Command, Finance/Administration, Logistics, Operations, and Planning/Intelligence) of the Incident Management System. (pp. 369–378)
3. Differentiate between singular and unified command and identify when each is most applicable. (pp. 371–372)
4. Describe the role of Command, the need for proper command transfer, and procedures for transferring it. (pp. 369, 373–375)
5. List and describe the functions of the following groups and leaders in the IMS as it pertains to EMS incidents:

   a. Safety Officer (p. 376)
   b. Logistics Section (p. 378)
   c. Rehabilitation (REHAB) (p. 390)
   d. Staging Area (p. 388)
   e. Treatment Unit or Branch (pp. 386–387)

TOTAL TEACHING TIME: 8.17 HOURS

The total teaching time is only a guideline based on the didactic and practical lab averages in the National Standard Curriculum. Instructors should take into consideration such factors as: the pace at which students learn, the size of the class, and breaks. The actual time devoted to teaching objectives is the responsibility of the instructor.

    f. Triage Unit or Branch (pp. 380–386)
    g. Transportation Unit or Branch (pp. 388–389)
    h. Extrication/Rescue Unit or Branch (p. 389)
    i. Disposition of Deceased (Morgue Unit) (p. 386)
    j. Communications Unit (pp. 373, 390)

6. Describe the methods and rationale for identifying specific functions and leaders for the functions in an IMS. (pp. 369–391)

7. Describe essential elements of the scene size-up when arriving at a potential mass/multiple-casualty incident (MCI). (pp. 370–371)

8. Define the terms *Mass/Multiple-Casualty Incident (MCI)*, *disaster management*, *open or uncontained incident*, and *closed or contained incident*. (pp. 364, 371, 391)

9. Describe the role of the paramedics and EMS system in planning for MCIs and disasters. (pp. 366–369, 378, 391)

10. Explain the local/regional threshold for establishing Command and implementation of an Incident Management System, including MCI declaration. (pp. 364–365, 369)

11. Describe the role of both Incident Command Posts and Mutual Aid Coordination Centers (MACCs) in MCI and disaster management. (pp. 368, 369, 373–374, 391)

12. Describe the role of the on-scene physician at Mass/Multiple-Casualty Incidents. (p. 387)

13. Define *triage* and describe the principles of triage. (pp. 380–386)

14. Describe the START (simple triage and rapid transport) and JumpSTART (START for pediatric patients) methods of initial triage. (pp. 380–384)

15. Given color-coded tags and numerical priorities, assign the following terms to each:

    a. Immediate
    b. Delayed
    c. Minimal
    d. Expectant (pp. 380–385)

16. Define primary, secondary, and ongoing triage and their implementation techniques. (pp. 380–385)

17. Describe techniques used to allocate patients to hospitals and track them. (pp. 388–389)

18. Describe the techniques used in tracking patients during mass/multiple-casualty incidents and the need for such techniques. (pp. 384–385, 388–389)

19. Describe modifications of telecommunications procedures during mass/multiple-casualty incidents. (pp. 373, 390)

20. List and describe the essential equipment to provide logistical support to MCI operations to include:

    a. Airway, respiratory, and hemorrhage control
    b. Burn management
    a. Patient packaging/immobilization (p. 387)

21. Describe the role of mental health support in MCIs. (pp. 377, 390, 393–394)

22. Describe the role of the following exercises in preparation for MCIs:

    a. Tabletop exercises
    b. Small and large MCI drills (pp. 392–393)

Skill Objective

23. Given several incident scenarios with preprogrammed patients, provide the appropriate triage, treatment, and transport options for MCI operations based on local resources and protocols. (pp. 364–394)

FRAMING THE LESSON

Select a variety of photos of mass/multiple-casualty incidents and disasters. If possible, have at least some of them represent local events. Have the students look at the photos, consider the cases (such as chain-reaction vehicular collisions, fire in a hospital or school, earthquake, tornado, or even mass shooting or bombing), and think about the following issues that are critical to medical incident command:

- The complexities of responding as EMS providers to situations in which there are many patients scattered over the scene and patients range from the slightly physically injured to the dying or deceased
- The need to collaborate efficiently with firefighters, police, or other officials
- The problems that operating in an unsafe or hazardous environment may present

CONSIDERING THE CASE STUDY

Ask a volunteer to read aloud the Case Study that begins on text page 362. Suggest that students close their eyes as the scenario is read to help them mentally visualize the events described in it. You can use the following questions as a starting point for teaching the chapter—a sort of chapter preview in a functional setting.

When the chapter is completed, you may wish to return to the Case Study and encourage further discussion aimed at answering the questions or solving the problems.

CASE STUDY DISCUSSION QUESTIONS (AND ANSWERS)

1. What is the Incident Commander looking for during the perimeter walk?
   (A 360-degree perimeter walk of the scene is conducted to assess the entire area, surveying for hazards to responders, rescue problems, and locations for the future staging of incoming resources.)
2. What are the initial duties of the Triage Officer?
   (After donning appropriate personal protective equipment [PPE], the Triage Officer obtains a patient count, then, using a tool such as START or JumpSTART, quickly moves from patient to patient, conducting a rapid assessment and triage tagging of each patient.)
3. What is a Mutual Aid Coordination Center (MACC)?
   (Key elements in the management of any incident that spans jurisdictions are the Mutual Aid Coordination Centers [MACCs], formerly referred to as Emergency Operations Centers (EOCs). The MACC is a site from which civil government officials [e.g., municipal, county, state, and/or federal] exercise direction and control in an emergency or disaster. Where possible, the MACC should be located in a secure and protected location.)

4. What are the roles of the Safety Officer, Treatment Group Supervisor, and Transportation Unit Leader?

(The Safety Officer monitors all on-scene actions and ensures that they do not create any potentially harmful conditions. The Safety Officer has the authority to stop any action that is deemed an immediate life threat with no further action needed.

The Treatment Group Supervisor controls all actions in the Treatment Group/Sector. As patients arrive in the treatment area, the Treatment Group Supervisor should conduct or oversee secondary triage to determine if their status has changed. Patients should then be separated into functional treatment areas based on their category: red [immediate, P-1], yellow [delayed, P-2], or green [minimal, P-3].

The Transportation Unit Supervisor coordinates operations with the Staging Officer and the Treatment Supervisor. His job is to get patients into the ambulances and routed to hospitals.)

TEACHING STRATEGIES

People learn in a variety of ways. Some do better with the spoken word, while others prefer the written. Some prefer to work alone, whereas others profit from working in groups. Recognizing these different ways of acquiring knowledge, the authors of this *Instructor's Resource Manual* have provided a variety of teaching strategies for the different types of learners. These strategies are intended to foster higher-level cognitive skills and encourage creative learning and problem solving.

For greatest effectiveness, incorporate these strategies into your class lecture. Marginal notes in the Teaching Outline indicate the points at which various exercises might be most appropriate. Other strategies can be used to preview the lesson or to summarize it.

The following strategies are keyed to specific sections of the lesson:

1. Fire Service Guest Speaker. Most classes would be served well by inviting a fire official to teach the concept of Incident Command. The fire department has been using this system of incident management on every call for many years, whereas EMS has really just begun using Incident Command. Often, inviting an expert in a subject attracts the students' attention for a subject they might otherwise see as boring.

2. Reviewing Command Structures. To emphasize the difference between unified and singular command, have students report on a notable incident of each type cited in the media or from your local area. Ask them to compare and contrast the types of incident and the manner in which they were handled. This activity reinforces research and oral presentation skills while clarifying these concepts.

3. Recognizing Roles in MCIs. Describe different activities involved in an MCI and have students identify which officer would be responsible for handling each task. If possible, identify titles ahead of time and have students role-play the situation so that they actually have a chance to act in the assigned role. This kinesthetic activity helps students perform behaviors required of the assigned role, improving the likelihood of responding correctly in the future.

4. Triage Practice. Create packages of paper-doll patients to be triaged by students. If possible, color in the injuries on one side of the doll and describe their situation on the back. For the less artistically inclined, make the doll a silhouette of color construction paper and describe the patient's condition on the back. Have students triage their victims using the START triage system.

5. Recognizing Disaster Management Factors. Place the names of several potential disasters on strips of paper and place them in a hat. Have small groups of students draw a disaster and identify mitigating factors for their chosen disaster. If these factors do not exist in your community, brainstorm solutions and share important ideas with people who can make a difference, in the form of a letter to your councilperson, fire chief, city planner, and so on. This activity lends realism to the disaster management concepts and promotes community activism.

The following strategy relates to Special Features in the student textbook and can be used to enhance the student's understanding:

Legal Notes: National Incident Management System (NIMS). Have the students do a Web search for information on NIMS. Sites might include the U.S. Department of Homeland Security, U.S. Fire Administration, and Federal Emergency Management Agency. Students can do a report, either for the instructor or presented to the class.

The following strategies can be used at various points throughout the lesson or to help summarize and demonstrate what students have learned:

Reviewing MCIs. Retrieve records of MCIs handled locally or regionally or create one or more scenarios. Discuss them with the students after you teach the lesson, asking them about their roles as paramedics, as well as the overall roles of other emergency personnel at the scene. Get them to synthesize the material taught in the chapter as they discuss triage and rescue, treatment and transport, and so on. Make sure they know the proper names of the different roles involved, because they will need to know them in the case of an actual MCI emergency.

Field Trips. If an MCI occurred locally and the scene conveys some sense of what the incident was like (perhaps a local stretch of highway where a chain reaction occurred in blizzard conditions), visit the scene. Discuss how EMS and other types of personnel would have covered the scene, negotiated any hazards, and fulfilled their roles as part of the overall incident team.

Participating in MCI Drills. Nearly every health department in the United States requires at least annual mass/multiple-casualty drills. Obtain the schedule and have your class included. When possible, have them integrated into the responding unit crews. If it is not possible for students to play patient care roles, be sure they are included as victims. Even observing a large-scale drill will be educational. Asking to participate in an already scheduled drill will save you the enormous effort required to stage a drill of your own. Additionally, students will have an opportunity to work side by side with professionals in their chosen field during the drill.

TEACHING OUTLINE

Chapter 9 is the ninth lesson in Volume 5, *Special Considerations/Operations.* Distribute Handout 9-1. If students have any questions about the objectives, answer them at this time.

Then present the chapter. One possible lecture outline follows. In the outline, the parenthetical references in regular type are references to text pages; those in bold type are to figures, tables, or procedures.

I. Introduction. As a paramedic, you will be involved in a wide variety of responses, including single-patient incidents, such as a cardiac patient or simple trauma patient; small-scale multiple-patient incidents, such as motor vehicle crashes, house fires, or gang activity; and large-scale mass/multiple-casualty incidents (MCIs), such as airplane crashes and natural disasters. (pp. 364–365)

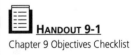
HANDOUT 9-1
Chapter 9 Objectives Checklist

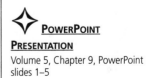
POWERPOINT PRESENTATION
Volume 5, Chapter 9, PowerPoint slides 1–5

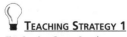

II. Origins of emergency incident management. (pp. 366–369) (Fig. 9-1; Fig. 9-2; Fig. 9-3; Fig. 9-4; Fig. 9-5)

   A. Evolution of the Incident Management System (IMS) from various earlier versions of Incident Command Systems (ICSs) (p. 366)
   B. National Incident Management System (NIMS) (p. 366)
   C. Regulations and standards (pp. 366–368)
   D. A uniform, flexible system (C-FLOP) (pp. 368–369)
      1. Mutual Aid Coordination Centers (MACCs)
      2. C-FLOP
         a. C—Command
         b. F—Finance/Administration
         c. L—Logistics
         d. O—Operations
         e. P—Planning

III. Command. (pp. 369–375)

   A. Concept of command as most important functional area (p. 369)
   B. Span of control
   C. Establishing command (p. 369) **(Fig. 9-6)**
   D. Incident size-up (pp. 370–371)
      1. Life safety
      2. Incident stabilization
         a. Open incident
         b. Closed incident
      3. Property conservation
   E. Singular vs. unified command (pp. 371–372)
   F. Identifying a staging area (p. 372)
   G. Incident communications (p. 373)
   H. Resource utilization (p. 373)
   I. Command procedures (pp. 373–375) **(Fig. 9-7; Fig. 9-8)**
   J. Termination of command (p. 375)

IV. Support of Incident Command. (pp. 375–378) **(Fig. 9-9)**

   A. Command staff (pp. 376–377)
      1. Safety Officer (SO)
      2. Liaison Officer (LO)
      3. Information Officer (IO)
      4. Mental health support
         a. Small incidents
         b. Major incidents/disasters
   B. Finance/Administration (pp. 377–378)
   C. Logistics (p. 378)
   D. Operations (p. 378)
   E. Planning/Intelligence (p. 378)
      1. Incident Action Plan (IAP)

V. Division of functions. (pp. 378–380)

   A. Branches (p. 379) **(Fig. 9-10)**
      1. Branch Director
   B. Groups and divisions (p. 380)
      1. Supervisor
   C. Units (p. 380)
      1. Unit Leader
   D. Sectors (p. 380)
      1. Sector Officer

VI. Functional groups within an EMS branch. (pp. 380–391) **(Fig. 9-9)**

A. Triage (pp. 380–386)
   1. Primary triage
   2. Secondary triage
   3. The START system **(Fig. 9-11)**
      a. Ability to walk
      b. Respiratory effort
      c. Pulse/perfusion
      d. Neurologic status
   4. The JumpSTART system **(Fig. 9-12; Fig. 9-13)**
      a. Optimizes the primary triage of injured children in the MCI setting
      b. Enhances the effectiveness of resource allocation for all MCI victims
      c. Reduces the emotional burden on triage personnel
   5. Triage tagging/labeling **(Fig. 9-14)**
   6. The need for speed
B. Morgue (p. 386)
C. Treatment (pp. 386–387) **(Fig. 9-15)**
   1. Red treatment unit
   2. Yellow treatment unit
   3. Green treatment unit
   4. Supervision of treatment units
D. On-scene physicians (p. 387)
E. Staging (p. 388) **(Fig. 9-16)**
F. Transport Unit (pp. 388–389)
G. Extrication/Rescue Unit (p. 389) **(Fig. 9-17)**
H. Rehabilitation (REHAB) Unit (p. 390)
I. Communications (pp. 390–391)
   1. EMS communications officer
   2. Alternative means of communication

VII. Disaster Management. (pp. 391–392)

A. Mitigation (p. 391)
B. Planning (p. 391)
C. Response (pp. 391–392)
D. Recovery (p. 392)

VIII. Meeting the challenge of mass/multiple-casualty incidents.
(pp. 392–394)

A. Common problems (p. 392)
B. Preplanning, drills, and critiques (pp. 392–393) **(Fig. 9-18)**
C. Disaster mental health services (pp. 393–394)
   1. Psychological first aid to meet providers' emotional needs
   2. Screening of rescuers and victims for abnormal signs and symptoms of traumatic stress

IX. Summary. Preparedness for a mass/multiple-casualty incident involves not only paramedic skills but thorough knowledge of the IMS. Familiarize yourself with all pertinent local protocols and follow them at every multiple-patient, multiple-unit response. (p. 394)

YOU MAKE THE CALL

Review student responses to the You Make the Call scenario on text pages 394–395. Suggested responses to the questions that follow the scenario are given below. Point out to students that these are acceptable answers but not necessarily the

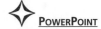
POWERPOINT
PRESENTATION
Volume 5, Chapter 9, PowerPoint slides 41–61

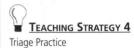
TEACHING STRATEGY 4
Triage Practice

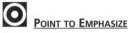
POINT TO EMPHASIZE
All personnel should be trained in triage techniques, and all response units should carry triage equipment.

POINT TO EMPHASIZE
The routing of patients to hospitals is as important as getting them into an ambulance.

SLIDES/VIDEOS
"Aeromedical Evacuation." *Pulse: Emergency Medical Update,* Aug. 1997.

TEACHING STRATEGY 5
Recognizing Disaster Management Factors

POWERPOINT
PRESENTATION
Volume 5, Chapter 9, PowerPoint slide 62

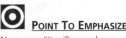
POINT TO EMPHASIZE
Never say, "It will never happen here."

only ones. Discuss with students the pros and cons of points where their responses differ from these.

1. What two roles in the Incident Management System will you and your partner fill, as you are first on-scene?
(Initially, you as the Senior Paramedic are the Incident Commander. You, as the IC, can assign any position or IMS role to your partner but in most systems, he or she would be the Triage Officer.)

2. How would you size up the incident?
(This incident has the potential to severely tax your resources and generate a large volume of potentially critical burn and smoke inhalation patients. The potential requires that you activate as many resources as you can as early as you can to assure a proper level of response.)

3. What additional resources would you anticipate, and what instructions would you provide for them?
(At a minimum, you need additional ambulances and more EMS-trained personnel. You should active any local MCI plans and consider activation of regional plans if they are availed to you.)

4. How would you use the Incident Management System to organize this incident?
(As units arrive, you as the initial IC need to transfer command to a fire agency representative. Once this is done you will likely assume the role of EMS Operations Chief since the first priority of this incident will be rescue and removal of victims for care. You will work hand in hand with the Operations Section Chief, who will in all likelihood be a representative of the fire agency as well. As more and more units arrive, more and more positions in the IMS system will be filled by the IC on an as-needed basis based on the needs of the incident.)

5. What problems would you anticipate, and how would you protect against them?
(Responses might vary due to the capabilities of the area. Have students discuss the local, regional, state, and federal resources that might be requested.)

6. What would your initial radio report sound like in this incident?
(Your report should state exactly what you see in a brief and concise matter. Something to the effect of "Hall County EMS 1 to Hall County, we have a motel with a fire in the rear. The Manager reports at least 20 possible victims in the area of the fire. Notify the fire department to prepare for rescues.")

ASSIGNMENTS

Assign students to complete Chapter 9 of the Workbook. Also assign them to read Chapter 10, "Rescue Awareness and Operations," of the textbook before the next class.

EVALUATION

Chapter Quiz and Scenario   Distribute copies of the Chapter Quiz provided in Handout 9-2 to evaluate student understanding of this chapter. Make sure each student reads the scenario to reinforce critical thinking on the scene. Remind students not to use their notes or textbooks while taking the quiz.

Student CD   Quizzes for every chapter are contained on the dynamic and highly visual in-text student CD.

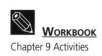
WORKBOOK
Chapter 9 Activities

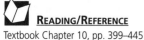
READING/REFERENCE
Textbook Chapter 10, pp. 399–445

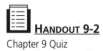
HANDOUT 9-2
Chapter 9 Quiz

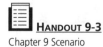
HANDOUT 9-3
Chapter 9 Scenario

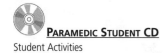
PARAMEDIC STUDENT CD
Student Activities

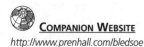
COMPANION WEBSITE
http://www.prenhall.com/bledsoe

©2009 Pearson Education, Inc.
Paramedic Care: Principles & Practice, Vol. 5, 3rd. Ed.

Companion Website Additional quizzes for every chapter are contained on this exciting website.

TestGen You may wish to create a custom-tailored test using *Prentice Hall TestGen for Paramedic Care: Principles & Practice,* 3rd edition, to evaluate student understanding of this chapter.

Online Test Preparation (for students and instructors) Additional test preparation is available through Brady's new online product, EMT Achieve: Paramedic Test Preparation, at *http://www.prenhall.com/emtachieve.* Instructors can also monitor student mastery online.

Success! for the Paramedic Keyed to *Paramedic Care: Principles & Practice* and *Essentials of Paramedic Care,* this comprehensive exam review contains hundreds of test questions and rationales.

REINFORCEMENT

Handouts If classroom discussion or performance on the quiz indicates that some students have not fully mastered the chapter content, you may wish to assign some or all of the Reinforcement Handouts for this chapter.

Student CD (for students) A wide variety of material on this CD-ROM will reinforce and also expand student knowledge and skills.

PowerPoint Presentation (for instructors) The PowerPoint material developed for this chapter offers useful reinforcement of chapter content.

Companion Website (for students) Additional review quizzes and links to EMS resources will contribute to further reinforcement of the chapter.

OneKey Online support is offered for this course on one of three platforms: CourseCompass, Blackboard, or WebCT. Includes the IRM, PowerPoints, Test Manager, and Companion Website for instruction. Ask your local sales representative for more information.

Brady Skills Series: Advanced Life Skills (Video or CD) Have your students watch the skills come to life on VHS or CD-ROM, or they can purchase the highly visual, full-color text with step-by-step procedures with rationales.

Paramedic National Standards Self-Test Another comprehensive review manual containing hundreds of review questions with page references keyed to several Brady texts.

TestGen
Volume 5, Chapter 9

**EMT Achieve:
Paramedic Test Preparation**
Mistovich & Beasley. *EMT Achieve: Paramedic Test Preparation,* http://www.prenhall.com/emtachieve

**Success! for the
Paramedic**
Cherry. *SUCCESS! for the Paramedic,* 4th edition

Handouts 9-4 to 9-7
Reinforcement Activities

Paramedic Student CD
Student Activities

**PowerPoint
Presentation**
Volume 5

Companion Website
http://www.prenhall.com/bledsoe

OneKey
Volume 5, Chapter 9

**Advanced Life
Support Skills**
Larmon & Davis. *Advanced Life Support Skills*

**Advanced Life
Skills Review**
Larmon & Davis. *Advanced Life Skills Review*

**Brady Skills
Series: ALS**
Larmon & Davis.
Brady Skills Series: ALS

**Paramedic National
Standards Self-Test**
Miller. *Paramedic National Standards Self-Test,* 5th edition

Student's Name _____

CHAPTER 9 OBJECTIVES CHECKLIST

Knowledge Objective	Date Mastered
1. Explain the need for the Incident Management System (IMS)/Incident Command System (ICS) in managing emergency medical services (EMS) incidents.	
2. Describe the functional components (Command, Finance/Administration, Logistics, Operations, and Planning/Intelligence) of the Incident Management System.	
3. Differentiate between singular and unified command and identify when each is most applicable.	
4. Describe the role of Command, the need for proper command transfer, and procedures for transferring it.	
5. List and describe the functions of the following groups and leaders in the IMS as it pertains to EMS incidents:	
a. Safety Officer	
b. Logistics Section	
c. Rehabilitation (REHAB)	
d. Staging Area	
e. Treatment Unit or Branch	
f. Triage Unit or Branch	
g. Transportation Unit or Branch	
h. Extrication/Rescue Unit or Branch	
i. Disposition of Deceased (Morgue Unit)	
j. Communications	
6. Describe the methods and rationale for identifying specific functions and leaders for the functions in an IMS.	
7. Describe essential elements of the scene size-up when arriving at a potential mass/multiple-casualty incident (MCI).	
8. Define the terms *Mass/Multiple-Casualty Incident (MCI)*, *disaster management*, *open or uncontained incident*, and *closed or contained incident*.	

©2009 Pearson Education, Inc.
Paramedic Care: Principles & Practice, Vol. 5, 3rd. Ed.

Knowledge Objective	Date Mastered
9. Describe the role of the paramedics and EMS system in planning for MCIs and disasters.	
10. Explain the local/regional threshold for establishing Command and implementation of an Incident Management System, including MCI declaration.	
11. Describe the role of both Incident Command Posts and Mutual Aid Coordination Centers (MACCs) in MCI and disaster management.	
12. Describe the role of the on-scene physician at Mass/Multiple-Casualty Incidents.	
13. Define *triage* and describe the principles of triage.	
14. Describe the START (simple triage and rapid transport) and JumpSTART (START for pediatric patients) methods of initial triage.	
15. Given color-coded tags and numerical priorities, assign the following terms to each:	
a. Immediate	
b. Delayed	
c. Minimal	
d. Expectant	
16. Define primary, secondary and ongoing triage and their implementation techniques.	
17. Describe techniques used to allocate patients to hospitals and track them.	
18. Describe the techniques used in tracking patients during multiple-casualty incidents and the need for such techniques.	
19. Describe modifications of telecommunications procedures during multiple-casualty incidents.	
20. List and describe the essential equipment to provide logistical support to MCI operations to include:	
a. Airway, respiratory, and hemorrhage control	
b. Burn management	
c. Patient packaging/immobilization	
21. Describe the role of mental health support in MCIs.	

OBJECTIVES

OBJECTIVES

Knowledge Objective	Date Mastered
22. Describe the role of the following exercises in preparation for MCIs:	
a. Table top exercises	
b. Small and large MCI drills	

Skill Objective	Date Mastered
23. Given several incident scenarios with preprogrammed patients, provide the appropriate triage, treatment, and transport options for MCI operations based on local resources and protocols.	

©2009 Pearson Education, Inc.
Paramedic Care: Principles & Practice, Vol. 5, 3rd. Ed.

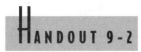

Student's Name _____

CHAPTER 9 QUIZ

Write the letter of the best answer in the space provided.

_____ 1. The individual who runs the management of a mass/multiple-casualty incident (MCI) and has ultimate authority for decision making is called the:
  A. Incident Senior Official.   C. Incident Coordinator.
  B. Incident Commander.   D. Incident Manager.

_____ 2. Incident priorities during scene size-up include all of the following EXCEPT:
  A. life safety.   C. incident containment.
  B. incident stabilization.   D. property conservation.

_____ 3. In all cases of a(n) _____, it is better to request more resources than are needed rather than to request an insufficient amount.
  A. multiple-casualty incident   C. open incident
  B. closed incident   D. unified incident

_____ 4. Incident Commanders should radio a brief progress report roughly every _____ minutes until the incident has been stabilized.
  A. 5   C. 15
  B. 10   D. 20

_____ 5. The use of _____ by the Incident Commander and other senior officers makes identification easier for incoming personnel.
  A. special reflective vests   C. special reflective jackets
  B. special reflective hats   D. special reflective tags on CP positions

_____ 6. At an MCI, the _____ monitors all actions to ensure no potentially harmful conditions are created.
  A. Scene Officer   C. Size-Up Officer
  B. Hazards Officer   D. Safety Officer

_____ 7. The functions of the EMS branch of operations include all of the following EXCEPT:
  A. triage.   C. staging.
  B. treatment.   D. transport.

_____ 8. In triage, the highest priority is given to patients tagged with the color:
  A. black.   C. green.
  B. yellow.   D. red.

_____ 9. Under the START triage system, the first distinction among patients is based on their:
  A. ability to tell you their name.
  B. ability to walk.
  C. ability to follow a simple command.
  D. ability to breathe spontaneously at a rate of 30 breaths per minute or less.

_____ 10. In triage, the best way to assess perfusion is:
  A. capillary refill.   C. radial pulse.
  B. carotid pulse.   D. assessment of mental status.

_____ 11. The JumpSTART triage tool is developed specifically for the triage of:
  A. adult MCI patients.   C. pregnant MCI patients.
  B. geriatric MCI patients.   D. pediatric MCI patients.

_____ **12.** Use of triage tags provides quick recognition of:
   A. who did the triage.
   B. priority of patient treatment.
   C. the patient's name.
   D. the facility to which the patient should be sent.

_____ **13.** Medical materials that should be carried by the triage officer include all of the following, EXCEPT:
   A. a bag-valve-mask (BVM) device.   **C.** oral airways.
   B. infection control supplies.   **D.** trauma dressings.

_____ **14.** Ideally, it should take _____ to triage each patient.
   A. less than 20 seconds   **C.** roughly 30 to 45 seconds
   B. less than 30 seconds   **D.** roughly 45 to 60 seconds

_____ **15.** Patients who are deceased are triaged as:
   A. red.   **C.** yellow.
   B. white.   **D.** black.

©2009 Pearson Education, Inc.
Paramedic Care: Principles & Practice, Vol. 5, 3rd. Ed.

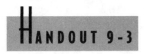

HANDOUT 9-3

Student's Name _____

CHAPTER 9 SCENARIO

Review the following real-life situation. Then answer the questions that follow.

You and your partner are called out at 9:07 P.M. for a motor vehicle collision involving two cars, injuries unknown. The night is foggy, and you have to drive fairly slowly. Fortunately, the scene is only minutes away from your station and the two cars are clearly visible in the right lane and shoulder of the highway. You park in front of the cars and set your lights to bright flashers so the scene will be as visible as possible to oncoming traffic. No other responders are on the scene yet, and there are no bystanders.

A quick survey of the two cars reveals one rear-ended the other, sending the first car into the sign for an exit ramp. The driver of the second car is sitting, apparently stunned, in his seat. You note that he looks up as you approach, that there is no visible blood, and that he is wearing his seat belt. The car, which is an older model, does not have an airbag. The driver's side door appears to be intact.

The first car is significantly more damaged, with rear-end damage from the collision and a broken windshield from the impact with the exit sign. The driver is sitting in her seat, contained between an airbag and the seat back. She is not moving and does not respond to your presence. She is clearly breathing. A young woman in the front passenger seat is also contained by an airbag. She is yelling "Help!" and trying to wipe blood and loose hair from her face. A toddler in the backseat is half in, half out of a car seat that has swung across the rear seat, and you can see bruising and abrasions on the side of her face that hit the side window. She is crying. The driver's side door appears to be intact, but the front passenger door has caved inward somewhat and the highway sign has been bent over the front bumper; it hangs over the windshield and the forward part of the passenger door. The rear doors appear to be intact. As you check the rear doors of the car, you realize that there is a faint smell of gasoline.

1. Does this appear to be a mass/multiple-casualty incident (MCI)? If so, what type?

2. What roles should the EMS responders assume, and what should they do next?

3. Should they call in more resources as they size up the scene? If so, what resources?

4. A police cruiser pulls up while the Incident Commander is on the radio. What, if any, briefing and instructions should the commander give the officers?

CHAPTER 9 REVIEW

Write the word or words that best complete each sentence in the space(s) provided.

1. Whenever _____ or more units respond to an emergency, it is a sound idea to implement IMS.

2. The standardized, national structure used to handle large-scale emergencies is called the _____ _____ _____ (_____), and it covers coordination of response elements such as triage, treatment, transport, and staging.

3. A key element in the management of any incident that spans jurisdictions is the _____ _____ _____ _____, which is a site from which civil government officials (e.g., municipal, county, state, and/or federal) exercise direction and control in an emergency or disaster.

4. The major elements of IMS can be remembered with the mnemonic C-FLOP: C for _____, F for _____/_____, L for _____, O for _____, and P for _____.

5. In _____ _____ , one individual is responsible for coordinating response to an incident, whereas managers from different jurisdictions such as law enforcement, fire, and EMS coordinate activity in the process of _____ _____.

6. Never forget the importance of assigning _____ early in the incident.

7. _____ forms the cornerstone of the Incident Management System (IMS).

8. Command is only transferred _____ -_____-_____, with a short but complete briefing on incident status.

9. At an MCI, the _____ _____ coordinates all operations that involve outside agencies.

10. The operations section at an MCI may have many _____, each of which represents one functional level based on role or geographic location.

11. _____ _____ takes place after patients have been moved to a treatment area and is done to determine any changes in status.

12. The four components of START are the signs/symptoms of _____ _____ _____, _____ _____, _____/_____, and _____ _____.

13. Any triage tags you use should meet these two criteria: easy to _____ and provide rapid visual identification of _____.

14. The routing of patients to _____ is as important as getting them to an ambulance.

15. The _____ area at an MCI is the location established to support on-scene rescuers, and the _____ _____ _____ is the ambulance crew dedicated to standing by to treat any ill or injured rescuer.

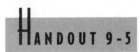
MEDICAL INCIDENT MANAGEMENT ABBREVIATIONS

Write the words represented by the following abbreviations in the spaces provided.

1. MCI _____

2. MVC _____

3. IMS _____

4. ICS _____

5. IC _____

6. CP _____

7. IO _____

8. CISM _____

9. START _____

10. NIMS _____

Student's Name _____

STRUCTURES OF THE INCIDENT MANAGEMENT SYSTEM

Each of the following diagrams represents a figure from the text that highlights key information about IMS. Fill in each box with the missing labels.

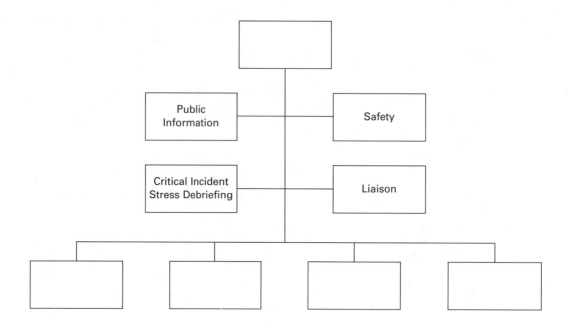

Public Information		Safety

Critical Incident Stress Debriefing		Liaison

Basic Elements of the Incident Management System

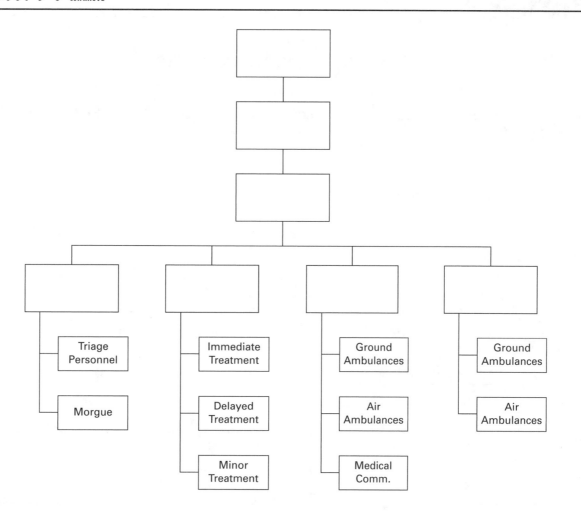

IMS EMS Branch

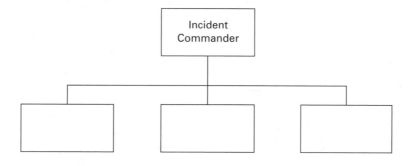

**Basic IMS Organization
EMS Operations**

HANDOUT 9-7

Student's Name ______________________________

THE START TRIAGE SYSTEM

The following diagram represents the operation of the START triage system. Fill in each missing label to complete the flow chart.

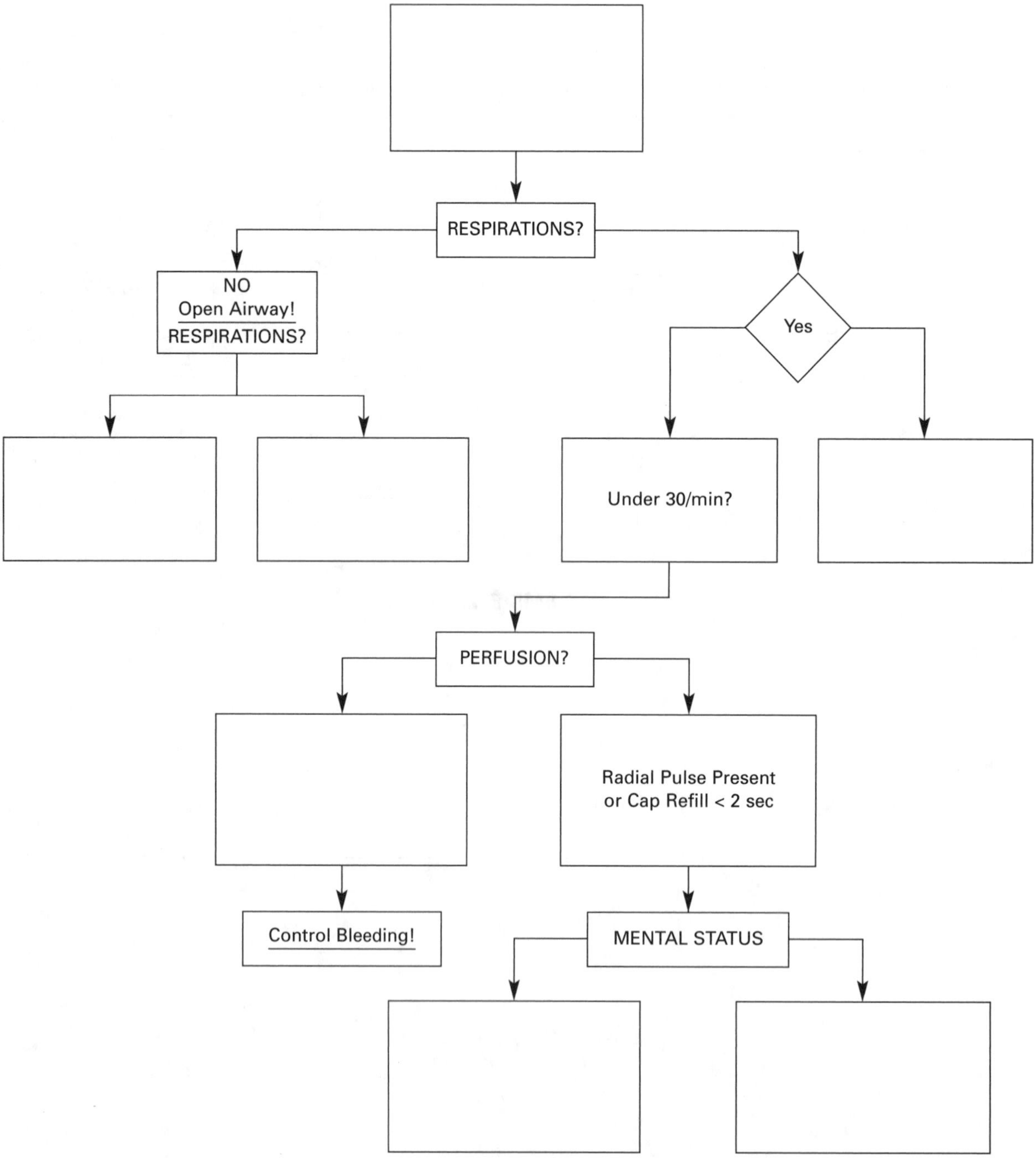
RESPIRATIONS?
NO
Open Airway!
RESPIRATIONS?
Yes
Under 30/min?
PERFUSION?
Radial Pulse Present
or Cap Refill < 2 sec
Control Bleeding!
MENTAL STATUS

Chapter 9 Answer Key

Handout 9-2: Chapter 9 Quiz

1. B	5. A	9. B	13. A
2. C	6. D	10. C	14. B
3. C	7. C	11. D	15. D
4. B	8. D	12. B	

Handout 9-3: Chapter 9 Scenario

1. This is a mass/multiple-casualty incident with four known victims. It is an uncontained (or open) incident because there is traffic on the highway, visibility is very poor, and thus there is real potential for additional collisions near or with the involved vehicles. IMS (Incident Management System) should be implemented because of the number of victims and the potential for more injuries from additional collisions or gasoline-related fire or explosion.

2. One provider should act as Incident Commander and size up the scene with three priorities:
   A. *Life safety.* Is there a visible gasoline spill, and what is the fire or explosion risk? What needs to be done to secure rescuer safety? Are there additional victims (perhaps from the second car) who are not in a car but are nearby and in need of help?
   B. *Incident stabilization.* The ambulance has already been parked in position to alert oncoming motorists to the accident. However, the second vehicle is still in the right travel lane.
   C. *Property conservation.* Not a primary issue during scene size-up on the highway.
   The other provider conducts triage of the four victims.

3. The Incident Commander needs to call dispatch and initiate IMS. At least one additional ambulance unit will be needed, dependent on the findings of the Triage Officer and the presence of any additional victims outside of the cars. Police will need to be on-scene to handle traffic and any bystanders who arrive, as well as to document any legal aspects of the collision. Fire will need to be called because of the possible gasoline leak, and there are also questions about possible need for extrication of at least one passenger (the young woman in the front passenger seat) from the first car.

4. The Incident Commander holds singular command unless the situation changes. He should direct the police to help stabilize the incident (by putting out flares and taking any other measures necessary to block off and protect the accident scene, making their own assessment of gasoline risk, and making a second check for other possible victims) and to make their initial report to their base command.

Handout 9-4: Chapter 9 Review

1. two
2. Incident Management System (IMS)
3. Mutual Aid Coordination Centers
4. Command, Finance/Administration, Logistics, Operations, Planning
5. Singular command, unified command
6. command
7. Communications
8. face-to-face
9. Liaison Officer
10. branches
11. Secondary triage
12. ability to walk, respiratory effort, pulses/perfusion, neurologic status
13. use, priorities
14. hospitals
15. rehabilitation, Rapid Intervention Team

Handout 9-5: Medical Incident Management Abbreviations

1. mass/multiple-casualty incident
2. motor vehicle collision
3. Incident Management System
4. Incident Command System
5. Incident Commander
6. Command post
7. Information Officer
8. Critical Incident Stress Management
9. Simple Triage and Rapid Transport
10. National Incident Management System

Handout 9-6: Structures of the Incident Management System

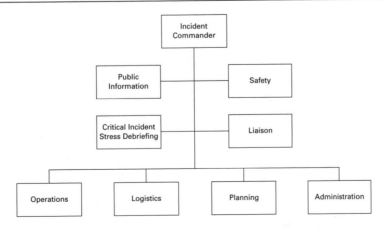

Basic Elements of the Incident Management System

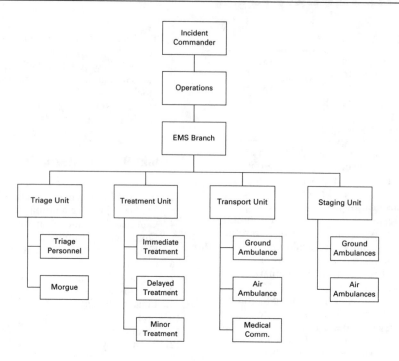

IMS EMS Branch

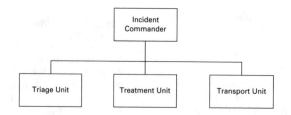

**Basic IMS Organization
EMS Operations**

©2009 Pearson Education, Inc.
Paramedic Care: Principles & Practice, Vol. 5, 3rd. Ed.

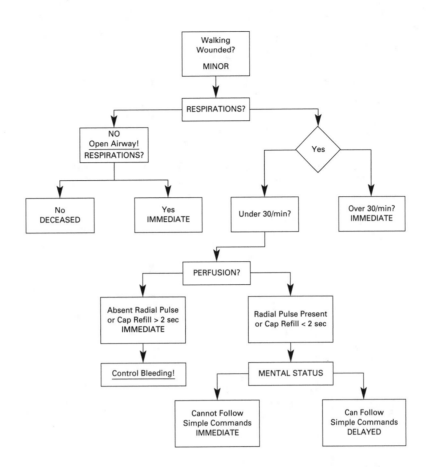

10 Rescue Awareness and Operations

INTRODUCTION

In almost all of the material your students have encountered so far in their course work, physical access to the patient has not been not an issue. The concept of rescue—that some victims need to be extricated before they can become patients who can be treated—was raised in Chapter 9 and is discussed in detail in this chapter. The goal of Chapter 10 is to give your students an "awareness level" of knowledge about rescues in different settings (namely, surface water, hazardous atmospheres, highway operations, and hazardous terrains) so that they can collaborate comfortably and efficiently with other personnel during a wide range of rescue operations.

CHAPTER OBJECTIVES

Knowledge Objectives

1. Define the term *rescue* and explain the medical and mechanical aspects of rescue operations. (pp. 402–403)
2. Describe the phases of a rescue operation, and the role of the paramedic at each phase. (pp. 409–416)
3. List and describe the personal protective equipment needed to safely operate in the rescue environment to include: (pp. 403–406)

    a. Head, eye, and hand protection
    b. Personal flotation devices
    c. Thermal protection/layering systems
    d. High-visibility clothing

4. Explain the risks and complications associated with rescues involving moving water, low head dams, flat water, trenches, motor vehicles, and confined spaces. (pp. 419–432)
5. Explain the effects of immersion hypothermia on the ability to survive sudden immersion and self-rescue. (pp. 417–418)
6. Explain the benefits and disadvantages of water entry or "go techniques" versus the reach-throw-row-go approach to water rescue. (pp. 418–419)
7. Explain the self-rescue position if unexpectedly immersed in moving water. (p. 421)

TOTAL TEACHING TIME: 35.99 HOURS

The total teaching time is only a guideline based on the didactic and practical lab averages in the National Standard Curriculum. Instructors should take into consideration such factors as: the pace at which students learn, the size of the class, and breaks. The actual time devoted to teaching objectives is the responsibility of the instructor.

8. Describe the use of apparatus placement, headlights and emergency vehicle lighting, cones and flare placement, and reflective and high-visibility clothing to reduce scene risk at highway incidents. (pp. 429–430)

9. List and describe the design element hazards and associated protective actions associated with autos and trucks, including energy-absorbing bumpers, air bag/supplemental restraint systems, catalytic converters, and conventional and nonconventional fuel systems. (pp. 430–432)

10. Given a diagram of a passenger auto, identify the A, B, C, and D posts, firewall, and unibody versus frame construction. (pp. 432–433)

11. Explain the difference between tempered and safety glass, identify its locations on a vehicle, and describe how to break it. (p. 432)

12. Explain typical door anatomy and methods to access through stuck doors. (p. 433)

13. Describe methods for emergency stabilization using rope, cribbing, jacks, spare tires, and come-alongs for vehicles found in various positions. (pp. 434–435)

14. Describe electrical and other hazards (above and below the ground) commonly found at highway incidents. (pp. 430–432)

15. Define low-angle rescue, high-angle rescue, belay, rappel, scrambling, and hasty rope slide. (pp. 436–438)

16. Describe the procedure for Stokes litter packaging for low-angle evacuations. (pp. 438–439)

17. Explain anchoring, litter/rope attachment, and lowering and raising procedures as they apply to low-angle litter evacuation. (pp. 437–438, 440)

18. Explain techniques used in nontechnical litter carries over rough terrain. (p. 439)

19. Explain nontechnical high-angle rescue procedures using aerial apparatus. (p. 440)

20. Explain assessment and care modifications (including pain medication, temperature control, and hydration) necessary for attending entrapped patients. (pp. 441–443)

21. List the equipment necessary for an "off-road" medical pack. (p. 442)

22. Explain the different types of Stokes or basket stretchers and the advantages and disadvantages associated with each. (pp. 438–439)

23. Given a list of rescue scenarios, provide the victim survivability profile and identify which are rescue versus body recovery situations. (pp. 402–443)

24. Given a series of pictures, identify those considered "confined spaces" and potentially oxygen deficient. (pp. 425–429)

FRAMING THE LESSON

Explore the variety of settings that require rescue. Have your students brainstorm about situations that might require victim rescue. Some examples, such as motor vehicle collisions, will come readily. Others, such as home occupants affected by carbon monoxide poisoning, children caught in a dry well or other confined space, or persons who fall through ice, may come only with prompting.

Try to get students to think of examples that fit the major categories discussed in the chapter: surface water (flat and moving water), hazardous atmospheres (trenches, incidents), highway operations (unstable vehicles, hazardous cargo,

©2009 Pearson Education, Inc.
Paramedic Care: Principles & Practice, Vol. 5, 3rd. Ed.

volatile fuel), and hazardous terrain (high-angle cliffs, off-road wilderness areas). Then get them to name the four major categories for themselves. Emphasize any categories of rescue that are particularly common in your area.

CONSIDERING THE CASE STUDY

Ask a volunteer to read aloud the Case Study that begins on text page 401. Suggest that students close their eyes as the scenario is read to help them visualize the events described in it. You can use the following questions as a starting point for teaching the chapter—a sort of chapter preview in a functional setting.

When the chapter is completed, you may wish to return to the Case Study and encourage further discussion aimed at answering the questions.

CASE STUDY DISCUSSION QUESTIONS (AND ANSWERS)

1. Name several elements of the emergency scene and its relationship to the ambulance station, ambulance, and paramedic conducting scene size-up that are important to the rescue and medical elements of this patient's case. *(Answers may include some or all of the following:*
   - *Distance of the scene from the station, necessitating nearly 30 minutes of time to reach the park*
   - *Inability to drive the ambulance to the patient, requiring one paramedic to go to the scene with limited supplies*
   - *Inability to reach dispatch from scene, requiring one paramedic to remain with ambulance and radio*
   - *Distance of size-up paramedic from patient and other climber, requiring a very remote assessment of medical condition [man lying still on a rock ledge roughly 55 feet below the trail—indicating a fall of considerable distance/significant mechanism of injury])*

2. What skills specific to this rescue situation do the backup paramedics demonstrate? *(Answers may include some or all of the following:*
   - *They have the knowledge and skill to ensure scene and personal safety.*
   - *They have the skill to gain direct access to the patient [rappel down the cliff face] and to ensure the safety of the uninjured climber [have him tie in for protection].*
   - *They have the skill to decide upon best method of extraction [removal in Stokes basket stretcher rather than direct helicopter evacuation].)*

3. How does the rescuer on the ledge adapt her medical treatment to the necessary delay in removal of the patient? *(Answers may include some or all of the following:*
   - *She collects additional history from the uninjured climber, who says he is a "best friend" [and therefore may have some knowledge of pertinent personal medical history as well as history of accident].*
   - *She conducts a detailed physical exam.*
   - *She renders needed immediate aid [cleans and dresses all wounds, splints all fractures] and sets up extended care [starts two IV lines and runs lactated Ringer's solution].)*

4. Is there any standard medical care you would expect to be given to a trauma patient that isn't specified in the case study? *(Although you are not told that the patient's neck and spine are immobilized before placement into the stretcher, you can assume that this was*

©2009 Pearson Education, Inc.
Paramedic Care: Principles & Practice, Vol. 5, 3rd. Ed.   CHAPTER 10 *Rescue Awareness and Operations* **303**

done to protect the patient. In addition, you can assume that the rescuer did ongoing assessment of the ABCs. You are not told if the rescuer could give oxygen supplementation to the patient, but it would have been done if possible.

The point of emphasis with this question is that standard care is always given when possible, but there may be circumstances in which certain equipment or procedures are not possible before rescue is complete.)

TEACHING STRATEGIES

People learn in a variety of ways. Some do better with the spoken word, while others prefer the written. Some prefer to work alone, whereas others profit from working in groups. Recognizing these different ways of acquiring knowledge, the authors of this *Instructor's Resource Manual* have provided a variety of teaching strategies for the different types of learners. These strategies are intended to foster higher-level cognitive skills and encourage creative learning and problem solving.

For greatest effectiveness, incorporate these strategies into your class lecture. Marginal notes in the Teaching Outline indicate the points at which various exercises might be most appropriate. Other strategies can be used to preview the lesson or to summarize it.

The following strategies are keyed to specific sections of the lesson:

1. Thinking about Rescue Equipment. Hold a "Protective Equipment Fashion Show." Among members of your class will be many who own or have access to specialized personal protective equipment for various rescue situations. Have them model the gear in class. An announcer can read from the script about the type of clothing, its protective function, and its availability. This activity involves all of the senses and learning domains and is great fun!

2. More on Rescue Equipment. Create a "treasure chest" of specialized clothing and equipment for your class to use. Be sure to include helmets, gloves, eye protection, personal protection equipment, turnout gear, body armor, and so on. When lab session scenarios present a hazardous situation, students can return to their vehicle (or your treasure chest) to don the appropriate gear. Remember, students will play like they practice, so it is your responsibility to instill good safety habits in the classroom.

3. Researching Rescue Situations. As an exercise in preplanning, have students research the training and gear required for various rescue situations. Be sure they learn the extent and technicality of the training, where to get this training, continuing education requirements, and the cost associated with the training. Ask that they identify an individual who has this training to interview for their experiences. Photos or brochures would be an added plus. This activity emphasizes research skills taught earlier in the program. Additionally, verbal communication skills are enhanced through the interview and report. Last, this activity lends realism to the adult learner by connecting with a professional or role model already trained in their topic area.

The following strategy relates to Special Features in the student textbook and can be used to enhance the student's understanding:

Legal Notes: Rescue Calls, Routine Calls, and Safety.   Contact your emergency services insurance carrier or the National Safety Council regarding programs related to emergency response. There are a variety of classroom and practical programs to assist the emergency vehicle operator.

The following strategies can be used at various points throughout the lesson or to help summarize and demonstrate what students have learned:

Wilderness Rescue. Two fantastic programs in Colorado exist as information sources and role models for a variety of wilderness medical topic areas. The Wilderness Medical Institute in Pitkin, Colorado, provides Wilderness EMT training and adventures. Colorado Mountain College in Breckenridge, Colorado, offers one of only three Wilderness Paramedic programs in the country. These programs teach the core EMT or Paramedic curricula along with special emphasis on backcountry survival, swift-water rescue, avalanche rescue, rock climbing and rappelling, and decision making in the absence of communication with medical direction.

River Rafting. A river rafting trip is a great way to teach the principles of swift-water rescue in a fun environment. Most states have day river trips for $20 to $50 per person. Make special arrangements so that the guide will allow stops to practice rescue techniques. You will likely be surprised at how much water safety the guide covers in the normal introduction. Whenever possible, bring students out of the classroom into the real world. Involvement of the senses engages the right brain and facilitates the learning of new ideas, concepts, and techniques.

Water Rescue. In most areas of the country, water rescue is a real possibility. Not every community is equipped with lifeguards for its pools, lakes, rivers, and oceans. Therefore, your students may be called upon to apply ground rescue techniques to the water. They will need practice in order to do this safely and effectively. Rent or borrow space at your local pool to practice spinal immobilization, wound care, airway management, and more in this new, wet, and relatively unstable environment.

TEACHING OUTLINE

Chapter 10 is the tenth lesson in Volume 5, *Special Considerations/Operations*. Distribute Handout 10-1. If students have any questions about the objectives, answer them at this time.

Then present the chapter. One possible lecture outline follows. In the outline, the parenthetical references in regular type are references to text pages; those in bold type are to figures, tables, or procedures.

I. Introduction. Rescue is the concept/definition of extrication and/or disentangling the victims who will become your patients after rescue is complete. (p. 402)

II. Role of the paramedic. (pp. 402–403)

A. The paramedic must have proficiency up to at least the "awareness level" for rescues involving (pp. 402–403)
  1. Surface water
  2. Hazardous atmospheres
  3. Highway operations
  4. Hazardous terrains (**Fig. 10-1**)

III. Protective equipment. (pp. 403–407)

A. Rescuer protection (pp. 403–406) (**Fig. 10-2**)
  1. Helmets (**Fig. 10-3**)
  2. Eye protection

POINT TO EMPHASIZE
The application of safety equipment—both to rescuers and patients—is paramount in any rescue situation.

HANDOUT 10-1
Chapter 10 Objectives Checklist

TEACHING STRATEGY 1
Thinking about Rescue Equipment

POWERPOINT PRESENTATION
Volume 5, Chapter 10, PowerPoint slides 1–3

HANDOUT 10-6
Rescuer Protective Equipment

TEACHING STRATEGY 2
More on Rescue Equipment

POWERPOINT PRESENTATION
Volume 5, Chapter 10, PowerPoint slides 7–11

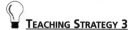

3. Hearing protection
4. Respiratory protection
5. Gloves
6. Foot protection
7. Flame/flash protection (**Fig. 10-4**)
8. Personal flotation devices
9. Lighting
10. Hazmat suits or SCBA (self-contained breathing apparatus)
11. Extended, remote, or wilderness protection

B. Patient protection (pp. 406–407)
1. Helmets
2. Eye protection
3. Hearing and respiratory protection
4. Protective blankets
5. Protective shielding

IV. Safety procedures. (pp. 407–409)

A. Rescue SOPs (p. 407)
B. Crew assignments (pp. 407–408) (**Fig. 10-5**)
C. Preplanning (pp. 408–409)

V. Rescue operations. (pp. 409–416)

A. Phase 1: Arrival and size-up (pp. 409–410) (**Fig. 10-6**)
B. Phase 2: Hazard control (pp. 410–411) (**Fig. 10-7**)
C. Phase 3: Patient access (pp. 411–412) (**Fig. 10-8**)
D. Phase 4: Medical treatment (pp. 412–414) (**Fig. 10-9**)
  1. Basic responsibilities
    a. Initiate patient assessment.
    b. Maintain patient care procedures.
    c. Accompany patient during removal and transport.
  2. Basic care steps
    a. Initial assessment of MS-ABCs
    b. Management of life-threatening ABC problems
    c. Spinal immobilization
    d. Splinting of major fractures
    e. Appropriate patient packaging
    f. Ongoing reassessment
E. Phase 5: Disentanglement (pp. 414–415) (**Fig. 10-10**)
  1. Basic responsibilities
    a. Skills to function in active rescue zone
    b. Readiness to provide prolonged patient care
    c. Ability to call for and use special rescue resources
F. Phase 6: Patient packaging (pp. 415–416) (**Fig. 10-11**)
G. Phase 7: Removal/Transport (p. 416) (**Fig. 10-12**)

VI. Surface water rescues. (pp. 416–425)

A. General background (pp. 417–419) (**Fig. 10-13**)
  1. Rescuers should know how to swim.
  2. Use PFDs.
  3. Water temperature
    a. Hypothermia
    b. HELP
    c. HUDDLE
  4. Basic rescue techniques (**Fig. 10-14**)
B. Moving water (pp. 419–421)
  1. Recirculating currents (**Fig. 10-15**)
  2. Strainers (**Fig. 10-16**)

3. Foot/extremity pins
4. Dams/hydroelectric intakes
5. Self-rescue techniques
   a. Cover mouth and nose during entry.
   b. Protect the head; keep face out of water.
   c. Do not attempt to stand in moving water.
   d. Float on back, feet downstream.
   e. Steer with feet.
   f. Remember that water moves faster around outside of a bend.
   g. Watch out for rocks and strainers.
   h. Watch for eddies.
   i. Be careful not to fall in in the first place.
C. Flat water (pp. 421–425) (**Fig. 10-17**)
   1. Factors affecting survival
   2. Personal flotation devices
   3. Cold protective response
   4. Location of submerged victims
   5. Rescue versus body recovery
   6. In-water patient immobilization (**Fig. 10-18**)
      a. Phase one: In-water spinal immobilization
      b. Phase two: Rigid cervical collar application
      c. Phase three: Back boarding and extrication from the water

VII. Hazardous atmosphere rescues. (pp. 425–429) (**Fig. 10-19**)

A. Confined-space hazards (pp. 425–427)
   1. Oxygen-deficient atmospheres
   2. Toxic or explosive chemicals (**Fig. 10-20**)
   3. Engulfment
   4. Machinery entrapment
   5. Electricity
   6. Structural concerns
B. Confined-space protections in the workplace (pp. 428–429)
C. Cave-ins and structural collapses (p. 428) (**Fig. 10-21**)
   1. Reasons for collapses/cave-ins
      a. Poor construction techniques
      b. Lip of trench caves in
      c. Wall shears away in entirety
      d. "Spoil pile" too close to edge of hole
      e. Water seepage, ground vibrations, intersecting trenches, disturbed soil
   2. Rescue from trenches/cave-ins

VIII. Highway operations and vehicle rescues. (pp. 429–436)

A. Hazards in highway operations (pp. 429–432)
   1. Traffic hazards
      a. Staging
      b. Positioning of apparatus
      c. Emergency lighting
      d. Redirection of traffic
      e. High visibility
   2. Other hazards
      a. Fire and fuel
      b. Alternative fuel systems
      c. Sharp objects
      d. Electric power (**Fig. 10-22**)
      e. Energy-absorbing bumpers
      f. Supplemental restraint systems (SRS)/air bags

READING/REFERENCE
Sargent, C. "Close Encounters: EMS at Confined Space Operations," *JEMS*, July 1999.

POINT TO EMPHASIZE
Suspect hazmat at any scene involving commercial vehicles.

      g. Hazardous cargoes
      h. Rolling vehicles
      i. Unstable vehicles

B. Auto anatomy (pp. 432–433)
   1. Basic constructions
   2. Firewall and engine compartment
   3. Glass
   4. Doors

C. Rescue strategies (pp. 433–434)
   1. Initial scene size-up
   2. Control hazards
   3. Assess the degree of entrapment and fastest means of extrication. (**Fig. 10-23**)
   4. Establish circles of operation.
   5. Treatment, packaging, removal

D. Rescue skills practice (pp. 434–436) (**Fig. 10-24; Table 10-1**)
   1. Hybrid vehicles (hybrid electric vehicles or HEVs) (**Fig. 10-25**)

IX. Hazardous terrain rescues. (pp. 436–443)

A. Types of hazardous terrain (p. 436)
B. Patient access in hazardous terrain (pp. 436–438)
   1. High-angle rescues (**Fig. 10-26**)
   2. Low-angle rescues (**Fig. 10-26**)
   3. Flat terrain with obstructions
C. Patient packaging for rough terrain (pp. 438–439) (**Fig. 10-27**)
D. Patient removal from hazardous terrain (pp. 439–440)
   1. Flat rough terrain
   2. Low-angle/high-angle evacuation
   3. Use of helicopters
   4. Packaging/evacuation practice (**Fig. 10-28**)
E. Extended care assessment and environmental issues (pp. 441–443)
   1. Need for protocols to address patient-related concerns and topics
      a. Long-term rehydration management
      b. Cleansing and care of wounds
      c. Removal of impaled objects
      d. Nonpharmacological pain management
      e. Pharmacological pain management
      f. Assessment/care of head and spine injuries
      g. Management of hypothermia or hyperthermia
      h. Termination of CPR
      i. Treatment of crush injury/compartment syndrome
   2. Environmental issues that can affect assessment
      a. Weather/temperature
      b. Limited patient access
      c. Difficulty transporting equipment
      d. Cumbersome PPE
      e. Patient exposure
      f. Use of ALS skills
      g. Patient monitoring
      h. Improvisation

X. Summary. Rescue operations, which are needed to extricate or disentangle someone who will become your patient, can be divided into at least seven phases: arrival and size-up, hazard control, patient access, medical treatment, disentanglement, patient packaging, and removal/transport. (p. 443)

SLIDES/VIDEOS

"Wilderness Rescue," *Pulse: Emergency Medical Update,* Aug. 1997.

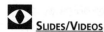

SLIDES/VIDEOS

"Packaging a Patient for Litter Evacuation," *Pulse: Emergency Medical Update,* Apr. 1996.

POWERPOINT
PRESENTATION
Volume 5, Chapter 10, PowerPoint slide 66

YOU MAKE THE CALL

Review student responses to the You Make the Call scenario on text page 443. Suggested responses to the questions that follow the scenario are given below. Point out to students that these are acceptable answers but not necessarily the only ones. Discuss with students the pros and cons of points where their responses differ from these.

1. What are your immediate considerations as you size up the scene? *(Immediate considerations include safety, hazards, number of patients, control of traffic and bystanders, and need for additional resources [implementation of IMS].)*

2. Why would you consider this a rescue operation? *(Because the patient is unconscious and entrapped in a potentially unstable vehicle/environment.)*

3. What additional resources would you request? *(Additional resources might include police, fire department, another EMS unit, and possibly a low-angle rescue team to help move the patient up the embankment.)*

ASSIGNMENTS

Assign students to complete Chapter 10 of the Workbook. Also assign them to read Chapter 11, "Hazardous Materials Incidents," of the textbook before the next class.

EVALUATION

Chapter Quiz and Scenario   Distribute copies of the Chapter Quiz provided in Handout 10-2 to evaluate student understanding of this chapter. Make sure each student reads the scenario to reinforce critical thinking on the scene. Remind students not to use their notes or textbooks while taking the quiz.

Student CD   Quizzes for every chapter are contained on the dynamic and highly visual in-text student CD.

Companion Website   Additional quizzes for every chapter are contained on this exciting website.

TestGen   You may wish to create a custom-tailored test using *Prentice Hall TestGen for Paramedic Care: Principles & Practice*, 3rd edition, to evaluate student understanding of this chapter.

Online Test Preparation (for students and instructors)   Additional test preparation is available through Brady's new online product, *EMT Achieve: Paramedic Test Preparation*, at *http://www.prenhall.com/emtachieve*. Instructors can also monitor student mastery online.

Success! for the Paramedic   Keyed to *Paramedic Care: Principles & Practice* and *Essentials of Paramedic Care*, this comprehensive exam review contains hundreds of test questions and rationales.

REINFORCEMENT

Handouts   If classroom discussion or performance on the quiz indicates that some students have not fully mastered the chapter content, you may wish to assign some or all of the Reinforcement Handouts for this chapter.

WORKBOOK
Chapter 10 Activities

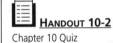
READING/REFERENCE
Textbook Chapter 11, pp. 446–477

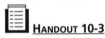
HANDOUT 10-2
Chapter 10 Quiz

HANDOUT 10-3
Chapter 10 Scenario

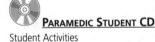
PARAMEDIC STUDENT CD
Student Activities

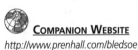
COMPANION WEBSITE
http://www.prenhall.com/bledsoe

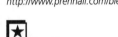
TESTGEN
Volume 5, Chapter 10

**EMT ACHIEVE:
PARAMEDIC TEST PREPARATION**
Mistovich & Beasley. *EMT Achieve: Paramedic Test Preparation*, *http://www.prenhall.com/emtachieve*

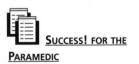
SUCCESS! FOR THE PARAMEDIC
Cherry. *SUCCESS! for the Paramedic*, 4th edition

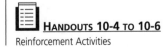
HANDOUTS 10-4 TO 10-6
Reinforcement Activities

PARAMEDIC STUDENT CD
Student Activities

POWERPOINT PRESENTATION
Volume 5

COMPANION WEBSITE
http://www.prenhall.com/bledsoe

ONEKEY
Volume 5, Chapter 10

ADVANCED LIFE SUPPORT SKILLS
Larmon & Davis. *Advanced Life Support Skills*

ADVANCED LIFE SKILLS REVIEW
Larmon & Davis. *Advanced Life Skills Review*

BRADY SKILLS SERIES: ALS
Larmon & Davis. *Brady Skills Series: ALS*

PARAMEDIC NATIONAL STANDARDS SELF-TEST
Miller. *Paramedic National Standards Self-Test*, 5th edition

Student CD (for students)   A wide variety of material on this CD-ROM will reinforce and also expand student knowledge and skills.

PowerPoint Presentation (for instructors)   The PowerPoint material developed for this chapter offers useful reinforcement of chapter content.

Companion Website (for students)   Additional review quizzes and links to EMS resources will contribute to further reinforcement of the chapter.

OneKey   Online support is offered for this course on one of three platforms: CourseCompass, Blackboard, or WebCT. Includes the IRM, PowerPoints, Test Manager, and Companion Website for instruction. Ask your local sales representative for more information.

Brady Skills Series: Advanced Life Skills (Video or CD)   Have your students watch the skills come to life on VHS or CD-ROM, or they can purchase the highly visual, full-color text with step-by-step procedures with rationales.

Paramedic National Standards Self-Test   Another comprehensive review manual containing hundreds of review questions with page references keyed to several Brady texts.

©2009 Pearson Education, Inc.
Paramedic Care: Principles & Practice, Vol. 5, 3rd. Ed.

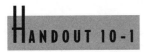

Student's Name _____

CHAPTER 10 OBJECTIVES CHECKLIST

Knowledge Objective	Date Mastered
1. Define the term *rescue* and explain the medical and mechanical aspects of rescue operations.	
2. Describe the phases of a rescue operation and the role of the paramedic at each phase.	
3. List and describe the personal protective equipment needed to safely operate in the rescue environment, to include:	
a. Head, eye, and hand protection	
b. Personal flotation devices	
c. Thermal protection/layering systems	
d. High-visibility clothing	
4. Explain the risks and complications associated with rescues involving moving water, low head dams, flat water, trenches, motor vehicles, and confined spaces.	
5. Explain the effects of immersion hypothermia on the ability to survive sudden immersion and self-rescue.	
6. Explain the benefits and disadvantages of water-entry or "go techniques" versus the reach-throw-row-go approach to water rescue.	
7. Explain the self-rescue position if unexpectedly immersed in moving water.	
8. Describe the use of apparatus placement, headlights and emergency vehicle lighting, cones and flare placement, and reflective and high-visibility clothing to reduce scene risk at highway incidents.	
9. List and describe the design element hazards and associated protective actions associated with autos and trucks, including energy-absorbing bumpers, air bag/supplemental restraint systems, catalytic converters, and conventional and nonconventional fuel systems.	
10. Given a diagram of a passenger auto, identify the A, B, C, and D posts, firewall, and unibody versus frame construction.	
11. Explain the difference between tempered and safety glass, identify its locations on a vehicle, and describe how to break it.	

OBJECTIVES

Knowledge Objective	Date Mastered
12. Explain typical door anatomy and methods to access through stuck doors.	
13. Describe methods for emergency stabilization using rope, cribbing, jacks, spare tires, and come-alongs for vehicles found in various positions.	
14. Describe electrical and other hazards (above and below the ground) commonly found at highway incidents.	
15. Define low-angle rescue, high-angle rescue, belay, rappel, scrambling, and hasty rope slide.	
16. Describe the procedure for Stokes litter packaging for low-angle evacuations.	
17. Explain anchoring, litter/rope attachment, and lowering and raising procedures as they apply to low-angle litter evacuation.	
18. Explain techniques used in nontechnical litter carries over rough terrain.	
19. Explain nontechnical high-angle rescue procedures using aerial apparatus.	
20. Explain assessment and care modifications (including pain medication, temperature control, and hydration) necessary for attending entrapped patients.	
21. List the equipment necessary for an "off-road" medical pack.	
22. Explain the different types of Stokes or basket stretchers and the advantages and disadvantages associated with each.	
23. Given a list of rescue scenarios, provide the victim survivability profile and identify which are rescue versus body recovery situations.	
24. Given a series of pictures, identify those considered "confined spaces" and potentially oxygen deficient.	

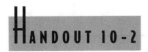

Student's Name _____

CHAPTER 10 QUIZ

Write the letter of the best answer in the space provided.

_____ 1. The use of _____ is paramount in any rescue situation.
   A. appropriately skilled personnel
   B. safety equipment
   C. appropriate time-saving measures
   D. portable medical equipment and supplies

_____ 2. Vital rescuer protective equipment includes all of the following EXCEPT:
   A. protective shielding.   C. hearing protection.
   B. respiratory protection.   D. a helmet.

_____ 3. The presence of electrical wires at the rescue scene indicates a possible threat of:
   A. fire.   C. shock.
   B. explosion.   D. both A and C.

_____ 4. Hazards that may not be visible during scene size-up include all of the following EXCEPT the presence of:
   A. infected material.
   B. poisonous substances.
   C. potential sources of violence or emotional trauma.
   D. a potentially unstable environment.

_____ 5. The goals of rescue assessment include all of the following EXCEPT:
   A. identification and care for existing patient problems.
   B. anticipation of changes in patient condition.
   C. anticipation of changes in physical environment.
   D. advance determination of needed assistance and equipment.

_____ 6. Because of the possibility of extended time in the field, for rescue patients you must be prepared to provide:
   A. ongoing assessment.   C. treatment protocols.
   B. stabilization techniques.   D. psychological support.

_____ 7. The use of force to free a patient from entrapment is called:
   A. extrication.   C. release.
   B. disentrapment.   D. removal.

_____ 8. Methods used to disentangle the patient must constantly be analyzed:
   A. to look for the shortest method of release.
   B. on a risk-to-benefits basis.
   C. to look for the technique that allows greatest paramedic access.
   D. to look for the methods safest for rescuers and the patient.

_____ 9. It is paramount that the rescuer know how to prevent further patient injury by adapting techniques of:
   A. disentanglement.   C. packaging.
   B. removal.   D. transport.

_____ 10. While en route to the hospital, you should perform ongoing assessments at these intervals if the patient is stable/unstable:
   A. 3 minutes/5 minutes.   C. 5 minutes/15 minutes.
   B. 5 minutes/10 minutes.   D. 5 to 7 minutes/17 to 20 minutes.

_____ 11. HELP (Heat Escape Lessening Position) is an in-water position designed to reduce heat loss by as much as:
A. 40 percent.
B. 60 percent.
C. 75 percent.
D. 90 percent.

_____ 12. Factors contributing to the death of a hypothermic patient include all of the following EXCEPT:
A. inability to grasp a line or flotation device.
B. inability to follow simple directions.
C. bronchospasm, which increases risk of drowning.
D. laryngospasm, which increases risk of drowning.

_____ 13. Recirculating currents, strainers, foot/extremity pins, and dams/hydroelectric intakes are examples of what type of scenario?
A. freshwater
B. swift-water
C. water obstacle
D. hazardous water

_____ 14. General factors in a person's survivability profile for a water accident include all of the following EXCEPT:
A. age.
B. lung volume.
C. water temperature.
D. use of alcohol and/or other drugs.

_____ 15. One of the MOST serious threats in a confined-space rescue is:
A. physical instability.
B. presence of toxic or caustic substances.
C. oxygen deficiency.
D. the presence of sharp or otherwise hazardous objects.

©2009 Pearson Education, Inc.
Paramedic Care: Principles & Practice, Vol. 5, 3rd. Ed.

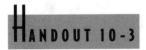
HANDOUT 10-3

Student's Name _____

EVALUATION

CHAPTER 10 SCENARIO

Review the following real-life situation. Then answer the questions that follow.

It is 10:40 P.M., and you and your partner are about to finish your shift on this pleasantly cool summer night. Then dispatch calls and sends you to a nearby residential neighborhood for "a woman who fell in a swimming pool."

You and your partner grab your personal flotation jackets as you leave the ambulance. When you arrive at the pool area, you find a middle-aged man standing by lawn chairs. When you look in the water, you see a woman on the far side of the pool crying and struggling to hold onto a ladder. She repeatedly tries to climb up the ladder but appears unable to coordinate her movements enough to get out of the pool.

Your partner jogs to the far side of the pool toward the woman while you turn toward the man. You notice he is dressed in light summer clothing, not swimwear, and there is a distinct odor of alcohol. He quickly tells you the woman is his wife and she fell in the swimming pool while they were walking to the house from the garage. "Got home from a party," he says. "She just lost her balance. Stupid, really."

He sits in a pool chair while you join your partner. A quick scan of the scene shows no flotation devices or other floatable object for you to throw or hand to the woman. The area around the pool is dry and level. There is nothing visible in the pool except the woman, who you notice is struggling to hold the ladder with one hand and pull up a skirt with the other. Your partner, who has knelt beside her, tells you her name is Frances and she is unable to say what happened except that she feels sick and can't pull herself up and out of the pool. She has blood dripping from the left temple and what appears to be the beginning of a black eye on the same side. You don't see any other obvious injuries, but the lighting is poor. She is spitting out some water but appears to be breathing relatively easily.

1. Is this a rescue situation? Do you see any potential hazards during your scene size-up?

2. Do you need any additional resources, and, if so, what?

3. What should be done to care for the patient while you wait for additional help (if you decide to wait)?

4. What steps will you need to take to remove the woman safely from the pool when the proper time comes?

©2009 Pearson Education, Inc.
Paramedic Care: Principles & Practice, Vol. 5, 3rd. Ed.   **CHAPTER 10** *Rescue Awareness and Operations* **315**

Student's Name _____

CHAPTER 10 REVIEW

Write the word or words that best complete each sentence in the space(s) provided.

1. The checklist for backcountry work includes protective equipment for _____ _____, provisions for personal _____ _____, snacks, temporary _____, _____ lighter, and redundant _____.

2. Most rescue calls have at least seven defined phases: _____ and size-up, _____ control, _____ access, _____ _____, _____, patient _____, and _____ and transport.

3. _____ triggers the technical beginning of the rescue.

4. During the fourth rescue phase, medical treatment, the paramedic has three responsibilities: initiation or _____ _____, maintenance of _____ _____ procedures during disentanglement, and accompaniment of the patient during _____ and _____.

5. The area in which special rescue teams operate is known as the _____ _____ _____.

6. Actions to delay hypothermia include use of _____ _____ _____ (_____), use of _____ _____ _____ _____ (_____), and _____ _____.

7. The water rescue model is called _____-_____-_____-_____.

8. _____ plays a role in many water accidents, including nearly 50 percent of fatal boating accidents.

9. Always put on a(n) _____ whenever you approach water.

10. Water rescue patients are never dead until they are _____ and _____.

11. The three phases of in-water patient immobilization are in-water _____ _____, _____ _____ _____ application, and _____ _____, and extrication from the water.

12. It only takes one spark to trigger an explosion: Always be careful of all potential sources of _____.

13. If a collapsed trench or cave-in has caused a burial, a _____ _____ is likely.

14. _____ _____ is the largest single hazard associated with EMS highway operations.

15. Do not _____ a vehicle until you have ruled out all electrical hazards.

16. For rescuer safety, suspect _____ _____ at any scene involving commercial vehicles.

17. _____ glass can produce glass dust or fracture into long shards, whereas _____ glass fractures into many small beads of glass.

18. Three types of hazardous terrain are _____-_____ terrain, _____-_____ terrain, and _____ _____ with obstructions.

19. Be aware of the _____ in mission, crew training, and capabilities of helicopters that do air medical care and those of helicopters that do rescue.

20. Good _____ skills are mandatory in hazardous terrains, but limit _____ skills to those that are really needed: Do not complicate any already complicated operation.

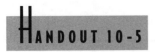

Student's Name _____

RESCUE AWARENESS TRUE OR FALSE

Indicate whether the following statements are true or false by writing T or F in the space provided.

_____ **1.** Failure to train paramedics in rescue awareness will eventually end in the injury or death of EMS personnel, patients, or both.

_____ **2.** In general, all paramedics should have the training and personal protective equipment to allow them to access and assess the patient and establish Incident Command.

_____ **3.** Personal flotation devices only need to be worn if you operate in water.

_____ **4.** Personnel screening for rescue unit training should include physical and psychological testing.

_____ **5.** Practice exercises with clear protocols and simulated patients will give you and your unit ample opportunity to train and to utilize IMS in rescue situations.

_____ **6.** If you are the first unit on-scene, be careful not to underestimate your ability to handle a rescue situation: Remember not to stretch resources farther than necessary.

_____ **7.** During the access phase, key medical, technical, and other personnel should confer with the Incident Commander on the safest strategy to accomplish the rescue.

_____ **8.** Disentanglement may be the most technical and time-consuming portion of the rescue.

_____ **9.** Nearly all incidents in and around water are preventable.

_____ **10.** Water causes heat loss 10 times faster than air.

_____ **11.** Water entry is a last-resort measure.

_____ **12.** It is always unsafe to walk in fast-moving water over midcalf depth because of the danger of entrapping a foot or extremity.

_____ **13.** The mammalian diving reflex is more pronounced in adults than in children.

_____ **14.** Confined space is defined as any space with limited access/egress that is not designed for human occupation.

_____ **15.** Over half of all fatalities associated with confined spaces are rescuers, not the original victim(s).

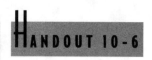
RESCUER PROTECTIVE EQUIPMENT

- **Helmets:** The best helmets have a four-point, nonelastic suspension system. Avoid helmets with nonremovable "duck bills" in back because they can compromise your ability to wear the helmet in tight spaces. A compact firefighting helmet that meets NFPA standards is adequate for most vehicle and structural applications.

- **Eye protection:** Two essential pieces of eye gear include goggles (vented to prevent fogging) and industrial safety glasses. These should be ANSI approved. Do not rely on the face shields found in fire helmets. They usually provide inadequate eye protection.

- **Hearing protection:** High-quality earmuff styles provide the best hearing protection. However, you must take into account other factors such as practicality, convenience, availability, and environmental considerations. In high-noise areas, for example, you might use the multibaffled rubber earplugs used by the military or the sponge-like disposable earplugs.

- **Respiratory protection:** Surgical masks or commercial dust masks prove adequate for most occasions. These should be routinely carried on all EMS units.

- **Gloves:** Leather gloves usually protect against cuts and punctures. They allow for free movement of the fingers and ample dexterity. As a rule, heavy, gauntlet-style gloves are too awkward for most rescue work.

- **Foot protection:** As a rule, the best general boots for EMS work are high-top, steel-toed and/or shank boots with a coarse lug sole to provide traction and prevent slipping. For rescue operations, lace-up boots offer greater stability and better ankle support by limiting the range of motion. They also don't come off as easily as pull-on boots when walking through deep mud.

- **Flame/flash protection:** Whenever there is the potential for fire, turnout gear, coveralls, and jumpsuits all offer some arm and leg protection and help prevent damage to your uniform. They also have the added advantage of quick and easy application. For protection against the sharp, jagged metal or glass found at many motor vehicle collisions or structural collapses, turnout gear generally works best.

- **Personal flotation devices (PFDs):** If your service includes areas where water emergencies can result, your unit should carry PFDs that meet the U.S. Coast Guard standards for flotation. They should be worn whenever operating in or around water. You should also attach a knife, strobe light, and whistle to the PFD so that they are easily accessible.

- **Lighting:** Depending upon the type and location of the rescue, you might also consider portable lighting. Many rescuers carry at least a flashlight or, better yet, a headlamp that can be attached to a helmet for hands-free operation.

- **Hazmat suits or SCBA (self-contained breathing apparatus):** These items should only be made available to the personnel trained to use them.

- **Extended, remote, or wilderness protection:** If your unit provides service to a remote or wilderness area, you would be advised to have a backcountry survival pack as part of your gear. This backpack should be loaded with PPE for inclement weather, provisions for personal drinking water (iodine tablets/water filter), snacks for a few hours, temporary shelter, butane lighter, and some redundancy in lighting in case of light-source failure.

Chapter 10 Answer Key

©2009 Pearson Education, Inc.
Paramedic Care: Principles & Practice, Vol. 5, 3rd. Ed.

Handout 10-2: Chapter 10 Quiz

1.	B	**5.**	C	**9.**	C	**13.**	B
2.	A	**6.**	D	**10.**	C	**14.**	D
3.	D	**7.**	A	**11.**	B	**15.**	C
4.	D	**8.**	B	**12.**	C		

Handout 10-3: Chapter 10 Scenario

1. This is a rescue situation because the woman is unable to get herself out of the pool and she has traumatic injury, although you can't yet determine the specifics. The presence of an early black eye and bleeding from the left temple suggests the possibility of a head injury.

   You should examine the rest of the pool perimeter for potential safety hazards, as well as for evidence of where she fell into the pool (perhaps the presence of blood at the edge of the pool, if she hit her head while falling into the pool).

   There is already evidence of potential hazard at the scene: The man is under the influence of alcohol and shows no concern about his wife. Not only has he not been helpful, he is a potential risk to you and your partner. The situation also has some suggestions of possible domestic violence, which further complicates matters for you and your partner and suggests the woman may have injuries unrelated to her exposure in the pool.

2. You should call for immediate police backup and consider a second EMS unit to help you evaluate the woman's condition in the pool and assist in her rescue.

3. While you wait for the scene to be secured, your partner should continue to talk with her to get any historical information about the incident or admission of complicating factors (namely, she didn't fall into the pool on her own) and as part of an ongoing assessment of mental status. You also need to monitor for any signs of hypothermia or other change in condition that would override a delay in removal until the scene is clearly secured and sufficient help is on hand.

4. When the scene has been secured for your safety, you will need to perform in-water spinal immobilization, apply a rigid cervical collar, and apply a spine board before removing the patient from the water.

Handout 10-4: Chapter 10 Review

1. inclement weather, drinking water, shelter, butane, lighting
2. arrival, hazard, patient, medical treatment, disentanglement, packaging, removal
3. Access
4. patient assessment, patient care, removal, transport
5. active rescue zone
6. personal flotation devices (PFDs), Heat Escape Lessening Position (HELP), huddling together
7. reach-throw-row-go
8. Alcohol
9. PFD
10. warm, dead
11. spinal immobilization, rigid cervical collar, back boarding
12. electricity
13. secondary collapse
14. Traffic flow
15. touch
16. hazardous materials
17. Safety, tempered
18. low-angle, high-angle, flat terrain
19. differences
20. BLS, ALS

Handout 10-5: Rescue Awareness True or False

1.	T	**6.**	F	**11.**	T
2.	F	**7.**	F	**12.**	F
3.	F	**8.**	T	**13.**	F
4.	T	**9.**	T	**14.**	T
5.	F	**10.**	F	**15.**	T

11

Hazardous Materials Incidents

INTRODUCTION

Students were introduced to the concept of EMS calls related to toxic materials in Volume 3 of this series, where they read about toxicological and environmental emergencies (Chapters 8 and 10, respectively). This chapter expands on that base to discuss incidents in which hazardous materials are spilled or released as a result of an accident, equipment failure, human error, or intentional actions designed to skirt regulations regarding such compounds. Students will learn about the role of the paramedic in such hazardous materials (hazmat) incidents as well as specifics about medical care for patients contaminated with a hazardous material.

CHAPTER OBJECTIVES

Knowledge Objectives

1. Explain the role of the paramedic/EMS responder at the hazardous material incident in terms of the following:
   a. Incident size-up (pp. 451–461)
   b. Assessment of toxicological risk (pp. 454–459, 463–467)
   c. Appropriate decontamination methods (pp. 468–471)
   d. Treatment of semi-decontaminated patients (pp. 465–467, 471)
   e. Transportation of semi-decontaminated patients (p. 471)

2. Identify resources for substance identification, decontamination, and treatment information. (pp. 456–459)

3. Identify primary and secondary decontamination risk. (pp. 463–464)

4. Describe topical, respiratory, gastrointestinal, and parenteral routes of exposure. (p. 464)

5. Explain acute and delayed toxicity, local versus systemic effects, dose response, and synergistic effects. (pp. 464–465)

6. Explain how the substance and route of contamination alters triage and decontamination methods. (pp. 468–470)

7. Explain the employment and limitations of field decontamination procedures. (pp. 470–471)

8. Explain the use and limitations of personal protective equipment (PPE) in hazardous material situations. (pp. 471–473)

 TOTAL TEACHING TIME: 12.50 HOURS
The total teaching time is only a guideline based on the didactic and practical lab averages in the National Standard Curriculum. Instructors should take into consideration such factors as: the pace at which students learn, the size of the class, and breaks. The actual time devoted to teaching objectives is the responsibility of the instructor.

9. List and explain the common signs, symptoms, and treatment of the following substances:

   a. Corrosives (acids/alkalis) (p. 465)
   b. Pulmonary irritants (ammonia/chlorine) (pp. 465–466)
   c. Pesticides (carbamates/organophosphates) (p. 466)
   d. Chemical asphyxiants (cyanides/carbon monoxide) (pp. 466–467)
   e. Hydrocarbon solvents (xylene, methylene chloride) (p. 467)

10. Describe the characteristics of hazardous materials and explain their importance to the risk assessment process. (pp. 449, 469–471)

11. Describe the hazards and protection strategies for alpha, beta, and gamma radiation. (pp. 462–463)

12. Define the toxicological terms and their use in the risk assessment process. (p. 463)

13. Given a specific hazardous material, research the appropriate information about its physical and chemical properties and hazards, suggest the appropriate medical response, and determine the risk of secondary contamination. (pp. 454–459)

14. Identify the factors that determine where and when to treat a hazardous material incident patient. (pp. 460–461, 469–471)

15. Determine the appropriate level of PPE for various hazardous material incidents including:

    a. Types, application, use, and limitations
    b. Use of a chemical compatibility chart (pp. 471–473)

16. Explain decontamination procedures including:

    a. Critical patient rapid two-step decontamination process (p. 470)
    b. Noncritical patient eight-step decontamination process (pp. 470–471)

17. Identify the four most common solutions used for decontamination. (p. 470)

18. Identify the body areas that are difficult to decontaminate. (p. 470)

19. Explain the medical monitoring procedures for hazardous material team members. (pp. 473–474)

20. Explain the factors that influence the heat stress of hazardous material team personnel. (p. 474)

21. Explain the documentation necessary for hazmat medical monitoring and rehabilitation operations. (pp. 473–474)

22. Given a simulated hazardous substance, use reference material to determine the appropriate actions. (pp. 456–459)

23. Integrate the principles and practices of hazardous materials response in an effective manner to prevent and limit contamination, morbidity, and mortality. (pp. 449–474)

24. Size up a hazardous material (hazmat) incident and determine:

    a. Potential hazards to the rescuers, public, and environment (pp. 451–461)
    b. Potential risk of primary contamination to patients (p. 463)
    c. Potential risk of secondary contamination to rescuers (pp. 463–464)

25. Given a contaminated patient, determine the level of decontamination necessary and:

    a. Level of rescuer PPE (pp. 471–473)
    b. Decontamination methods (pp. 468–471)
    c. Treatment (pp. 465–467)
    d. Transportation and patient isolation techniques (p. 471)

©2009 Pearson Education, Inc.
Paramedic Care: Principles & Practice, Vol. 5, 3rd. Ed.

26. Determine the hazards present to the patient and paramedic given an incident involving a hazardous material. (pp. 449–474)

FRAMING THE LESSON

Where do you find hazardous materials? Ask students to list situations in which an EMS responder might find hazardous materials. Get students to list examples of the three major settings: residential, industrial, transportation, and then have them work to identify specific local sites that might be considered at high risk for a hazmat incident if an accident or terrorist act occurred there. Examples might include home fires, gas explosion, gasoline vapor inhalation from a ruptured container, industrial manufacturing settings (as well as industries that use chemicals, which range from photo development sites to dry cleaners to hair parlors), buried pipelines, bombings or fires, and highway accidents and train derailments.

CONSIDERING THE CASE STUDY

Ask a volunteer to read aloud the Case Study on text pages 448–449. Suggest that students close their eyes as the scenario is read to help them mentally visualize the events described in it. You can use the following questions as a starting point for teaching the chapter—a sort of chapter preview in a functional setting.

When the chapter is completed, you may wish to return to the Case Study and encourage further discussion aimed at answering the questions or solving the problems.

CASE STUDY DISCUSSION QUESTIONS (AND ANSWERS)

1. What elements of this incident are you already familiar with based on Chapter 9, "Medical Incident Command Management"?
   (Answers may include any of the following:
   - *Multiple casualties [six patients]*
   - *Scene size-up with one paramedic acting as Incident Commander and one acting as Triage Officer*
   - *Implementation of IMS with request for additional resources*
   - *Evaluation of incident as open or closed [closed: ammonia source has been eliminated as threat]*
   - *Transfer of command to supervisor*
   - *EMS work [as rehabilitation/rapid intervention team for hazmat crew])*

2. What elements of this incident and its management distinguish it as a hazmat incident?
   (Answers may include any of the following:
   - *Dispatch call for a chemical burn at an industrial plant signals possible hazmat incident*
   - *Field decontamination of patients with removal of clothing [with personal items] and gross decontamination measures*
   - *EMS completion of decontamination before treatment by ambulance crew*
   - *Support of hazmat team by first-response crew with preentry and postexit documentation of vitals and condition of each team member)*

3. What information that might be helpful is missing from the Case Study as printed?

(Answers may include any of the following:

- *Who confirmed that none of the bystanders or the security guard was exposed to the hazardous material?*
- *Could any of the bystanders who were helping the patient with eye injuries have been contaminated themselves [secondary contamination]?*
- *Is anhydrous ammonia a gas, a fluid, or a fluid with gas vapors?*
- *What routes of exposure are involved—respiratory, surface absorption, or both?*
- *What is the recommended decontamination for anhydrous ammonia? Where might you find that information at the plant [MSDS]?*
- *Were personal items [such as watches] removed with clothing, and how and by whom were they catalogued, cleaned, and retained safely?)*

TEACHING STRATEGIES

People learn in a variety of ways. Some do better with the spoken word, while others prefer the written. Some prefer to work alone, whereas others profit from working in groups. Recognizing these different ways of acquiring knowledge, the authors of this *Instructor's Resource Manual* have provided a variety of teaching strategies for the different types of learners. These strategies are intended to foster higher-level cognitive skills and encourage creative learning and problem solving.

For greatest effectiveness, incorporate these strategies into your class lecture. Marginal notes in the Teaching Outline indicate the points at which various exercises might be most appropriate. Other strategies can be used to preview the lesson or to summarize it.

The following strategies are keyed to specific sections of the lesson:

1. *Using Guidebooks.* Be sure to have a library of guidebooks available for student reference because most will be used too infrequently to warrant a purchase by the students. The library should include the following guidebooks: *Hazardous Waste Operations and Emergency Response Standard, NFPA 473: Standard for Competencies for EMS Personnel Responding to Hazardous Materials Incidents,* and the *North American Emergency Response Guidebook.* Encourage students to establish their own reference library as well as use your school's professional library. This demonstrates a commitment to lifelong learning that is important in prehospital care.

2. *Reviewing the Curriculum.* If they aren't already, be sure the hazmat awareness competencies are included in your core curriculum. Not only are they the standard for all emergency personnel, the information is imperative to your students' future personal safety.

3. *Hazmat Simulator.* Large or well-endowed fire departments possess simulators for hazmat operations much the way EMS does for rhythm generation and ACLS. Borrow or buy time with one of these simulators to give students a more realistic vision of the types of hazmat incidents they may encounter. The simulators use a mix of video and computer graphics to show the scene, victims, and even smoke, fumes, and fire. When using the simulator or other scenarios, be sure to focus on the paramedics' approach to the incident. Emphasize the difference in tactics used when the EMS responder is responsible for patient care versus hazmat operations in which the responder might be acting with the fire department.

©2009 Pearson Education, Inc.
Paramedic Care: Principles & Practice, Vol. 5, 3rd. Ed.

4. *Tabletop Scenarios.* Use your tabletop town for hazmat scenarios. Use toy or cardboard buildings and small cars to simulate hazmat incidents involving tanker trucks, school buses, farm equipment, and cargo trains. When you use your imagination, your students will too, improving their creative problem-solving skills.

5. *Thinking about Hazards.* Map out the block on which your school sits. Have students identify, by either educated guess or actual investigation, the hazardous materials that exist in each building or space. Whether you are on a college campus, in a hospital, or on a block with a hair salon, you are likely to have numerous hazardous materials lurking around your building. Facilitate a discussion about how those materials would need to be handled if an incident occurred at one of those facilities. You might even use your *Emergency Response Guidebook* to identify the proper decontamination and secure handling required in the event of an incident.

6. *Hazmat Placards.* Make your class a set of "placard flash cards" with colored cardstock. The symbols and numbers can be changed by affixing Velcro to them. When doing hazmat simulations or scenarios, use your placards. Similarly, drill the recall of the colors and numbers by using your placard flash cards for review.

7. *Assigned Reading.* *Vector* by Robin Cook is a novel based in reality and research that addresses the use and danger of biological weapons. Invite students to read the book and report on the themes. Or buy several paperback copies and use them as prizes when playing review games in class. Robin Cook has many books out that address particular medical topics, such as food-borne illness, cancer treatments, and female reproductive issues.

The following strategy relates to Special Features in the student textbook and can be used to enhance the student's understanding:

Patho Pearls: Hazmats and Terrorism. Your state emergency management agency can provide materials, education programs, and emergency operations information regarding hazardous materials and bioterrorism.

The following strategy can be used at various points throughout the lesson or to help summarize and demonstrate what students have learned:

Field Trip. If a hazmat incident occurred in your area, consider a field trip to the site, preferably in the company of an EMS provider who served there. Discuss relevant details on the nature of the hazardous substance; the degree of contamination of persons, equipment, and environment; and the medical care provided on site and during transportation (including decontamination on site and precautions taken against secondary contamination during packaging and transport). If there is no appropriate local site, consider use of photos as a case study aid.

TEACHING OUTLINE

Chapter 11 is the eleventh lesson in Volume 5, *Special Considerations/Operations.* Distribute Handout 11-1. If students have any questions about the objectives, answer them at this time.

Then present the chapter. One possible lecture outline follows. In the outline, the parenthetical references in regular type are references to text pages; those in bold type are to figures, tables, or procedures.

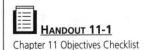
HANDOUT 11-1
Chapter 11 Objectives Checklist

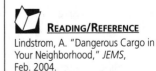
READING/REFERENCE
Lindstrom, A. "Dangerous Cargo in Your Neighborhood," *JEMS,* Feb. 2004.

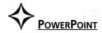

PowerPoint

PRESENTATION

Volume 5, Chapter 11, PowerPoint
slides 1–4

PowerPoint

PRESENTATION

Volume 5, Chapter 11, PowerPoint
slides 5–8

Teaching Strategy 1

Using Guidebooks

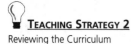

Patho Pearls

Hazmats and Terrorism, p. 450

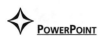

Teaching Strategy 2

Reviewing the Curriculum

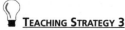

PowerPoint

PRESENTATION

Volume 5, Chapter 11, PowerPoint
slides 9–28

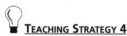

Teaching Strategy 3

Hazmat Simulator

Teaching Strategy 4

Tabletop Scenarios

Point to Emphasize

Placards may only provide minimal
information about a hazardous
substance. Some materials, when
shipped in smaller quantities, may
not require a placard at all.

PowerPoint

PRESENTATION

Volume 5, Chapter 11, PowerPoint
slides 29–30

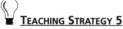

Teaching Strategy 5

Thinking about Hazards

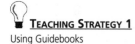

Teaching Strategy 6

Hazmat Placards

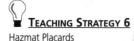

Teaching Strategy 7

Assigned Reading

I. Introduction. Hazardous materials (hazmat) are very common in all regions and in all settings. Definition per DOT is "any substance which may pose an unreasonable risk to health and safety of operating or emergency personnel, the public, and/or the environment if not properly controlled during handling, storage, manufacture, processing, packaging, use, disposal, or transportation." (p. 449) (**Fig. 11-1**)

II. Role of the paramedic. (pp. 450–451)

A. If first responders, roles include (p. 450)
   1. Scene size-up
   2. Assessment of toxicological risk
   3. Activation of IMS
   4. Establishment of command
B. Requirements and standards: Become familiar with publications (p. 450)
   1. OSHA
   2. EPA
   3. NFPA
C. Levels of training (p. 451)
   1. Awareness Level
   2. EMS Level 1
   3. EMS Level 2

III. Incident size-up. (pp. 451–461)

A. IMS and hazmat emergencies (pp. 451–452)
B. Incident awareness (pp. 452–454) (**Fig. 11-2**)
   1. Transportation (**Fig. 11-3**)
   2. Fixed facilities
   3. Terrorism
C. Recognition of hazards (pp. 454–456)
   1. Placard classifications (**Fig. 11-4; Fig. 11-5; Table 11-1**)
   2. NFPA 704 system (**Fig. 11-6**)
D. Identification of substances (pp. 456–459)
   1. *Emergency Response Guidebook* (ERG) (**Fig. 11-7**)
   2. Shipping papers
   3. Material safety data sheets (MSDS) (**Fig. 11-8**)
   4. Monitors and testing
   5. Other sources of information
E. Hazardous materials zones (pp. 459–460) (**Fig. 11-9**)
   1. Hot (red or exclusionary) zone
   2. Warm (yellow or contamination reduction) zone
   3. Cold (green or safe) zone

IV. Specialized terminology. (pp. 461–463)

A. Terms for medical hazmat operations (pp. 461–463)
   1. Boiling point
   2. Flammable/explosive limits
   3. Flash point
   4. Ignition temperature
   5. Specific gravity
   6. Vapor density
   7. Vapor pressure
   8. Water solubility
   9. Alpha radiation (**Fig. 11-10**)
   10. Beta radiation
   11. Gamma radiation

B. Toxicological terms (p. 463)
    1. Threshold limit value/time weighted average (TLV/TWA)
    2. Threshold limit value/short-term exposure limit (TLV/STEL)
    3. Threshold limit value/ceiling level (TLV/CL)
    4. Lethal concentration/lethal dose (LCt/LD)
    5. Parts per million/parts per billion (ppm/ppb)
    6. Immediately dangerous to life and health (IDLH)

V. Contamination and toxicology review. (pp. 463–467)

A. Types of contamination (pp. 463–464)
    1. Primary
        a. Direct exposure to a hazardous substance
    2. Secondary
        a. Transfer of a hazardous substance to a noncontaminated person via contact with someone or something already contaminated
B. Routes of exposure (p. 464)
    1. Respiratory
    2. Topical
    3. Parenteral
    4. Gastrointestinal
C. Cycles and actions of poisons (pp. 464–465)
    1. Acute effects
        a. Signs and symptoms displayed rapidly on exposure to a substance
    2. Delayed effects
        a. Signs and symptoms that develop well after exposure
    3. Local effects
        a. Effects involving the area around the immediate site of exposure
    4. Systemic effects
        a. Effects that occur throughout the body after exposure to a toxic substance
D. Treatment of common exposures (pp. 465–467)
    1. Corrosives
    2. Pulmonary irritants
    3. Pesticides
    4. Chemical asphyxiants
        a. Cyanide exposure
            i. Cyanide antidote kit (also called a Pasadena, Lilly, or Taylor kit)
            ii. Hydoxocobalamin (Cyanokit®)
    5. Hydrocarbon solvents

VI. Approaches to decontamination. (pp. 468–471)

A. Methods of decontamination (p. 468)
    1. Dilution
    2. Absorption
    3. Neutralization
    4. Isolation/disposal
B. Decontamination decision making (pp. 469–470)
    1. Modes of operation
        a. Fast-break decision making
        b. Long-term decision making
C. Field decontamination (pp. 470–471)
    1. Two-step process
        a. Removal of clothing and personal effects
        b. Gross decontamination (two times)

 POINT TO EMPHASIZE
At a hazmat incident, keep a bad situation from becoming worse by evacuating uncontaminated people from the area around the incident.

 POWERPOINT
PRESENTATION
Volume 5, Chapter 11, PowerPoint slides 31–47

 POWERPOINT
PRESENTATION
Volume 5, Chapter 11, PowerPoint slides 48–59

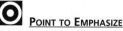 **POINT TO EMPHASIZE**
If life threat exists, the patients come first, environmental considerations last.

2. Eight-step process
   a. *Step 1*: Workers enter decon area and mechanically remove contaminants from victims.
   b. *Step 2*: Drop equipment in tool-drop area; remove outer gloves.
   c. *Step 3*: Decon personnel showers for victims and rescuers.
   d. *Step 4*: Removal and isolation of SCBA.
   e. *Step 5*: Removal of all protective clothing.
   f. *Step 6*: Removal of personal clothing from victims and rescuers.
   g. *Step 7*: Full-body wash for rescuers and victims.
   h. *Step 8*: Assessment and transport of victims; monitoring of rescuers.
3. Transportation considerations

POWERPOINT

PRESENTATION

Volume 5, Chapter 11, PowerPoint slides 60–66

VII. Hazmat protection equipment. (pp. 471–473) **(Fig. 11-12)**

A. Level A (p. 471)
   1. Highest-level respiratory and splash protection
   2. Sealed, impenetrable, fully encapsulating hazmat suits
B. Level B (pp. 471–473)
   1. Full respiratory protection
   2. Nonencapsulating but chemical resistant
C. Level C (pp. 473)
   1. Nonpermeable suit with air-purifying respirator
D. Level D (p. 473)
   1. Turnout gear

VIII. Medical monitoring and rehabilitation. (pp. 473–474)

A. Entry readiness (p. 473)
B. Post-exit "rehab" (p. 473) **(Fig. 11-13)**
C. Heat stress factors (p. 474)

IX. Importance of practice. (p. 474)

A. Potential incident scene activities
   1. Establish command
   2. Make the first incident decisions
   3. Help protect all on-scene personnel

POINT TO EMPHASIZE

If you observe anything abnormal during preentry medical monitoring, do not allow the hazmat team member to attempt a rescue.

B. To achieve proficiency, paramedics must become actively involved in drills and exercises to prepare for a hazardous materials incident.
C. Become involved with local emergency operations planning.

X. Summary. It is critically important that the paramedic be prepared for a hazmat incident. Become involved with the planning and practicing of hazmat operations plans within your jurisdiction. (p. 474)

POWERPOINT

PRESENTATION

Volume 5, Chapter 11, PowerPoint slide 67

YOU MAKE THE CALL

Review student responses to the You Make the Call scenario on text page 475. Suggested responses to the questions that follow the scenario are given below. Point out to students that these are acceptable answers but not necessarily the only ones. Discuss with students the pros and cons of points where their responses differ from these.

1. What do you suspect has happened based on your quick scene size-up?
   (You suspect hazardous materials are involved in the incident. The tractor-trailer is carrying a placard, it is leaking some kind of liquid, and occupants are drooling, tearing, sweating, and experiencing respiratory distress.)

2. What are your initial priorities?
(Your incident priorities include life safety, incident stabilization, and property conservation.)

3. How will you identify the substance involved in the accident?
(Identification of the substance can be performed through use of the placard, which indicates some kind of poison. An NAERG will identify the specific chemical. Based on the poison placard and the SLUDGE symptoms exhibited by the occupants of the truck, you suspect an organophosphate insecticide. Positive identification can be made using the shipping papers found with the driver of the truck or in the cab. You might also consult one or more of the computerized data banks or telephone hotlines mentioned in this chapter.)

4. What additional resources would you request?
(You will ask for a hazmat team and special fire apparatus. These units will be needed for entry, removal of the patient from the car, hazard control, and decontamination. You will also request three additional ambulances. Counting your unit, there will be one ambulance for each patient and one for the hazardous materials team.)

5. Is this a fast-break or a long-term incident? Explain.
(This is a fast-break incident. Two patients exhibiting critical symptoms have self-rescued and brought themselves to your ambulance.)

6. What are your first actions?
(Your first actions are to secure the scene, set up a perimeter to prevent further contamination, and request assistance. Upon arrival of fire apparatus, available PPE can be donned and two-step decontamination performed on the two occupants of the truck who are near your ambulance.)

ASSIGNMENTS

Assign students to complete Chapter 11 of the Workbook. Also assign them to read Chapter 12, "Crime Scene Awareness," of the textbook before the next class.

EVALUATION

Chapter Quiz and Scenario Distribute copies of the Chapter Quiz provided in Handout 11-2 to evaluate student understanding of this chapter. Make sure each student reads the scenario to reinforce critical thinking on the scene. Remind students not to use their notes or textbooks while taking the quiz.

Student CD Quizzes for every chapter are contained on the dynamic and highly visual in-text student CD.

Companion Website Additional quizzes for every chapter are contained on this exciting website.

TestGen You may wish to create a custom-tailored test using *Prentice Hall TestGen for Paramedic Care: Principles & Practice*, 3rd edition, to evaluate student understanding of this chapter.

Online Test Preparation (for students and instructors) Additional test preparation is available through Brady's new online product, *EMT Achieve: Paramedic Test Preparation*, at *http://www.prenhall.com/emtachieve*. Instructors can also monitor student mastery online.

WORKBOOK
Chapter 11 Activities

READING/REFERENCE
Textbook, pp. 478–499

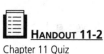
HANDOUT 11-2
Chapter 11 Quiz

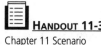
HANDOUT 11-3
Chapter 11 Scenario

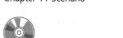
PARAMEDIC STUDENT CD
Student Activities

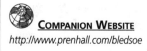
COMPANION WEBSITE
http://www.prenhall.com/bledsoe

TESTGEN
Volume 5, Chapter 11

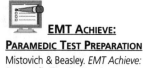
EMT ACHIEVE: PARAMEDIC TEST PREPARATION
Mistovich & Beasley. *EMT Achieve: Paramedic Test Preparation*, *http://www.prenhall.com/emtachieve*.

SUCCESS! FOR THE PARAMEDIC
Cherry. *SUCCESS! for the Paramedic,* 4th edition

HANDOUTS 11-4 TO 11-6
Reinforcement Activities

PARAMEDIC STUDENT CD
Student Activities

POWERPOINT PRESENTATION
Volume 5

COMPANION WEBSITE
http://www.prenhall.com/bledsoe

ONEKEY
Volume 5, Chapter 11

ADVANCED LIFE SUPPORT SKILLS
Larmon & Davis. *Advanced Life Support Skills*

ADVANCED LIFE SKILLS REVIEW
Larmon & Davis. *Advanced Life Skills Review*

BRADY SKILLS SERIES: ALS
Larmon & Davis. *Brady Skills Series: ALS*

PARAMEDIC NATIONAL STANDARDS SELF-TEST
Miller. *Paramedic National Standards Self-Test,* 5th edition

Success! for the Paramedic   Keyed to *Paramedic Care: Principles & Practice* and *Essentials of Paramedic Care,* this comprehensive exam review contains hundreds of test questions and rationales.

REINFORCEMENT

Handouts   If classroom discussion or performance on the quiz indicates that some students have not fully mastered the chapter content, you may wish to assign some or all of the Reinforcement Handouts for this chapter.

Student CD (for students)   A wide variety of material on this CD-ROM will reinforce and also expand student knowledge and skills.

PowerPoint Presentation (for instructors)   The PowerPoint material developed for this chapter offers useful reinforcement of chapter content.

Companion Website (for students)   Additional review quizzes and links to EMS resources will contribute to further reinforcement of the chapter.

OneKey   Online support is offered for this course on one of three platforms: CourseCompass, Blackboard, or WebCT. Includes the IRM, PowerPoints, Test Manager, and Companion Website for instruction. Ask your local sales representative for more information.

Brady Skills Series: Advanced Life Skills (Video or CD)   Have your students watch the skills come to life on VHS or CD-ROM, or they can purchase the highly visual, full-color text with step-by-step procedures with rationales.

Paramedic National Standards Self-Test   Another comprehensive review manual containing hundreds of review questions with page references keyed to several Brady texts.

©2009 Pearson Education, Inc.
Paramedic Care: Principles & Practice, Vol. 5, 3rd. Ed.

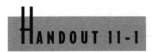
CHAPTER 11 OBJECTIVES CHECKLIST

Knowledge Objective	Date Mastered
1. Explain the role of the paramedic/EMS responder at the hazardous material incident in terms of the following:	
a. Incident size-up	
b. Assessment of toxicological risk	
c. Appropriate decontamination methods	
d. Treatment of semi-decontaminated patients	
e. Transportation of semi-decontaminated patients	
2. Identify resources for substance identification, decontamination, and treatment information.	
3. Identify primary and secondary decontamination risk.	
4. Describe topical, respiratory, gastrointestinal, and parenteral routes of exposure.	
5. Explain acute and delayed toxicity, local versus systemic effects, dose response, and synergistic effects.	
6. Explain how the substance and route of contamination alters triage and decontamination methods.	
7. Explain the employment and limitations of field decontamination procedures.	
8. Explain the use and limitations of personal protective equipment (PPE) in hazardous material situations.	
9. List and explain the common signs, symptoms, and treatment of the following substances:	
a. Corrosives (acids/alkalis)	
b. Pulmonary irritants (ammonia/chlorine)	
c. Pesticides (carbamates/organophosphates)	
d. Chemical asphyxiants (cyanides/carbon monoxide)	
e. Hydrocarbon solvents (xylene, methylene chloride)	

OBJECTIVES

Knowledge Objective	Date Mastered
10. Describe the characteristics of hazardous materials and explain their importance to the risk assessment process.	
11. Describe the hazards and protection strategies for alpha, beta, and gamma radiation.	
12. Define the toxicological terms and their use in the risk assessment process.	
13. Given a specific hazardous material, research the appropriate information about its physical and chemical properties and hazards, suggest the appropriate medical response, and determine the risk of secondary contamination.	
14. Identify the factors that determine where and when to treat a hazardous material incident patient.	
15. Determine the appropriate level of PPE for various hazardous material incidents including:	
a. Types, application, use, and limitations	
b. Use of a chemical compatibility chart	
16. Explain decontamination procedures including:	
a. Critical patient rapid two-step decontamination process	
b. Noncritical patient eight-step decontamination process	
17. Identify the four most common solutions used for decontamination.	
18. Identify the body areas that are difficult to decontaminate.	
19. Explain the medical monitoring procedures for hazardous material team members.	
20. Explain the factors that influence the heat stress of hazardous material team personnel.	
21. Explain the documentation necessary for hazmat medical monitoring and rehabilitation operations.	
22. Given a simulated hazardous substance, use reference material to determine the appropriate actions.	
23. Integrate the principles and practices of hazardous materials response in an effective manner to prevent and limit contamination, morbidity, and mortality.	

Knowledge Objective	Date Mastered
24. Size up a hazardous material (hazmat) incident and determine:	
a. Potential hazards to the rescuers, public, and environment	
b. Potential risk of primary contamination to patients	
c. Potential risk of secondary contamination to rescuers	
25. Given a contaminated patient, determine the level of decontamination necessary and:	
a. Level of rescuer PPE	
b. Decontamination methods	
c. Treatment	
d. Transportation and patient isolation techniques	
26. Determine the hazards present to the patient and paramedic given an incident involving a hazardous material.	

Student's Name _____

CHAPTER 11 QUIZ

Write the letter of the best answer in the space provided.

_____ 1. Roles of EMS providers who are the first responders to a hazmat incident include all of the following EXCEPT:
   A. assessment of toxicological risk.
   B. activation of IMS.
   C. initial containment procedures.
   D. establishment of Incident Command.

_____ 2. The three levels of training that an EMS provider may acquire include all of the following EXCEPT:
   A. awareness level.   C. operations level.
   B. supervisory level.   D. technician level.

_____ 3. The transportation warning placard for a flammable gas will have:
   A. red or green color and a flame symbol.
   B. red or green color and a ball-on-fire symbol.
   C. orange color and a flame symbol.
   D. yellow color and a ball-on-fire symbol.

_____ 4. At fixed facilities, the diamond segments of the hazmat placard give information on all of the following EXCEPT:
   A. health hazards.   C. fire hazards.
   B. explosion hazards.   D. reactivity.

_____ 5. CHEMTREC is an example of a:
   A. telephone hotline.   C. printed reference book.
   B. computerized database.   D. poison control center.

_____ 6. At a fixed facility, suggested emergency first-aid treatment may be found:
   A. at a central safety office.   C. on the container label.
   B. on the NFPA placard.   D. on a material safety data sheet.

_____ 7. Colorimetric tubes are used to:
   A. measure approximate pH of a liquid.
   B. measure approximate concentration of a given gas in the air.
   C. search air for specific chemicals.
   D. measure approximate concentration of oxygen in air.

_____ 8. Early in scene size-up of a hazmat incident, make sure to:
   A. evacuate all people from the scene of the incident.
   B. evacuate uncontaminated people from the region around the incident.
   C. rescue uncontaminated people from the scene of the incident.
   D. triage contaminated people at the scene of the incident.

_____ 9. The lowest temperature at which a liquid will give off enough vapors to ignite is called the:
   A. lower ignition limit.   C. ignition temperature.
   B. flash point.   D. vapor density temperature.

_____ 10. The most hazardous type of radiation is called:
   A. alpha radiation.   C. delta radiation.
   B. beta radiation.   D. gamma radiation.

©2009 Pearson Education, Inc.
Paramedic Care: Principles & Practice, Vol. 5, 3rd. Ed.

_____ **11.** The toxicological term used to express the level of exposure safe for someone with full-time occupational exposure is abbreviated as:
    A. LD.
    B. TLV/CL.
    C. TLV/TWA.
    D. IDLH.

_____ **12.** Secondary contamination is quite likely with:
    A. liquids and particulates.
    B. gases and liquids.
    C. gases, liquids, and particulates.
    D. liquids only.

_____ **13.** In hazmat incidents, the least common route of exposure is:
    A. respiratory inhalation.
    B. topical absorption.
    C. gastrointestinal ingestion.
    D. parenteral injection.

_____ **14.** Decontamination for pesticide exposure features:
    A. topical administration of water and green soap.
    B. oral administration of water.
    C. inhalation administration with high-flow oxygen.
    D. IV administration of sodium nitrite.

_____ **15.** Among the general methods of decontamination, the one almost never used by EMS personnel is:
    A. dilution.
    B. absorption.
    C. isolation/disposal.
    D. neutralization.

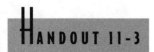

EVALUATION

Student's Name _____

CHAPTER 11 SCENARIO

Review the following real-life situation. Then answer the questions that follow.

You and your partner are called to an area near the railroad tracks that is frequented by homeless adults. The dispatcher tells you a small fire has been reported and there may be casualties.

When you arrive, you and your partner walk through a dumping area to reach a sheltered area near a bridge. Firefighters have already doused the fire, which burned down a makeshift tent made of cardboard and plastic sheeting. Two adults are sitting on a pile of tires near the fire scene: Each has visibly labored breathing, leaning forward and straining to breathe. One man looks as if he is barely conscious. A firefighter runs up to tell you that the two men stayed in the shelter after it started to burn because it was so cold outside. He moved them to their current position. He is concerned about smoke inhalation injury and possible hypothermia.

1. During initial scene size-up, what, if any, clues are present that might indicate a hazmat incident?

2. What needs to be done to confirm scene and personal safety?

3. Assume there is no evidence of hazardous substances other than those to which the men were exposed while they were in the burning shelter. What decontamination and treatment steps do you take?

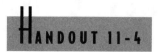

ANDOUT 11-4

Student's Name _____

REINFORCEMENT

CHAPTER 11 REVIEW

Write the word or words that best complete each statement in the space(s) provided.

1. Even a small-scale hazmat incident may turn into a multijurisdictional event, triggering use of the
_____ _____ _____ (_____).

2. The federal agencies that have published the most important requirements and standards are
_____ and _____.

3. Never compromise _____ _____ during the early phase of a hazmat operation or you risk becoming a patient yourself.

4. Basic IMS structure at a hazmat incident includes a(n) _____ _____,
a(n) _____ _____, and a(n) _____ _____.
Be sure you establish backup plans in case wind conditions or other environmental factors change quickly.

5. Hazardous materials may be present in any setting: residential, business, or highway. If you suspect hazmat, use _____ to inspect the scene from a distance.

6. When hazardous materials are transported in _____ _____, the use of a placard may not be required.

7. With the NFPA system, the scale of 0 to 4 represents _____ _____ on one end of the scale and _____ _____ on the other end.

8. After you have determined that one or more hazardous materials is present at a scene, you need to find _____ or more concurring reference sources regarding identification before taking any specific actions.

9. Two limitations of the *North American Emergency Response Guidebook* (ERG) are the presence of only _____ information on medical treatment and the fact that more than one _____ may have the same UN number.

10. The three control zones at a hazmat incident are coded as red (hot, exclusionary) zone,
_____ (_____, _____) zone, and
_____ (_____, _____) zone.

11. Unless you or your crew have appropriate training, support, and equipment, you should remain inside the _____ zone.

12. Specific gravity compares a chemical with _____, whereas vapor density compares a chemical with _____.

13. Two sets of terms used to describe the action of a poison are _____ or
_____ effects and _____ or _____ effects.

14. Primary respiratory exposure cannot be decontaminated; however, you should _____
_____ _____ and _____ _____ to release any trapped gas.

15. Assess patients with smoke inhalation for these two by-products of combustion: _____
_____ and _____.

16. The four general methods of decontamination are _____, _____,
_____, and _____/_____.

©2009 Pearson Education, Inc.
Paramedic Care: Principles & Practice, Vol. 5, 3rd. Ed.

CHAPTER 11 *Hazardous Materials Incidents* 337

17. The first rule of EMS in hazmat situations is DO NOT _____ _____ _____!

18. Fast-break decision making is often employed at incidents with _____ injured patients and unknown or life-threatening materials.

19. When possible, use _____-_____ decision making because of its many advantages.

20. The two measures in two-step decontamination are removal of _____ and _____ _____ and _____ _____.

21. The four most common decontamination solvents are _____, _____, _____ _____, and _____ _____.

22. Another term for a field-decontaminated patient is a _____-_____ patient.

23. A hazmat suit that offers full respiratory protection and chemically resistant material that is nonencapsulating is termed _____ _____.

24. For a hazmat incident, always remember that some level of protection is better than none: Use _____ gloves and wear _____ boots.

25. Be sure to document seven variables for each member of the hazmat team at preentry and at postexit: _____ _____, _____, _____ rate, _____, _____, _____, and _____/_____ status.

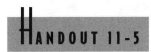

Student's Name _____

REINFORCEMENT

HAZMAT ABBREVIATIONS

Write out the term represented by each of the abbreviations used in Chapter 11.

1. DOT _____
2. IMS _____
3. OSHA _____
4. EPA _____
5. NFPA _____
6. MVC _____
7. WMD _____
8. UN _____
9. NA _____
10. ERG _____
11. CAMEO _____
12. CHEMTREC _____
13. CHEMTEL _____
14. MSDS _____
15. LEL _____
16. UEL _____
17. TLV/TWA _____
18. PEL _____
19. TLV/STEL _____
20. TLV/CL _____
21. LCt _____
22. LD _____
23. ppm _____
24. ppb _____
25. IDLH _____
26. SLUDGE _____
27. SCBA _____
28. APR _____

Handout 11-5

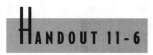

REINFORCEMENT

HANDOUT 11-6

Student's Name ______________________

HAZARDOUS MATERIALS REFERENCE TABLES

Complete the following tables and keep them for reference.

TABLE 1: HAZARD CLASSES AND PLACARD COLORS

Hazard Class	Hazard Type	Color Code
1		
2		
3		
4		
5		
6		
7		
8		
9		

TABLE 2: SYMBOLS FOR DIFFERENT TYPES OF HAZARDS

Hazard	Symbol
Flammable	
Oxidizer	
Radioactive	
Poisonous	
Reacts with water	

©2009 Pearson Education, Inc.

Chapter 11 Answer Key

Handout 11-2: Chapter 11 Quiz

1. C	**5.** A	**9.** B	**13.** C
2. B	**6.** D	**10.** D	**14.** A
3. A	**7.** C	**11.** C	**15.** D
4. B	**8.** B	**12.** A	

Handout 11-3: Chapter 11 Scenario

1. Fire always produces by-products, among them carbon monoxide and cyanides. Every patient with smoke inhalation has a possible exposure to one or both compounds. In addition, this fire involved burning plastic (a chemical compound) and may have involved one or more of the dumped items in the area. Thus, there is the potential for other hazardous substances to be present.

2. You should check with the firefighters to see what, if any, steps they took to identify possible hazards and remove them from the fire scene. Either you or your partner should make a quick scene check for possible hazardous substances while the other evaluates the two patients for possible surface contamination and then for medical needs. Both you and your partner should have donned personal protective gear including rubber boots and other protection (Level C or D gear, depending upon local protocol).

3. Both patients show respiratory distress or respiratory failure. Decontamination for carbon monoxide and cyanides would include immediate removal of clothing and personal items. (Watch for signs of hypothermia as you help them change into clean clothing.) Field medical treatment for carbon monoxide is oxygenation. Cyanide exposure is treated with use of a cyanide kit, which contains amyl nitrite, sodium nitrite, and sodium thiosulfate. Medical care still includes support of the ABCs, prevention or treatment of hypothermia, and any other needs suggested by patient assessment.

Handout 11-4: Chapter 11 Review

1. Incident Management System (IMS)
2. OSHA, EPA
3. scene safety
4. command post, staging area, decontamination corridor
5. binoculars
6. small quantities
7. no hazard, extreme hazard
8. two
9. general, chemical
10. yellow (warm, contamination reduction), green (cold, safe)
11. green
12. water, air
13. acute, delayed, local, systemic
14. remove all clothing, personal effects
15. carbon monoxide, cyanides
16. dilution, absorption, neutralization, isolation/disposal
17. become a patient
18. critically
19. long-term
20. clothing, personal effects, gross decontamination
21. water, green soap, isopropyl alcohol, vegetable oil
22. semi-decontaminated
23. Level B
24. nitrile, rubber
25. blood pressure, pulse, respiratory, temperature, body weight, ECG, mental/neurologic

Handout 11-5: Hazmat Abbreviations

1. Department of Transportation
2. Incident Management System
3. Occupational Safety and Health Administration
4. Environmental Protection Agency
5. National Fire Protection Association
6. motor vehicle collision
7. weapons of mass destruction
8. United Nations
9. North America(n)
10. *Emergency Response Guidebook*
11. Computer-Aided Management of Emergency Operations
12. Chemical Transportation Emergency Center
13. Chemical Telephone, Inc.
14. material safety data sheets
15. lower explosive limit
16. upper explosive limit
17. threshold limit value/time weighted average
18. permissible exposure limit
19. threshold limit value/short-term exposure limit
20. threshold limit value/ceiling limit
21. lethal concentration
22. lethal dose
23. parts per million
24. parts per billion
25. immediately dangerous to life and health
26. salivation, lacrimation, urination, diarrhea, gastrointestinal distress, emesis
27. self-contained breathing apparatus
28. air-purifying respirator

Handout 11-6: Hazardous Materials Reference Tables

Table 1: Hazard Classes and Placard Colors

Hazard Class	Hazard Type	Color Code
1	Explosives	Orange
2	Gases	Red or green
3	Liquids	Red
4	Solids	Red and white
5	Oxidizers and organic peroxides	Yellow
6	Poisonous and etiological agents	White
7	Radioactive materials	Yellow and white
8	Corrosives	Black and white
9	Miscellaneous	Black and white

Table 2: Symbols for Different Types of Hazards

Hazard	Symbol
Flammable	Flame
Oxidizer	Ball-on-fire
Radioactive	Propeller
Poisonous	Skull-and-crossbones
Reacts with water	W with a line through it

©2009 Pearson Education, Inc.
Paramedic Care: Principles & Practice, Vol. 5, 3rd. Ed.

12 Crime Scene Awareness

INTRODUCTION

Your students have already encountered the concepts of scene danger and of criminal activity in Chapters 4 and 9 (on abuse and neglect and IMS, respectively). This chapter discusses the possibility of danger in every setting, on every call, and it teaches safety strategies that your students can use throughout their working lives. In addition, the chapter explains basic guidelines for collaboration with law enforcement when EMS providers need to provide medical care at a crime scene. After reading this chapter, your students will understand the principles of evidence preservation and documentation.

CHAPTER OBJECTIVES

Knowledge Objectives

1. Explain how EMS providers are often mistaken for the police. (pp. 481, 486)
2. Explain specific techniques for risk reduction when approaching the following types of routine EMS scenes:
   a. Highway encounters (p. 484)
   b. Violent street incidents (pp. 484–486)
   c. Residences and "dark houses" (pp. 481–482)
3. Describe the warning signs of potentially violent situations. (pp. 481–482, 483–488)
4. Explain emergency evasive techniques for potentially violent situations, including: (pp. 484–494)
   a. Threats of physical violence
   b. Firearms encounters
   c. Edged-weapon encounters
5. Explain EMS considerations for the following types of violent or potentially violent situations:
   a. Gangs and gang violence (pp. 485–486)
   b. Hostages/sniper situations (pp. 491–494)
   c. Clandestine drug labs (pp. 487–488)
   d. Domestic violence (p. 488)
   e. Emotionally disturbed people (p. 488)

TOTAL TEACHING TIME: 5.39 HOURS
The total teaching time is only a guideline based on the didactic and practical lab averages in the National Standard Curriculum. Instructors should take into consideration such factors as: the pace at which students learn, the size of the class, and breaks. The actual time devoted to teaching objectives is the responsibility of the instructor.

6. Explain the following techniques: (pp. 490–491)

   a. Field "contact and cover" procedures during assessment and care
   b. Evasive tactics
   c. Concealment techniques

7. Describe police evidence considerations and techniques to assist in evidence preservation. (pp. 494–497)

Skill Objective

8. Given several crime scene scenarios, identify potential hazards and determine if the scene is safe to enter, then provide care, preserving the crime scene as appropriate. (pp. 480–497)

FRAMING THE LESSON

What makes up a dangerous situation? Have students recollect case studies from previous chapters of this book, as well as previous discussions in class, that focus on personal and scene safety. Students should recollect the chapter on abuse and neglect, as well as mention personal safety in the setting of major multiple-casualty incidents and in settings of violence (such as hostage/sniper incidents and terrorist acts). Some students may bring up environmental hazards such as highway accidents and physically unstable scenes and other rescue (or potential rescue) settings.

Get your students to see that potential dangers exist in almost every call and that it becomes crucial to have safety strategies in mind each time dispatch sends out their unit. Teach them that good safety skills may avert violence or save them from it and that the same types of awareness and tactical skills will help them to collaborate effectively with police when they need to give medical care at a crime scene.

CONSIDERING THE CASE STUDY

Ask a volunteer to read aloud the Case Study that begins on text page 479. Suggest that students close their eyes as the scenario is read to help them mentally visualize the events described in it. You can use the following questions about the Case Study as a starting point for teaching the lesson—a sort of chapter preview in a functional setting.

When the chapter is completed, you may wish to return to the Case Study and encourage further discussion aimed at answering the questions. Some questions, for instance those on provider roles on-scene, will make far more sense to students after they read the chapter.

CASE STUDY DISCUSSION QUESTIONS
(AND ANSWERS)

1. Walk through the Case Study with students. Ask them for material that relates specifically to safety.
   (Answers should include the following:
   - *Recognition at time of dispatch of geographic region of city in which call site is located ["well-kept part of the city"]*
   - *Actions taken at arrival to downplay visibility of ambulance [turning off lights at entrance to street, stopping two houses from the call house]*

©2009 Pearson Education, Inc.
Paramedic Care: Principles & Practice, Vol. 5, 3rd. Ed.

- *Request for additional information, notation of CAD information on that address*
- *Moving rig closer quietly*
- *Exiting with minimal equipment and taking separate, unpredictable paths to residence*
- *Looking in front window before approaching door)*

2. If you delete that material, what distinguishes this Case Study from others on medical emergencies?
(Nothing, and this is the point of the Case Study. Every call has the potential to be one, or become one, of violence toward your patient or you and your colleagues. The skills learned in this chapter and incorporated into your work life will help you to distinguish situations of potential danger as early as possible and to develop effective tactics when you find yourself in a situation that compromises your personal safety.)

TEACHING STRATEGIES

People learn in a variety of ways. Some do better with the spoken word, while others prefer the written. Some prefer to work alone, whereas others profit from working in groups. Recognizing these different ways of acquiring knowledge, the authors of this *Instructor's Resource Manual* have provided a variety of teaching strategies for the different types of learners. These strategies are intended to foster higher-level cognitive skills and encourage creative learning and problem solving.

For greatest effectiveness, incorporate these strategies into your class lecture. Marginal notes in the Teaching Outline indicate the points at which various exercises might be most appropriate. Other strategies can be used to preview the lesson or to summarize it.

The following strategies are keyed to specific sections of the lesson:

1. ***Restudying Scenarios.*** Have students look at situations with new eyes. Tell them to review earlier case studies and chapter scenarios such as those for Chapter 4 of this volume (on abuse and neglect), looking for instances in which personal danger was present for the EMS provider or could have developed. Have your students review their impressions of those cases in light of the awareness developed in previewing this chapter.

2. ***Developing Checklists.*** As you look at a typical call in your local area from time of dispatch to time of return, get students to develop a checklist of physical and mental actions they should take at every step. The list should cover each time point from dispatch (full information on call/caller, location of call) to scene arrival (inconspicuous arrival, initial scene size-up before leaving ambulance) to patient transport (watching family, bystanders for signs of incipient violence or threat, requesting backup if necessary).

3. ***Verbal Judo.*** "Verbal Judo" is a program that specializes in using verbal and body language to mitigate the potential for violent behavior in emergency situations. There is a full course offered by certified professionals in this program, as well as a book by the same name and a website at *www.verbaljudo.com*.

4. ***Gang Awareness.*** Most law enforcement agencies have a division or officer who specializes in gang intelligence. If you live in a small or rural area, call upon the services of your nearest urban law enforcement agency for this expertise. They will be able to share with students critical information about gang identification, behavior, and danger. Do not underestimate the penetration of gangs into your area, no matter how small or rural your community. Additionally, many students may go on to practice in cities beyond the immediate community.

If this information is omitted from your curriculum, your students will be ill-prepared in potentially dangerous situations.

5. *Identifying Hazards.* Many reality crime and law enforcement shows exist on television today. Select a few clips to show in class so that students can identify possible hazards and mitigation or safety approaches to the situation. This visual activity can be done as a cooperative learning exercise. Students will be amazed at how poor their memory is and how many details they miss. You may have to replay the tape several times before all hazards can be identified. Be sure to discuss the consequences of careless scene safety practices specific to the clips you are showing.

6. *Preserving Evidence.* Invite a crime scene technician or medical examiner to speak to your class about the preservation of evidence. Many students will be impressed by the type of evidence that can solve a case or lead to a conviction. Most will have a new respect for the consideration of evidence when treating persons involved in a crime. Few things will make as strong an impression as a trip to the morgue to watch a medical examiner gather the forensic evidence. Try arranging this with your ME office.

The following strategy relates to Special Features in the student textbook and can be used to enhance the student's understanding:

Legal Notes: Preserving Evidence at a Crime Scene. Invite a crime scene technician from your state police to speak on evidence, evidence collection, and how EMS can manage patient care while maintaining evidence integrity.

The following strategies can be used at various points throughout the lesson or to help summarize and demonstrate what students have learned:

Tactical Training. Borrow a tactical training area to run simulations for a day. A CONTOMS, TEMS, SWAT or other law enforcement academy will likely have a mock city area in which to practice scenarios that mimic crime scenes. Your students will benefit from getting out of the classroom, where they can actually approach an area from the side yard, peer through windows, and find areas of cover; all concepts you have taught in this chapter. This change of environment will definitely prepare students better than the standard classroom scenario situations.

Self-Defense. Offer a personal safety or self-defense course to your students after class or on a weekend. While this type of skill is not necessarily a psychomotor objective of the curriculum, many of the principles of personal safety are applicable. Most of these programs are low cost and can be contracted through a health club, gym, or law enforcement agency.

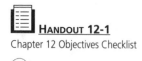

HANDOUT 12-1
Chapter 12 Objectives Checklist

TEACHING STRATEGY 1
Restudying Scenarios

TEACHING STRATEGY 2
Developing Checklists

POWERPOINT PRESENTATION
Volume 5, Chapter 12, PowerPoint slides 1–3

TEACHING OUTLINE

Chapter 12 is the twelfth lesson in Volume 5, *Special Considerations/Operations.* Distribute Handout 12-1. If students have any questions about the objectives, answer them at this time.

Then present the chapter. One possible lecture outline follows. In the outline, the parenthetical references in regular type are references to text pages; those in bold type are to figures, tables, or procedures.

I. Introduction. Violence is widespread, and you may be caught up in it during EMS calls. Learn safety tactics, know your local area, and familiarize yourself with protocols for handling dangerous situations and interacting with police. (p. 480)

II. Approach to the scene. Begin consideration of safety strategies at the time of dispatch (pp. 480–483)

   A. Possible scenarios (pp. 481–483)
      1. Advised of danger en route (**Fig. 12-1**)
      2. Observing danger upon arrival (**Fig. 12-2; Fig. 12-3; Fig. 12-4**)
      3. Eruption of danger during care or transport

III. Specific dangerous scenes. (pp. 483–488)

   A. Highway encounters (p. 484)
   B. Violent street incidents (pp. 484–486)
      1. Murder, assault, robbery
      2. Dangerous crowds and bystanders
         a. Signs of danger
            i. Shouts or loud voices
            ii. Pushing or shoving
            iii. Hostilities toward anyone on-scene
            iv. Rapid increase in crowd size
            v. Inability of law officers to control crowd
      3. Street gangs
         a. Appearance
         b. Graffiti
         c. Tattoos
         d. Hand signals/language
   C. Drug-related crimes (pp. 486–487) (**Fig. 12-5**)
      1. Signs of drug involvement
         a. Prior history of drugs in neighborhood of call
         b. Clinical evidence that patient used drugs
         c. Drug-related comments by bystanders
         d. Drug paraphernalia at scene
   D. Clandestine drug laboratories (pp. 487–488) (**Fig. 12-6**)
      1. Actions to take on discovering a clandestine drug lab
         a. Leave area immediately.
         b. Do not touch anything.
         c. Do not stop chemical reactions in process.
         d. Do not smoke or bring a source of flame into lab.
         e. Notify police.
         f. Initiate ICS and hazmat procedures.
         g. Consider evacuation.
   E. Domestic violence (p. 488)

IV. Tactical considerations. (pp. 488–494)

   A. Safety tactics (pp. 488–491)
      1. Retreat (**Fig. 12-7**)
      2. Cover and concealment (**Fig. 12-8**)
      3. Distraction and evasion
      4. Contact and cover (**Table 12-1**)
      5. Warning signals and communication
   B. Tactical patient care (pp. 491–494)
      1. Body armor (**Fig. 12-9**)
      2. Tactical EMS
         a. Members and organizations
             i. TEMS
            ii. SWAT-Medics
            iii. EMT-Tacticals
            iv. CONTOMS
            v. NTOA

POWERPOINT

PRESENTATION
Volume 5, Chapter 12, PowerPoint slides 4–10

POWERPOINT

PRESENTATION
Volume 5, Chapter 12, PowerPoint slides 11–20

POINT TO EMPHASIZE
There is no such thing as a dead hero!

POINT TO EMPHASIZE
In most cases, you can legally leave behind a patient when there is a documented danger.

TEACHING STRATEGY 3
Verbal Judo

TEACHING STRATEGY 4
Gang Awareness

READING/REFERENCE
Meade, D. M., and K. Dernocoeur. "The Art of Crowd Control," *EMS*, Sept. 1998.

TEACHING STRATEGY 5
Identifying Hazards

POWERPOINT

PRESENTATION
Volume 5, Chapter 12, PowerPoint slides 21–37

POINT TO EMPHASIZE
Nothing in the ambulance is worth your life. Retreat by foot or whatever means possible to avoid violence that threatens your life.

READING/REFERENCE
Meade, D. M., and K. Dernocoeur. "Cover and Concealment," *EMS*, Apr. 1998.

TEACHING STRATEGY 6
Preserving Evidence

LEGAL NOTES
Preserving Evidence at a Crime Scene, p. 495

POWERPOINT PRESENTATION
Volume 5, Chapter 12, PowerPoint slides 38–44

READING/REFERENCE
MacKay, D. W. "Evidence Preservation and Collection," *EMS*, Nov. 1997.

Cid, D., et al. "Integrating Criminal Investigation into EMS Scenes," *JEMS*, Jan. 1999.

POINT TO EMPHASIZE
If you must touch or move an item, remember to tell police.

POWERPOINT PRESENTATION
Volume 5, Chapter 12, PowerPoint slide 45

WORKBOOK
Chapter 12 Activities

READING/REFERENCE
Textbook Chapter 13, pp. 500–523

HANDOUT 12-2
Chapter 12 Quiz

HANDOUT 12-3
Chapter 12 Scenario

PARAMEDIC STUDENT CD
Student Activities

COMPANION WEBSITE
http://www.prenhall.com/bledsoe

b. Possible scenarios
   i. Raids on clandestine drug labs
   ii. EMS in barricade situations
   iii. Wounding by weapons or booby traps
      • Special gear for tactical operations
   iv. Use of CS, OC, or other gas
   v. Blank-firing weapons
   vi. Helicopter operations
   vii. Pyrotechnics
   viii. Extreme conditions
   ix. Firefighting and hazmat operations

V. EMS at crime scenes. (pp. 494–497)

A. EMS and police operations (p. 494) (**Fig. 12-10**)
B. Preserving evidence (pp. 495–497)
   1. Types of evidence
      a. Prints
      b. Blood and body fluids
      c. Particulate evidence
      d. On-scene observations
   2. Documenting evidence

VI. Summary. Your first priority at any crime scene is your own safety, and development of crime scene awareness is vital. When you treat patients at crime scenes, remember that you must work with police to preserve evidence. (p. 497)

YOU MAKE THE CALL

Review student responses to the You Make the Call scenario on text page 498. Suggested responses to the questions that follow the scenario are given below. Point out to students that these are acceptable answers but not necessarily the only ones. Discuss with students the pros and cons of points where their responses differ from these.

1. What is your evaluation of this situation from a safety perspective?
(There is a significant potential for danger. The son's apparent intoxication combined with the patient's warning that he "isn't quite right when he's drinking" clearly indicate the need for immediate action.)

2. What are your options?
(The two immediate options both involve retreat. You retreat either with the patient or without the patient. In this case, both you and the son want the same thing—you to leave. However, unless you can calm down the son, you may have to leave the patient behind, at least temporarily. Even though this action may be tactically and legally correct, thoughts of abandonment charges can be haunting. You may try to buy some time until the police arrive, but your main priority is personal safety. You also know that further agitation may only worsen the patient's condition. No matter how unsatisfactory, you may have to leave the scene until the police arrive to take charge of the situation.)

ASSIGNMENTS

Assign students to complete Chapter 12 of the Workbook. Also assign them to read Chapter 13, "Rural EMS," of the textbook before the next class.

EVALUATION

Chapter Quiz and Scenario Distribute copies of the Chapter Quiz provided in Handout 12-2 to evaluate student understanding of this chapter. Make sure each student reads the scenario to reinforce critical thinking on the scene. Remind students not to use their notes or textbooks while taking the quiz.

Student CD Quizzes for every chapter are contained on the dynamic and highly visual in-text student CD.

Companion Website Additional quizzes for every chapter are contained on this exciting website.

TestGen You may wish to create a custom-tailored test using *Prentice Hall TestGen for Paramedic Care: Principles & Practice*, 3rd edition, to evaluate student understanding of this chapter.

Online Test Preparation (for students and instructors) Additional test preparation is available through Brady's new online product, *EMT Achieve: Paramedic Test Preparation*, at *http://www.prenhall.com/emtachieve*. Instructors can also monitor student mastery online.

Success! for the Paramedic Keyed to *Paramedic Care: Principles & Practice* and *Essentials of Paramedic Care*, this comprehensive exam review contains hundreds of test questions and rationales.

REINFORCEMENT

Handouts If classroom discussion or performance on the quiz indicates that some students have not fully mastered the chapter content, you may wish to assign some or all of the Reinforcement Handouts for this chapter.

Student CD (for students) A wide variety of material on this CD-ROM will reinforce and also expand student knowledge and skills.

PowerPoint Presentation (for instructors) The PowerPoint material developed for this chapter offers useful reinforcement of chapter content.

Companion Website (for students) Additional review quizzes and links to EMS resources will contribute to further reinforcement of the chapter.

OneKey Online support is offered for this course on one of three platforms: CourseCompass, Blackboard, or WebCT. Includes the IRM, PowerPoints, Test Manager, and Companion Website for instruction. Ask your local sales representative for more information.

Brady Skills Series: Advanced Life Skills (Video or CD) Have your students watch the skills come to life on VHS or CD-ROM, or they can purchase the highly visual, full-color text with step-by-step procedures with rationales.

Paramedic National Standards Self-Test Another comprehensive review manual containing hundreds of review questions with page references keyed to several Brady texts.

TestGen
Volume 5, Chapter 12

**EMT Achieve:
Paramedic Test Preparation**
Mistovich & Beasley. *EMT Achieve: Paramedic Test Preparation,*
http://www.prenhall.com/emtachieve.

Success! for the Paramedic
Cherry. *SUCCESS! for the Paramedic,* 4th edition

Handouts 12-4 to 12-6
Reinforcement Activities

Paramedic Student CD
Student Activities

PowerPoint Presentation
Volume 5

Companion Website
http://www.prenhall.com/bledsoe

OneKey
Volume 5, Chapter 12

Advanced Life Support Skills
Larmon & Davis. *Advanced Life Support Skills*

Advanced Life Skills Review
Larmon & Davis. *Advanced Life Skills Review*

Brady Skills Series: ALS
Larmon & Davis. *Brady Skills Series: ALS*

Paramedic National Standards Self-Test
Miller. *Paramedic National Standards Self-Test,* 5th edition

Student's Name _____

CHAPTER 12 OBJECTIVES CHECKLIST

OBJECTIVES

Knowledge Objective	Date Mastered
1. Explain how EMS providers are often mistaken for the police.	
2. Explain specific techniques for risk reduction when approaching the following types of routine EMS scenes:	
a. Highway encounters	
b. Violent street incidents	
c. Residences and "dark houses"	
3. Describe the warning signs of potentially violent situations.	
4. Explain emergency evasive techniques for potentially violent situations, including:	
a. Threats of physical violence	
b. Firearms encounters	
c. Edged-weapon encounters	
5. Explain EMS considerations for the following types of violent or potentially violent situations:	
a. Gangs and gang violence	
b. Hostages/sniper situations	
c. Clandestine drug labs	
d. Domestic violence	
e. Emotionally disturbed people	
6. Explain the following techniques:	
a. Field "contact and cover" procedures during assessment and care	
b. Evasive tactics	
c. Concealment techniques	
7. Describe police evidence considerations and techniques to assist in evidence preservation.	

Skill Objective	Date Mastered
8. Given several crime scene scenarios, identify potential hazards and determine if the scene is safe to enter, then provide care, preserving the crime scene as appropriate.	

OBJECTIVES

Student's Name _____

CHAPTER 12 QUIZ

Write the letter of the best answer in the space provided.

_____ 1. Arrest rates for violent crime have risen most in which age group?
A. 10 to 20 years   C. 15 to 34 years
B. 15 to 25 years   D. 35 to 50 years

_____ 2. Safety information about a location for an upcoming call commonly comes from all of the following EXCEPT:
A. information from CAD on the location.
B. information from law enforcement officers on the location.
C. your familiarity with the neighborhood.
D. your experience (or lack of it) at that address.

_____ 3. Signs of impending danger in the setting of a crowd include all of the following EXCEPT:
A. hostilities toward anyone on the scene.
B. increasingly loud voices.
C. inability of police to control bystanders.
D. rapid decrease in crowd size.

_____ 4. The difference between cover and concealment relates to the degree to which you:
A. can rapidly exit if needed.
B. are protected from bullets.
C. can be seen by others.
D. can be identified by law enforcement.

_____ 5. Common safety tactics include all of the following EXCEPT:
A. contact and cover.   C. distraction and evasion.
B. retreat.   D. persuasion and retreat.

_____ 6. Your physical well-being is key to which tactic?
A. distraction and evasion   C. contact and cover
B. retreat   D. cover and concealment

_____ 7. With the use of contact and cover, the contact provider is responsible for all of the following EXCEPT:
A. initiating direct patient care.
B. providing limited function such as handling equipment.
C. performing patient assessment.
D. handling most interpersonal contacts at the scene.

_____ 8. Differences in care offered by a TEMS unit and a standard EMS unit include all of the following EXCEPT:
A. the major priority of patient extraction from the hot zone.
B. the fact that trauma patients are more frequently encountered than medical patients.
C. the use of metal clipboards and chemical agents.
D. consultation with Incident Commander regarding treatment and transport.

_____ 9. The best material in which to collect potential evidence is:
A. a plastic bag.   C. any airtight container.
B. a brown paper bag.   D. a glass container.

_____ **10.** Evidence that you may be asked to provide includes all of the following EXCEPT:
  A. clothing or other personal items you removed from the patient.
  B. your scene size-up regarding possible safety threats.
  C. your on-scene observations of setting and persons present.
  D. precautions you took to preserve blood evidence.

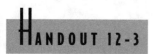

Student's Name _____

CHAPTER 12 SCENARIO

Review the following real-life situation. Then answer the questions that follow.

Dispatch calls at 10:43 P.M. on a hot summer night with a call for "person down in the street" in an area of the city you know well during daylight hours: a neighborhood with two hospitals, medical offices, and other businesses. The dispatcher has no additional information on the call because the caller hung up before she could ask any questions.

As your partner drives down a main street in the neighborhood, you notice how few people are walking by. There isn't much vehicular traffic, either. When your partner turns into the street given in the call, you don't see any cars or pedestrians and almost all of the buildings are completely dark.

Partway down the block, a young man runs into the street and starts waving his arms. You decide to get out and approach the man by walking up the opposite sidewalk. Your partner agrees to park on that side of the street near the corner. He will radio for police backup and come out to cover you from the street if you signal him. If you feel the scene is insecure, you are to retreat toward him and he'll drive forward to pick you up.

The young man looks frightened and is waving his arms frantically. "Hurry up, man. He's bleeding. You've got to help him." He points to a figure slumped on the sidewalk in the shadow of an office building.

You turn toward your partner and use your agreed-upon signal that he should call for police backup, move the ambulance somewhat closer, and then get out to cover you. The young man says "Thanks, man," touches your shoulder gently, and moves toward the figure, whom you see is another young man in similar clothes. The second man looks up, sees you, and says, "Please help me. He stuck me with a knife. I'm bleeding."

1. List the information given in the case study that would raise your suspicion of the possibility of danger at the scene or the possibility that the call involves violent crime.

2. The paramedic crew chose to use contact and cover as a safety tactic. Do you agree or disagree with their choice? Explain.

3. Is there any additional information that might have been available to the paramedics that might have influenced their choice of tactic?

©2009 Pearson Education, Inc.
Paramedic Care: Principles & Practice, Vol. 5, 3rd. Ed.

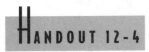

Student's Name _____

CHAPTER 12 REVIEW

Write the word or words that best complete each sentence in the space(s) provided.

1. Your most important safety tactic is an ability to identify _____ _____
   _____ as soon as possible.

2. A(n) _____ _____ (_____) unit is designed and staffed to
   handle on-site medical support to law enforcement.

3. Never follow a(n) _____ _____ to the scene of a call: Use lights and siren
   _____.

4. Two factors that might lead bystanders to confuse EMS providers with police officers are use of
   _____ and _____ on a vehicle and similarity in _____ or
   _____.

5. Potentially dangerous scenes include _____, _____, _____,
   and _____, to name a few.

6. _____ _____ should be well thought out in advance of the response to a
   hate crime.

7. Remember that EMS and law enforcement officials are on the same side: Be sure to have good
   _____ _____ with law enforcement.

8. Types of evidence include _____, _____, and _____.

9. Record only the _____ at the scene of a crime, and record them accurately.

10. If you must _____ or _____ an item at a crime scene, remember to tell
    the police.

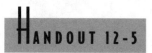
Student's Name _____

CRIME SCENE AWARENESS TRUE OR FALSE

Indicate whether each statement is true or false by writing T or F in the space provided.

_____ **1.** Because a significant number of people do not report violent crime to the police, an EMS provider may be the only contact a victim has with a professional who can intervene to prevent further harm.

_____ **2.** On arrival at a scene, you should rule out all immediate hazards before you knock on a door for entrance.

_____ **3.** Remember that there are only a few cases in which you can legally and ethically retreat without taking the patient with you.

_____ **4.** If you have to limit assessment and proceed with rapid transport of a patient because of on-scene danger, be sure to document your reasons for acting quickly.

_____ **5.** Retreat signals the end of the call: Thorough documentation will reduce liability and refute charges of abandonment.

_____ **6.** The effectiveness of body armor is largely unaffected by wetness or temperature, although it can get uncomfortably warm when worn in hot conditions.

_____ **7.** Never jeopardize patient care for the sake of evidence, but do treat every object that may be important as potential evidence in your handling and documentation.

_____ **8.** Remember that everything that you and your EMS colleagues see or hear can become evidence in a criminal case.

_____ **9.** If you have to move a gun, do not handle it on the grips or handles because you will destroy potentially valuable fingerprints.

_____ **10.** Most current body armor will prevent many types of penetration and severe cavitation.

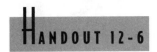

HANDOUT 12-6

Student's Name _____

REINFORCEMENT

CRIME SCENE AWARENESS REFERENCE SHEET

Some potential warning signs of danger in a vehicle include:

- Violent or abusive behavior
- An altered mental state
- Grabbing or hiding items from inside the vehicle
- Arguing or fighting among passengers
- Lack of activity where activity is expected
- Physical signs of alcohol or drug abuse—namely, liquor bottles, beer cans, or syringes
- Open or unlatched trunks—a potential hiding spot for people or weapons
- Differences among stories told by occupants

To make a safe approach to a vehicle at a roadside emergency, follow these steps:

- Park the ambulance in a position that provides safety from traffic.
- Notify dispatch of the situation, location, the vehicle make and model, and the state and number of the license plate.
- Use a one-person approach. The driver should remain in the ambulance, which is elevated and provides greater visibility.
- The driver should remain prepared to radio for immediate help and to back or drive away rapidly once the other medic returns.
- At nighttime, use the ambulance lights to illuminate the vehicle. However, do not walk between the ambulance and the other vehicle. You will be backlit, forming an easy target.
- Since police approach vehicles from the driver's side, you should approach from the passenger's side—an unexpected route.
- Use the A, B, and C door posts for cover.
- Observe the rear seat. Do not move forward of the C post unless you are sure there are no threats in the rear seat or foot wells.
- Retreat to the ambulance (or another strategic position of cover) at the first sign of danger.
- Make sure you have mapped out your intended retreat and escape with the ambulance driver.

In responding to the scene of any violent crime, keep these precautions in mind:

- Dangerous weapons may have been used in the crime.
- Perpetrators may still be on-scene or could return to the scene.
- Patients may sometimes exhibit violence toward EMS, particularly if they risk criminal penalties as a result of the original incident.

Whenever a crowd is present, look for these warning signs of impending danger:

- Shouts or increasingly loud voices
- Pushing or shoving

©2009 Pearson Education, Inc.
Paramedic Care: Principles & Practice, Vol. 5, 3rd. Ed.

CHAPTER 12 *Crime Scene Awareness* **357**

- Hostilities toward anyone on-scene, including the perpetrator of a crime, the victim, the police, and so on
- Rapid increase in crowd size
- Inability of law enforcement officials to control bystanders

Commonly observed gang characteristics include the following:

- *Appearance*—Gang members frequently wear unique clothing specific to the group. Because the clothing is often a particular color, even a bandana can signify gang membership. Within the gang itself, members sometimes wear different articles to signify rank.
- *Graffiti*—Gangs have definite territories, or "turfs." Members often mark their turf with graffiti broadcasting the gang's logo, warning away intruders, bragging about crimes, insulting rival gangs, or taunting police.
- *Tattoos*—Many gang members wear tattoos or other body markings to identify their gang affiliations. Some gangs even require these tattoos. The tattoos will be in the gang's colors and often contain the gang's motto or logo.
- *Hand signals/language*—Gangs commonly create their own methods of communication. They give gang-related meanings to everyday words or create codes. Hand signals provide quick identification among gang members, warn of approaching law enforcement, or show disrespect to other gangs. Gang members often perform signals so quickly that an uninformed outsider may not spot them, much less understand them.

There are a number of signs that can alert you to the involvement of drugs at an EMS call. These include the following:

- Prior history of drugs in the neighborhood of the call
- Clinical evidence that the patient has used drugs of some kind
- Drug-related comments by bystanders
- Drug paraphernalia visible at the scene such as
  - tiny zip-top bags or vials
  - sandwich bags with the corners torn off (indicating drug packaging) or untied corners of sandwich bags (indicating drug use)
  - syringes or needles
  - glass tubes, pipes, or homemade devices for smoking drugs
  - chemical odors or residues

If you ever come upon a clandestine laboratory, take these actions:

- Leave the area immediately.
- Do not touch anything.
- Never stop any chemical reactions already in progress.
- Do not smoke or bring any source of flame near the lab.
- Notify the police.
- Initiate IMS and hazmat procedures.
- Consider evacuation of the area.

Chapter 12 Answer Key

Handout 12-2: Chapter 12 Quiz

1.	C	**3.**	D	**5.**	D	**7.**	B	**9.**	B
2.	B	**4.**	B	**6.**	A	**8.**	C	**10.**	B

Handout 12-3: Chapter 12 Scenario

1. Answers include the following:

   - The call to 911 itself is suspicious: It comes long after dark and notes only that a person is down in a nonresidential area. The dispatcher cannot elicit any details because the caller hangs up right away.
   - In addition, there may be an element of concern at time of dispatch that any possible crime would involve drugs, given that the area has hospitals and doctors' offices.
   - While driving to the scene, you note there are few vehicles or pedestrians, which means you are more isolated.
   - In addition, the street location itself has no vehicles or pedestrians and is deserted and dark.
   - At the scene, you see only one person, a young man (in the age group [15 to 34 years] most likely to commit violent crime) who is visibly distraught.
   - The apparent patient, described only as "bleeding," is in a poorly lit, isolated spot.
   - The patient is another young man wearing clothes similar to the distraught man's, which might signal possible gang involvement.
   - The patient says he was stabbed, which makes it a crime scene.

2. There is no one way to handle an incident, and often wisdom comes only with hindsight. In the scenario, the contact provider decided that the scene was sufficiently safe to initiate patient contact with appropriate cover given by his partner (and with the knowledge that police had been notified). He may have noted that the man in the street seemed genuinely frightened and concerned for the patient and showed no hostility or fear toward the paramedic. In fact, he seemed grateful for help.

   A more conservative option would have been to call for police backup and wait for its arrival before exiting the ambulance. The unit would then have been capable of quickest retreat. This option could have been justified on the basis of the following:

   - The isolated nature of the scene
   - The lack of bystanders
   - The darkness of the scene (which could have been concealing individuals intent on harming the paramedics or stealing drugs from the ambulance)
   - The possibility of street crime or gang involvement
   - The presence of a number of doctors' offices, any of which could have been robbed for drugs or medical equipment

3. Answers might include any of the following:

   - Information from the dispatcher (or personal knowledge) about whether there had been incidents of attacks/thefts from ambulance crews in the city, particularly in that neighborhood
   - Information from the dispatcher (or personal knowledge) about whether the area had a high incidence of street crime, gang-related violence, or drug-related violence
   - Information from the dispatcher (or personal knowledge) of average time for police backup to arrive in that area at that time of night

Handout 12-4: Chapter 12 Review

1. potentially violent situations
2. tactical EMS (TEMS)
3. police car, cautiously (if at all)
4. lights, siren, uniforms, badges
5. Any four of the following are acceptable: highway encounters, violent street incidents, murders/assaults/robberies, dangerous crowds, street gangs, drug-related crimes, clandestine drug labs, domestic violence
6. Crew assignments
7. ongoing communication
8. Any three of the following are acceptable: prints (fingerprints, footprints, tire prints, and so on), blood and blood splatter, body fluids, particulate evidence, on-scene EMS observations
9. facts
10. touch, move

Handout 12-5: Crime Scene Awareness True or False

1.	T	**3.**	F	**5.**	F	**7.**	T	**9.**	F
2.	F	**4.**	T	**6.**	F	**8.**	T	**10.**	F

13 Rural EMS

INTRODUCTION

Although much of the material your students have studied applies in any setting, there are some situations that are more common in urban or in rural areas. This chapter addresses the issues that face rural EMS units, such as the frequency of rescue situations and long transport times to an appropriate hospital facility, as well as specific problems such as agricultural accidents and farm-related hazmat incidents.

CHAPTER OBJECTIVES

Knowledge Objectives

*1. Identify situations and conditions unique to rural EMS. (pp. 502–505, 508–520)

*2. Discuss various challenges facing rural EMS providers. (pp. 502–505, 508–520)

*3. Describe some of the possible solutions to problems commonly faced by rural EMS units. (pp. 505–507)

*4. Differentiate between rural and urban EMS when considering treatment and response time. (pp. 502–505)

*5. Identify important issues when faced with agricultural emergencies. (pp. 511–520)

*6. Review typical rural EMS scenarios, and identify what decisions a rural EMS provider needs to consider. (pp. 510, 515, 518, 519–520)

Note: The objectives for this chapter are not included in the DOT Paramedic curriculum.

FRAMING THE LESSON

What makes rural settings different? Ask students to consider what makes rural EMS service different from that of urban or suburban areas.

• Answers relating to distance may include long distances between the EMS unit and the medical scene and between the scene and the nearest appropriate medical facility.

• Answers relating to staffing may include the rarity of properly trained specialty teams (for wilderness or water rescue, for certain hazmat incidents, for multiple-casualty incidents, tactical EMS, and so on) or ALS-trained units.

TOTAL TEACHING TIME
There is no specific time requirement for this topic in the National Standard Curriculum for Paramedic. Instructors should take into consideration such factors as: the pace at which students learn, the size of the class, and breaks. The actual time devoted to teaching objectives is the responsibility of the instructor.

- Answers relating to medical problems may include the specificity of agricultural accidents or trauma associated with livestock handling, as well as common problems (such as acute MI) that may not be able to be handled in the recommended way (for example, ability to come within the window for thrombolytic therapy).

Either as a frame for the lesson or as a closing exercise, ask students to consider what alternatives and solutions are available to rural providers. Have them consider conventional solutions (air transport, for example) as well as ones dependent on new technology (such as cell phones for communication, electronic transfer of ECGs to a distant center, Internet-based visual demonstration of a procedure transmitted from a distant center, and so on).

CONSIDERING THE CASE STUDY

Ask a volunteer to read aloud the Case Study that begins on text page 501. Suggest that students close their eyes as the scenario is read to help them visualize the events described in it. You can use the following questions as a starting point for teaching the chapter—a sort of chapter preview in a functional setting.

When the chapter is completed, you may wish to return to the Case Study and encourage further discussion aimed at answering the questions.

CASE STUDY DISCUSSION QUESTIONS (AND ANSWERS)

1. After reviewing the Case Study, what elements of this medical emergency are unique to a rural setting?
   (Answers may include the following:
   - *The presence of a local BLS unit, with your ALS unit acting as a regional backup*
   - *The relatively long distance/time between the two EMS units and the farm scene*
   - *The setting of the silo, which raises questions on mechanism of injury if the problem is related to a fall or to a toxic exposure*
   - *Requesting permission from medical direction for contingency procedures in case complications arise and there is a communications blackout en route to the hospital.)*

2. Considering the problems related to the rural setting of this emergency, what alternatives are available, if any, for each problem?
   (Answers might include the following:
   - *The role of the ALS unit as a backup is actually a solution to problems of adequate staffing in rural areas. If the area is truly understaffed with ALS-qualified providers, additional training of BLS-certified providers is an option.*
   - *The issue of distance/time both from base to scene and from scene to hospital has two possible solutions: ground transport (which was used) and air transport. If the patient's personal medical history indicated he was at risk for myocardial infarction and/or the ECG suggested ischemia or injury, the team could have discussed air transport with medical direction if this were needed to preserve the possibility of thrombolytic therapy.*

©2009 Pearson Education, Inc.
Paramedic Care: Principles & Practice, Vol. 5, 3rd. Ed.

- *The BLS unit leader's questions about scene safety probably reflected concerns about the possible presence of hazardous materials at the silo. Some chemicals and chemical reactions are common at farms, and the EMS providers of both units should have some familiarity with common materials in use in their area. Knowing what questions to ask is as important as knowing that questions should be asked.*
- *The request for contingency orders reflects prudent problem solving in an area where communications blackouts are possible. It may also be worthwhile for the administrators of the ALS unit and the hospital to explore other wireless communications options.)*

TEACHING STRATEGIES

People learn in a variety of ways. Some do better with the spoken word, while others prefer the written. Some prefer to work alone, whereas others profit from working in groups. Recognizing these different ways of acquiring knowledge, the authors of this *Instructor's Resource Manual* have provided a variety of teaching strategies for the different types of learners. These strategies are intended to foster higher-level cognitive skills and encourage creative learning and problem solving.

For greatest effectiveness, incorporate these strategies into your class lecture. Marginal notes in the Teaching Outline indicate the points at which various exercises might be most appropriate. Other strategies can be used to preview the lesson or to summarize it.

The following strategies are keyed to specific sections of the lesson:

1. Developing a Rural EMS System. Develop a rural EMS system in class. Assign students to create solutions to the problem areas identified in the book, such as distance and time, communication, recruitment and retention, training, funding, and medical direction. This cooperative learning exercise gives students practice in real-world problem solving that may come in handy when your students are in a position to administrate in a rural area.

2. Thinking about Medical Direction. It's a fact that in some areas of the rural United States medical direction calls are taken by a receptionist who phones the physician at home and relays a message to providers. Challenge students to find as many examples of "medical direction" as possible by interviewing providers, using the Internet, and reviewing journals for variants in medical direction practices.

3. Studying Expanded Scope of Practice. To give students a better idea of the increased responsibilities common in rural areas, present information about systems utilizing expanded scope of practice models such as those in Syracuse, New York, and Red River, New Mexico. Either have students research these systems as a project or invite a speaker from one of the systems. Professional journals also carry information about such systems as well. This activity utilizes research skills important for effective and efficient information gathering. This skill will be important when students become professionals in positions that require them to make decisions about system issues.

The following strategy relates to Special Features in the student textbook and can be used to enhance the student's understanding:

Patho Pearls: Quality Considerations in Rural EMS. Check with your local hospital or state department of public health for information on rural health initiatives in your area. These initiatives usually address both hospital and prehospital patient care in the rural community.

The following strategies can be used at various points throughout the lesson or to help summarize and demonstrate what students have learned:

Field Trip: EMS System.   If you teach in an urban area, this lecture will seem unimportant and possibly even foreign to your students. Lend a note of reality to it by arranging a class visit to a rural EMS system. Visit dispatch and arrange for ride-alongs if possible. Be sure to invite members of the rural service to share the experiences and challenges they face in EMS delivery in a rural area. Nearly half of all the people in the United States are treated by rural or volunteer providers, so the issues of EMS delivery in rural areas are very real and important to all providers, educators, and researchers.

Field Trip: Farm Visit.   Make arrangements with a local farmer to visit his property and view it and the type of equipment used in the enterprise. The farmer will be able to show the dangers of the equipment and may even be able to teach extrication from the hazards on the site. Many students, if they are from an urban area, will never have been on a farm, let alone seen the massive equipment that is used daily. This visit provides a stimulating environment in which to teach the objectives in this chapter, while employing all the senses of the students.

Volunteering in Rural EMS.   Encourage students to contribute to the profession by volunteering to provide EMS or education services to a rural area. Service to the profession is admirable and is much needed in these medically underserved areas. In addition, there are many principles of problem solving and decision making in the rural area that can enhance the urban paramedic's practice.

TEACHING OUTLINE

Chapter 13 is the thirteenth lesson in Volume 5, *Special Considerations/Operations*. Distribute Handout 13-1. If students have any questions about the objectives, answer them at this time.

Then present the chapter. One possible lecture outline follows. In the outline, the parenthetical references in regular type are references to text pages; those in bold type are to figures, tables, or procedures.

I. Introduction. The challenge for rural EMS providers is to give the same high-quality care possible in nonrural regions of the country (p. 502)

II. Practicing rural EMS. (pp. 502–507)

A. Special problems (pp. 503–505)
  1. Distance and time
  2. Communication difficulties (**Figs. 13-1; Fig. 13-2**)
  3. Enrollment shortages
  4. Training and practice
  5. Inadequate medical support
B. Creative problem solving (pp. 505–507)
  1. Improved communications
  2. Recruitment and certification (**Fig. 13-3; Fig. 13-4**)
  3. Improved medical support
  4. Ingenuity and increased responsibilities

III. Typical rural EMS situations and decisions. (pp. 508–518)

A. The distance factor (pp. 508–509) (**Table 13-1**)
B. Agricultural emergencies (pp. 511–518)

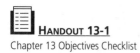

HANDOUT 13-1
Chapter 13 Objectives Checklist

READING/REFERENCE
Criss, E. "Rural Hospitals & Trauma Survival," *JEMS,* Sep 2002.

Garman, et al. "The Golden Rule: Do Unto Rural as You Do Unto Urban," *JEMS,* Dec. 2004.

Garza, M. "National EMS Survey Provides Data on Rural EMS," *JEMS,* Sept. 2002.

POWERPOINT
PRESENTATION
Volume 5, Chapter 13, PowerPoint slides 1–3

POWERPOINT
PRESENTATION
Volume 5, Chapter 13, PowerPoint slides 4–17

POINT TO EMPHASIZE
Every decision that a paramedic makes in a rural setting needs to be made with thoughts of distance in mind.

PATHO PEARLS
Quality Considerations in Rural EMS, p. 503

TEACHING STRATEGY 1
Developing a Rural EMS System

TEACHING STRATEGY 2
Thinking about Medical Direction

©2009 Pearson Education, Inc.
Paramedic Care: Principles & Practice, Vol. 5, 3rd. Ed.

1. Safety
   a. Farm machinery (**Fig. 13-5**)
   b. Hazardous materials (**Fig. 13-6; Fig. 13-7**)
2. Potential for trauma
3. Mechanisms of injury
   a. Wrap points (**Fig. 13-8**)
      i. Point where an appendage can get caught and significantly twisted
   b. Pinch points (**Proc. 13-1**)
      i. When two objects come together and catch a portion of the patient's body in between them
   c. Shear points
      i. When pinch points either meet or pass, causing amputation of a body part
   d. Crush points
      i. When two or more objects come together with enough weight or force to crush the affected appendage
4. Emergency medical care (**Fig. 13-9**)
C. Recreational emergencies (pp. 518–519) (**Fig. 13-10**)

IV. Summary. The unique challenges of rural EMS care have given rise to creative solutions in communication, transport, and staffing, and this problem-solving trend will continue. (p. 520)

YOU MAKE THE CALL

Review student responses to the You Make the Call scenario on text page 521. Suggested responses to the questions that follow the scenario are given below. Point out to students that these are acceptable answers, but not necessarily the only ones. Discuss with students the pros and cons of points where their responses differ from these.

1. What apparatus or support are you going to need to perform this rescue? *(As soon as the mechanism of injury and scene environment are known, additional personnel should be summoned. Because the water is surrounded by high cliffs and is remote, you should request a water rescue team. Following the request for adequate support and specialized rescue teams, you determine whether the patient should be transported by helicopter or ground unit. The transport time to the trauma center, the weather, the difficulty in assessing the patient, and the overall time from the onset of the injury should be considered. It is better to ask for help that you may not need than to need help and realize it has not been requested.)*

2. Based on the mechanisms of injury, what injuries should you suspect? *(The victim jumped into the water from a 50-foot cliff and landed in water of unknown depth, but apparently shallow. The history that he "jumped" in the water instead of "dove" into the water indicates that the patient may have lower extremity injuries in addition to head and chest injuries. Because the patient is unresponsive, it is likely that he has sustained a head injury. A chest injury is possible, as is the possibility of barotrauma if Todd held his breath when he jumped. If the patient landed on his feet, you should expect lower extremity injuries, including possible calcaneal fractures, lumbar spine fractures, and a cervical spinal injury. Always assume the worst and hope for the best.)*

3. What will you do to stabilize this patient? *(Stabilization of this patient is primarily surgical. However, you can attempt "field stabilization" while the rescue resources prepare for egress*

POWERPOINT
PRESENTATION
Volume 5, Chapter 13, PowerPoint slides 18–34

TEACHING STRATEGY 3
Studying Expanded Scope of Practice

SLIDES/VIDEOS
"Farm Emergencies," *Pulse: Emergency Medical Update,* Aug. 1997.
"Hunting Injuries," *Pulse: Emergency Medical Update,* Apr. 1997.
"Skiing Injuries," *Pulse: Emergency Medical Update,* Apr. 1997.

POWERPOINT
PRESENTATION
Volume 5, Chapter 13, PowerPoint slide 35

POINT TO EMPHASIZE
Paramedics who live or work in an agricultural area must familiarize themselves with the range of equipment used on farms or ranches.

from the quarry. The airway should be controlled if the GCS is less than or equal to 8. Full spinal immobilization should occur. Special attention should be paid to the chest because the patient is at risk for direct trauma and barotrauma. The on-scene time could be prolonged. Therefore, initiate fluid therapy per protocols and splint any fractures. If the patient has a neurologic deficit consistent with a spinal cord injury, consider beginning high-dose methylprednisolone therapy. Be sure to protect body temperature.)

4. What factors made it impossible for you to adhere to the axiom of the Golden Period?
(The location, mechanism of injury, required rescue resources, distance to the trauma center, and many other factors indicate that this patient will not be in a trauma center, much less an operating room, within an hour. You may have to provide extended care while the extrication is carried out. You have to do the best you can with what you have available. This victim undertook a high-risk exposure with some knowledge that the transport to a hospital might be quite prolonged. He has to accept those risks.)

ASSIGNMENTS

Assign students to complete Chapter 13 of the Workbook. Also assign them to read Chapter 14, "Responding to Terrorist Acts," of the textbook before the next class.

EVALUATION

Chapter Quiz and Scenario   Distribute copies of the Chapter Quiz provided in Handout 13-2 to evaluate student understanding of this chapter. Make sure each student reads the scenario to reinforce critical thinking on the scene. Remind students not to use their notes or textbooks while taking the quiz.

Student CD   Quizzes for every chapter are contained on the dynamic and highly visual in-text student CD.

Companion Website   Additional quizzes for every chapter are contained on this exciting website.

TestGen   You may wish to create a custom-tailored test using *Prentice Hall TestGen for Paramedic Care: Principles & Practice,* 3rd edition, to evaluate student understanding of this chapter.

Online Test Preparation (for students and instructors)   Additional test preparation is available through Brady's new online product, EMT Achieve: Paramedic Test Preparation, at *http://www.prenhall.com/emtachieve.* Instructors can also monitor student mastery online.

Success! for the Paramedic   Keyed to *Paramedic Care: Principles & Practice* and *Essentials of Paramedic Care,* this comprehensive exam review contains hundreds of test questions and rationales.

REINFORCEMENT

Handouts   If classroom discussion or performance on the quiz indicates that some students have not fully mastered the chapter content, you may wish to assign some or all of the Reinforcement Handouts for this chapter.

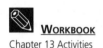 **WORKBOOK**
Chapter 13 Activities

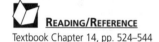 **READING/REFERENCE**
Textbook Chapter 14, pp. 524–544

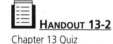 **HANDOUT 13-2**
Chapter 13 Quiz

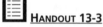 **HANDOUT 13-3**
Chapter 13 Scenario

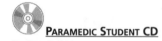 **PARAMEDIC STUDENT CD**
Student Activities

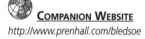 **COMPANION WEBSITE**
http://www.prenhall.com/bledsoe

 TESTGEN
Volume 5, Chapter 13

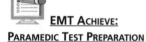 **EMT ACHIEVE:**
PARAMEDIC TEST PREPARATION
Mistovich & Beasley. *EMT Achieve: Paramedic Test Preparation,* http://www.prenhall.com/emtachieve.

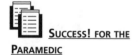 **SUCCESS! FOR THE PARAMEDIC**
Cherry. *SUCCESS! for the Paramedic,* 4th edition

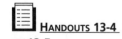 **HANDOUTS 13-4 TO 13-5**
Reinforcement Activities

Student CD (for students)   A wide variety of material on this CD-ROM will reinforce and also expand student knowledge and skills.

PowerPoint Presentation (for instructors)   The PowerPoint material developed for this chapter offers useful reinforcement of chapter content.

Companion Website (for students)   Additional review quizzes and links to EMS resources will contribute to further reinforcement of the chapter.

OneKey   Online support is offered for this course on one of three platforms: CourseCompass, Blackboard, or WebCT. Includes the IRM, PowerPoints, Test Manager, and Companion Website for instruction. Ask your local sales representative for more information.

Brady Skills Series: Advanced Life Skills (Video or CD)   Have your students watch the skills come to life on VHS or CD-ROM, or they can purchase the highly visual, full-color text with step-by-step procedures with rationales.

Paramedic National Standards Self-Test   Another comprehensive review manual containing hundreds of review questions with page references keyed to several Brady texts.

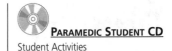
PARAMEDIC STUDENT CD
Student Activities

POWERPOINT PRESENTATION
Volume 5

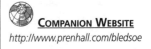
COMPANION WEBSITE
http://www.prenhall.com/bledsoe

ONEKEY
Volume 5, Chapter 13

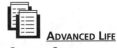
ADVANCED LIFE SUPPORT SKILLS
Larmon & Davis. *Advanced Life Support Skills*

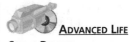
ADVANCED LIFE SKILLS REVIEW
Larmon & Davis. *Advanced Life Skills Review*

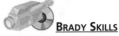
BRADY SKILLS SERIES: ALS
Larmon & Davis. *Brady Skills Series: ALS*

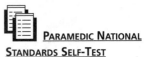
PARAMEDIC NATIONAL STANDARDS SELF-TEST
Miller. *Paramedic National Standards Self-Test,* 5th edition

Student's Name _____

OBJECTIVES

CHAPTER 13 OBJECTIVES CHECKLIST

Knowledge Objective	Date Mastered
*1. Identify situations and conditions unique to rural EMS.	
*2. Discuss various challenges facing rural EMS providers.	
*3. Describe some of the possible solutions to problems commonly faced by rural EMS units.	
*4. Differentiate between rural and urban EMS when considering treatment and response time.	
*5. Identify important issues when faced with agricultural emergencies.	
*6. Review typical rural EMS scenarios, and identify what decisions a rural EMS provider needs to consider.	

Note: The objectives for this chapter are not included in the DOT Paramedic Curriculum.

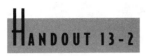
Student's Name _____

CHAPTER 13 QUIZ

Write the letter of the best answer in the space provided.

_____ **1.** Which of the following statements about rural U.S. settings is NOT true?
   A. Residents have a disproportionately high incidence of chronic medical conditions.
   B. There is a disproportionately low number of doctors who practice in the area.
   C. There is a higher level of mortality associated with trauma and medical emergencies.
   D. There is roughly the same age distribution of residents as found in urban/suburban areas.

_____ **2.** The high frequency of volunteer EMS squads correlates with all of the following EXCEPT:
   A. aggravation of the distance/time factor because volunteers must travel from home/work to the ambulance before leaving for the scene.
   B. squad makeup is more constant over time than in cities because of low turnover.
   C. ongoing training is paid by the volunteer, forcing a time and monetary sacrifice to remain up-to-date.
   D. low call volume may lead to inadequate experience with certain procedures to remain fully competent.

_____ **3.** Hospital agencies that provide limited care and nonemergent medical treatment are called:
   A. hospital satellites.   **C.** prompt care facilities.
   B. limited care facilities.   **D.** rural hospital affiliates.

_____ **4.** Reasons to consider putting a helicopter on standby include all of the following EXCEPT:
   A. mechanism of injury is a fall of 15 feet.
   B. mechanism of injury is ejection from a vehicle.
   C. a lengthy extrication is required.
   D. victim was in an unrestrained motor vehicle collision.

_____ **5.** One contraindication to helicopter transport is:
   A. high-altitude conditions, such as HAPE or HACE.
   B. posttrauma cardiac arrest.
   C. need for a hyperbaric chamber.
   D. smoke inhalation with altered level of consciousness.

_____ **6.** The safety tactic for eliminating accidental restart of farm machinery is called:
   A. equipment shut down.   **C.** equipment lock-out/tag-out.
   B. equipment power kill.   **D.** equipment stabilization.

_____ **7.** Possible hazards around grain tanks and silos include all of the following EXCEPT:
   A. presence of gases such as nitrogen oxides and methane.
   B. possible need for high-angle rescue.
   C. possible need for confined-space rescue.
   D. presence of chemicals used to preserve grain.

_____ **8.** The development of toxic shock in a patient who had circulation to a part of the body cut off for a period of time is called:
   A. anoxia syndrome.
   B. compartment syndrome.
   C. amputation syndrome.
   D. circulatory syndrome.

EVALUATION

_____ **9.** Common mechanisms of injury involving agricultural equipment include all of the following EXCEPT:
    A. pinch points.   **C.** crush points.
    B. shear points.   **D.** torque points.

_____ **10.** A tractor rollover may produce severe injury through the mechanism of:
    A. ejection.   **C.** exhaust inhalation.
    B. crush injury.   **D.** wrap injury.

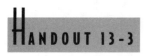

Student's Name _____

CHAPTER 13 SCENARIO

Review the following real-life situation. Then answer the questions that follow.

You work with a paramedic crew that serves as ALS backup for four local, volunteer EMS services. On a summer Sunday afternoon, you get a call simultaneously with one of the local units for a multivehicle collision on an interstate highway. As your partner checks the map, he says that you are probably 30 to 35 minutes from the accident scene. You will almost certainly be the first EMS responders because the local unit will not be able to roll until volunteers assemble, and the unit itself is garaged at least 20 to 25 minutes away from the scene.

As you drive to the accident location, the dispatcher comes back with additional information obtained by CB radio from a truck driver at the scene: The accident involved a tractor-trailer truck and two cars. The first car, which clipped the truck while trying to change lanes, has gone down a steep embankment but has not rolled. The trucker told the dispatcher two of the occupants seemed to be badly injured. The truck overturned and came to rest in the right travel lane and shoulder. The condition of the driver was not mentioned. The second car was traveling behind the truck and swerved off the road when trying to miss the colliding vehicles. It went down a less steep embankment and hit a tree before coming to rest. The trucker said the passengers in the front seats seemed to be badly injured, as well. He had no specifics on type of injury or whether the occupants of the truck and cars were still in their vehicles. He did add that a fluid was leaking from the truck, but he was unsure whether it was gasoline or something contained in the cargo tank.

1. Assume that you will not be able to obtain more information from the scene via CB radio or other means before your unit arrives. Your local protocol encourages implementation of IMS before arrival on-scene if you believe it highly likely this IMS is required based on dispatcher information. What is your size-up based on dispatcher information and what types of additional equipment, if any, do you activate before arrival?

2. What, if any, elements of this scenario are unique to rural EMS care?

CHAPTER 13 REVIEW

Write the word or words that best complete each sentence in the space(s) provided.

1. Every decision that a paramedic makes in a rural setting needs to be made with the thought of _____/_____ in mind.

2. Rural paramedics must think ahead and ask for orders in anticipation of medical conditions that might develop during a(n) _____ _____ _____.

3. Access to computers and the Internet enhances educational opportunities and medical care: _____ and _____ are two examples.

4. Rural paramedics can improve or maintain good communications with their hospitals by spending time there and requesting to sit in on relevant in-service _____ _____ for the hospital staff.

5. In wilderness rescues, _____ and _____ _____ play critical roles in your decision making.

6. Indiscriminate use of _____ can delay treatment time and, in some cases, cause further patient injury.

7. A rural paramedic whose territory includes a lake should be well versed in _____ emergencies.

8. _____ _____ occur when two objects come together and catch a portion of the patient's body between them.

9. The toxic fumes produced by the fermentation of grains in an enclosed space is known as _____ _____.

10. A basic safety principle to keep in mind when you are dealing with a patient injured by farm machinery is _____-_____/_____-_____.

©2009 Pearson Education, Inc.
Paramedic Care: Principles & Practice, Vol. 5, 3rd. Ed.

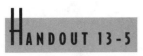

Student's Name _____

STEPS FOR REMOVAL FOR A PINCH-POINT INJURY PATIENT

1. Determine if machinery is operated by other equipment such as a tractor. If so, use the machinery to extricate the patient. Then lock-out/tag-out the appropriate levers or switches.

2. Stabilize both fractures and circulatory injuries during extrication.

3. Provide rapid treatment for shock, especially if the call for help was delayed for a lengthy period.

4. Package and transport to the nearest appropriate medical facility, using the most effective means of transport.

Chapter 13 Answer Key

1. D	**4.** A	**7.** D	**9.** D
2. B	**5.** B	**8.** B	**10.** B
3. C	**6.** C		

Handout 13-3: Chapter 13 Scenario

1. Size-up: IMS should be implemented based on multiple-vehicle, multiple-casualty accident. The number of patients is unknown, as is the nature and degree of injuries. The number of EMS units activated before assessment depends on the number of units covering the area and the local protocols for activation. Additional units that should be activated include police and fire units. One or more occupants of the cars may require mechanical extrication from the vehicle. In addition, low-angle rescue, high-angle rescue, or both may be required for one or more occupants. Air transport may be required for transport to a trauma center, and a hazmat team may be required to evaluate and handle the leaking fluid.

2. The elements of distance/time to the scene and to the trauma center are rural concerns, as is the low level of EMS coverage per geographic area. The volunteer nature of the BLS units compounds the problem of distance/time. In addition, it probably takes longer to assemble the required specialty teams (rescue hazmat), if appropriately trained personnel are available at all, than it would take in an urban setting.

Handout 13-4: Chapter 13 Review

1. distance/time
2. radio dead spot (or communications blackout, or similar wording)
3. any two of the following: distance learning, interagency interface/communication, networking, computer simulation software, interactive CD-ROM
4. training programs
5. distance, extrication time
6. helicopter (air transport)
7. water
8. Pinch points
9. silo gas
10. lock-out/tag-out

Chapter

14

Responding to Terrorist Acts

INTRODUCTION

The events of September 11, 2001, have greatly affected our society and our sensitivity to the threat of terrorist acts. This new awareness forces the EMS community to prepare itself to respond to acts of terrorism. Though the weapon of choice used by terrorist groups worldwide is the conventional explosive, it is clear that the 21st century will bring new terrorism threats using more unconventional means, such as commercial aircraft to bring down structures and weapons of mass destruction including nuclear, biological, and chemical weapons.

CHAPTER OBJECTIVES

Knowledge Objectives

*1. Identify the typical weapons of mass destruction likely to be used by terrorists. (pp. 527–539)

*2. Explain the mechanisms of injury associated with conventional and nuclear weapons of mass destruction. (pp. 527–530)

*3. Identify and describe the major subclassifications of chemical and biological weapons of mass destruction. (pp. 530–539)

*4. List the scene evidence that might alert the EMS provider to a terrorist attack that involves a weapon of mass destruction. (p. 540)

*5. Describe the special safety precautions and safety equipment appropriate for an incident involving nuclear, biological, or chemical weapons. (pp. 539, 540–541)

*6. Identify the assessment and management concerns for victims of conventional, nuclear, biological, and chemical weapons. (pp. 527–539)

*7. Given a narrative description of a conventional, nuclear, biological, or chemical terrorist attack, identify the elements of scene size-up that suggest terrorism, and identify the likely injuries and any special patient management considerations necessary. (pp. 526–541)

Note: The objectives for this chapter are not included in the DOT Paramedic curriculum.

TOTAL TEACHING TIME

There is no specific time requirement for this topic in the National Standard Curriculum for Paramedic. Instructors should take into consideration such factors as: the pace at which students learn, the size of the class, and breaks. The actual time devoted to teaching objectives is the responsibility of the instructor.

FRAMING THE LESSON

Briefly highlight recent incidents of WMD, including the anthrax-laced letters (2001), destruction of the World Trade Center Towers (2001), sarin gas release in the Tokyo Subway System (1996), Oklahoma City federal building bombing (1995), and first World Trade Center bombing (1993). Discuss that terrorism is a worldwide problem. During their careers in EMS, it is possible they will be called upon to respond to some type of terrorist act or mass/multiple-casualty incident (MCI).

CONSIDERING THE CASE STUDY

Ask a volunteer to read aloud the Case Study that begins on text page 525. Suggest that students close their eyes as the scenario is read to help them visualize the events described in it. You can use the following questions as a starting point for teaching the chapter—a sort of chapter preview in a functional setting.

When the chapter is completed, you may wish to return to the Case Study and encourage further discussion aimed at answering the questions.

CASE STUDY DISCUSSION QUESTIONS (AND ANSWERS)

1. What are the possible targets of foreign or domestic terrorists?
    (Answers may include some or all of the following:
    *   *Locations that are symbolic of the government*
    *   *Locations that represents the influence of our country*
    *   *Corporations or their executives who represent a threat to their cause*
    *   *Own employer or the public through their employer's products)*

2. What are your responsibilities at the scene of a potential terrorist incident?
    (Answer may include some or all of the following:
    *   *Ensure your own safety and that of your patient, other rescuers, and the public.*
    *   *Make certain all patients are properly decontaminated [if needed].*
    *   *Provide the appropriate emergency medical care.)*

3. How should various categories of terrorist incidents be managed?
    (Answers may include some or all of the following:
    *   *A nuclear incident is handled like a conventional explosion with a hazardous material [radiation] involved.*
    *   *A chemical agent incident is handled like a hazardous material incident.*
    *   *A biological weapon release is handled like an infectious disease outbreak.)*

TEACHING STRATEGIES

People learn in a variety of ways. Some do better with the spoken word, while others prefer the written. Some prefer to work alone, whereas others profit from working in groups. Recognizing these different ways of acquiring knowledge, the authors of this *Instructor's Resource Manual* have provided a variety of teaching strategies for the different types of learners. These strategies are intended to foster higher-level cognitive skills and encourage creative learning and problem solving.

©2009 Pearson Education, Inc.
Paramedic Care: Principles & Practice, Vol. 5, 3rd. Ed.

For greatest effectiveness, incorporate these strategies into your class lecture. Marginal notes in the Teaching Outline indicate the points at which various exercises might be most appropriate. Other strategies can be used to preview the lesson or to summarize it.

The following strategies are keyed to specific sections of the lesson:

1. *Thinking about Associated Dangers.* Have students consider the effects of an explosive agent in their own communities. Map out a section of the community in which your school stands. If possible, include both commercial and residential areas. Have students identify, either by educated guess or by actual investigation, the potential hazards that exist in each building or space. Facilitate a discussion about how those materials would need to be handled if a terrorist incident occurred at one of those buildings.

2. *Assigned Reading.* *Vector* by Robin Cook is one novel among many that addresses the use and danger of biological weapons. Encourage students to read one such book and report on the themes. Or buy several paperback copies and use them as prizes when playing review games in class.

3. *Assigned Viewing.* *Outbreak* (1995) by Warner Brothers is a movie that addresses the spread of an ebola outbreak from its African origins to a small California community. Encourage students to view this video and report on the themes.

4. *Guest Speaker: ESDA/OEM Official.* Consider inviting a representative from your area ESDA/OEM office to discuss response preparedness and EMS's roll.

5. *Tabletop Exercise.* Use a community layout and Matchbox-type vehicles to role-play management of a terrorist act on "Anywhere, USA." Students should use the Incident Command System (ICM) to manage the situation.

The following strategy relates to Special Features in the student textbook and can be used to enhance the student's understanding:

Legal Notes: Training for Nontraditional Roles in a WMD Attack. Invite a representative from your local emergency management agency to present information on the EMS role in the local emergency operations plan.

The following strategies can be used at various points throughout the lesson or to help summarize and demonstrate what students have learned:

Field Trip. If an explosive hazmat incident occurred in your area, consider a field trip to the site, preferably in the company of an EMS provider who served there. Discuss relevant details on the nature of the hazardous materials involved and the extent of contamination. Also consider the equipment and the medical care provided on-site and during transportation, including decontamination efforts and precautions taken against secondary contamination during packaging and transport.

Recognizing Disaster Management Factors. Write the names of several potential disasters on strips of paper and place them in a hat. Have small groups of students draw a disaster and identify mitigating factors. If these factors do not exist in your community, brainstorm solutions and share important ideas with people who can make a difference, such as by way of a letter to your council representative, fire chief, city planner, and so on. This activity lends realism to disaster management concepts and promotes community activism.

HANDOUT 14-1

Chapter 14 Objectives Checklist

TEACHING STRATEGIES

In addition to the Teaching Strategies listed at the beginning of this chapter, instructors should check with their local/state/federal emergency management agencies regarding supplemental information or to observe/participate in preparedness exercises.

POWERPOINT

PRESENTATION

Volume 5, Chapter 14, PowerPoint slides 1–5

READING/REFERENCE

Erich, J. "The Expert Take: Assessing the Terrorism Issues Facing EMS," *Emergency Medical Services*, Jan. 2002.

POWERPOINT

PRESENTATION

Volume 5, Chapter 14, PowerPoint slides 6–8

POWERPOINT

PRESENTATION

Volume 5, Chapter 14, PowerPoint slides 9–15

POWERPOINT

PRESENTATION

Volume 5, Chapter 14, PowerPoint slides 16–32

Participating in MCI Drills. Nearly every health department in the nation has annual mass casualty drills. Obtain the schedule and have your class included. When possible, have them integrated into the responding unit crews. If it is not possible for students to play patient care roles, be sure they are included as patients. Even observing a large-scale drill will be educational. Asking to participate in an already-scheduled drill will save you the enormous effort required to stage one of your own.

TEACHING OUTLINE

Chapter 14 is the fourteenth lesson in Volume 5, *Special Considerations/ Operations*. Distribute Handout 14-1. If students have any questions about the objectives, answer them at this time.

Then present the chapter. One possible lecture outline follows. In the outline, the parenthetical references in regular type are references to text pages; those in bold type are to figures, tables, or procedures.

I. Introduction. Terrorism threats may involve weapons of mass destruction (WMD) including nuclear, biological, and chemical (NBC) weapons. (pp. 526–527) (**Fig. 14-1**)

II. Explosive agents. (pp. 527–528) (**Fig. 14-2**)

A. Explosives (p. 527)
    1. Most likely method by which terrorists will strike
    2. Compression/decompression injuries
    3. Secondary explosions
B. Incendiary agents (p. 528)
    1. Less explosive power and greater heat and burn potential
C. Incorporating other agents with explosives (p. 528)

III. Nuclear detonation. (pp. 528–530) (**Fig. 14-3**)

A. Release of energy that is generated when heavy nuclei split (fission) or light nuclei combine (fusion) to form new elements (p. 528)
B. Nuclear radiation cannot be felt, seen, or otherwise detected by any of our senses. (p. 528)
C. Mechanisms of injury (pp. 528–529)
    1. Initial detonation
    2. Fallout
D. Nuclear incident response (pp. 529–530)
    1. First hour spent moving patients to safety
    2. Evacuation of fallout area
    3. Geiger counter
    4. Dosimeter
    5. Sodium iodine tablets
E. Nuclear contamination with "dirty bomb" (p. 530)
    1. Results in an explosion site, with radioactive material contaminating the immediate vicinity

IV. Chemical agents. (pp. 530–535)

A. Volatility (p. 531)
B. Specific gravity (p. 531)
C. Nerve agents (pp. 531–532)
    1. Nerve agents generally inhibit the degradation of a neurotransmitter (acetylcholine) and quickly cause a nervous system overload.

2. SLUDGE signs and symptoms
   a. Salivation
   b. Lacrimation
   c. Urination
   d. Diarrhea
   e. Gastrointestinal distress
   f. Emesis
3. Mark I Kit
   a. Atropine, 2 mg
   b. Pradoxime chloride, 600 mg
D. Vesicants (blistering agents) (p. 532)
   1. Agents that damage exposed tissue, frequently causing vesicles (blisters)
E. Pulmonary agents (chemical) (p. 533)
F. Biotoxins (p. 533)
G. Incapacitating agents (p. 534)
H. Other hazardous chemicals (p. 534)
I. Recognition of a chemical agent release (pp. 534–535)
J. Management of a chemical agent release (p. 535) (**Fig. 14-4**)

V. Biological agents. (pp. 535–539) (**Table 14-1**)

A. Pneumonia-like agents (pp. 537–538)
B. Encephalitis-like agents (p. 538)
C. Other agents (p. 538)
D. Protection against biological agent transmission (pp. 538–539) (**Fig. 14-5**)

VI. General considerations regarding terrorist attacks. (pp. 539–541)

A. Scene safety (p. 539)
B. Recognizing a terrorist attack (p. 540)
C. Responding to a terrorist attack (pp. 540–541)

VII. Summary. The EMS role in a nuclear, biological, or chemical release or exposure is generally limited to the awareness of such incident, reduction in exposure to responders and the general public, and treatment of those exposed to the substance. (p. 541)

READING/REFERENCE
Sachs, E. M. "The Bubonic Man: Lessons from a Bioterrorism Incident," *Emergency Medical Services*, Aug. 2000.

POWERPOINT
PRESENTATION
Volume 5, Chapter 14, PowerPoint slides 33–40

POWERPOINT
PRESENTATION
Volume 5, Chapter 14, PowerPoint slides 41–45

POWERPOINT
PRESENTATION
Volume 5, Chapter 14, PowerPoint slide 46

LEGAL NOTES
Training for Nontraditional Roles in a WMD Attack, p. 539

YOU MAKE THE CALL

Review student responses to the You Make the Call scenario on text page 541. Suggested responses to the questions that follow the scenario are given below. Point out to students that these are acceptable answers, but not necessarily the only ones. Discuss with students the pros and cons of points where their responses differ from these.

You are dispatched to "an explosion with possible injuries." You arrive as the first emergency vehicle to a Jewish synagogue with smoke pouring from broken windows and obviously injured people on the lawn.

1. What special safety considerations would you observe for this scene? *(After the initial explosion, associated dangers include structural collapse, fire, electrical hazard, and combustible or toxic gas hazards. Also be wary of secondary explosives set intentionally to disrupt rescue and to injure emergency responders.)*

2. What are the likely injuries to expect from this mechanism of injury? *(The blast pressure wave causes compression/decompression injury as it passes through the lungs, the ears, and other hollow, air-filled organs. This damage may be enhanced when the explosion occurs in a confined*

space, such as the interior of a building or other structure. Debris thrown by the blast produces penetrating or blunt injuries, and similar additional injury occurs as the victim is thrown by the blast wind. Secondary combustion induces burn injury, and structural collapse causes blunt and crushing injuries.)

3. Should you enter the synagogue?
   (Your first role in responding to a possible act of terrorism is to ensure your own safety and that of your patient, other rescuers, and the public. Once safety is ensured, make certain all patients are properly decontaminated [if need be], and then begin to provide the appropriate emergency medical care.)

WORKBOOK
Chapter 14 Activities

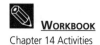
HANDOUT 14-2
Chapter 14 Quiz

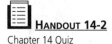
HANDOUT 14-3
Chapter 14 Scenario

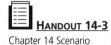
PARAMEDIC STUDENT CD
Student Activities

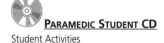
COMPANION WEBSITE
http://www.prenhall.com/bledsoe

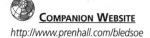
TESTGEN
Volume 5, Chapter 14

EMT ACHIEVE:
PARAMEDIC TEST PREPARATION
Mistovich & Beasley. *EMT Achieve: Paramedic Test Preparation,*
http://www.prenhall.com/emtachieve.

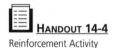
SUCCESS! FOR THE
PARAMEDIC
Cherry. *SUCCESS! for the Paramedic,* 4th edition

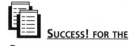
HANDOUT 14-4
Reinforcement Activity

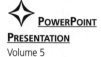
PARAMEDIC STUDENT CD
Student Activities

POWERPOINT
PRESENTATION
Volume 5

ASSIGNMENTS

Assign students to complete Chapter 14 of the Workbook.

EVALUATION

Chapter Quiz and Scenario   Distribute copies of the Chapter Quiz provided in Handout 14-2 to evaluate student understanding of this chapter. Make sure each student reads the scenario to reinforce critical thinking on the scene. Remind students not to use their notes or textbooks while taking the quiz.

Student CD   Quizzes for every chapter are contained on the dynamic and highly visual in-text student CD.

Companion Website   Additional quizzes for every chapter are contained on this exciting website.

TestGen   You may wish to create a custom-tailored test using *Prentice Hall TestGen for Paramedic Care: Principles & Practice,* 3rd edition, to evaluate student understanding of this chapter.

Online Test Preparation (for students and instructors)   Additional test preparation is available through Brady's new online product, EMT Achieve: Paramedic Test Preparation, at *http://www.prenhall.com/emtachieve.* Instructors can also monitor student mastery online.

Success! for the Paramedic   Keyed to *Paramedic Care: Principles & Practice* and *Essentials of Paramedic Care,* this comprehensive exam review contains hundreds of test questions and rationales.

REINFORCEMENT

Handouts   If classroom discussion or performance on the quiz indicates that some students have not fully mastered the chapter content, you may wish to assign some or all of the Reinforcement Handouts for this chapter.

Student CD (for students)   A wide variety of material on this CD-ROM will reinforce and also expand student knowledge and skills.

PowerPoint Presentation (for instructors)   The PowerPoint material developed for this chapter offers useful reinforcement of chapter content.

Companion Website (for students)   Additional review quizzes and links to EMS resources will contribute to further reinforcement of the chapter.

OneKey   Online support is offered for this course on one of three platforms: CourseCompass, Blackboard, or WebCT. Includes the IRM, PowerPoints, Test Manager, and Companion Website for instruction. Ask your local sales representative for more information.

Brady Skills Series: Advanced Life Skills (Video or CD)   Have your students watch the skills come to life on VHS or CD-ROM, or they can purchase the highly visual, full-color text with step-by-step procedures with rationales.

Paramedic National Standards Self-Test   Another comprehensive review manual containing hundreds of review questions with page references keyed to several Brady texts.

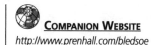
COMPANION WEBSITE
http://www.prenhall.com/bledsoe

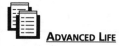
ONEKEY
Volume 2, Chapter 1

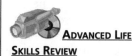
ADVANCED LIFE SUPPORT SKILLS
Larmon & Davis. *Advanced Life Support Skills*

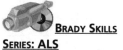
ADVANCED LIFE SKILLS REVIEW
Larmon & Davis. *Advanced Life Skills Review*

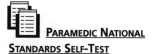
BRADY SKILLS SERIES: ALS
Larmon & Davis. *Brady Skills Series: ALS*

PARAMEDIC NATIONAL STANDARDS SELF-TEST
Miller. *Paramedic National Standards Self-Test,* 5th edition

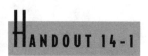

CHAPTER 14 OBJECTIVES CHECKLIST

Knowledge Objective	Date Mastered
*1. Identify the typical weapons of mass destruction likely to be used by terrorists.	
*2. Explain the mechanisms of injury associated with conventional and nuclear weapons of mass destruction.	
*3. Identify and describe the major subclassifications of chemical and biological weapons of mass destruction.	
*4. List the scene evidence that might alert the EMS provider to a terrorist attack that involves a weapon of mass destruction.	
*5. Describe the special safety precautions and safety equipment appropriate for an incident involving nuclear, biological, or chemical weapons.	
*6. Identify the assessment and management concerns for victims of conventional, nuclear, biological, and chemical weapons.	
*7. Given a narrative description of a conventional, nuclear, biological, or chemical terrorist attack, identify the elements of scene size-up that suggest terrorism, and identify the likely injuries and any special patient management considerations necessary.	

*Note: The objectives for this chapter are not included in the DOT Paramedic Curriculum.

©2009 Pearson Education, Inc.
Paramedic Care: Principles & Practice, Vol. 5, 3rd. Ed.

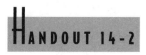 ANDOUT 14-2

Student's Name _____

EVALUATION

CHAPTER 14 QUIZ

Write the letter of the best answer in the space provided.

_____ 1. Which of the following is considered a weapon of mass destruction?
   A. nuclear bomb
   B. chemical weapon
   C. biological agent
   D. all of the above

_____ 2. Which one of the following injuries is NOT expected from a conventional explosive blast?
   A. blunt trauma
   B. penetrating trauma
   C. severe and extensive burns
   D. compression/decompression injury

_____ 3. Which one of the following is considered an incendiary agent?
   A. tularemia
   B. napalm
   C. sarin
   D. ebola

_____ 4. The danger that separates the conventional from the nuclear detonation is:
   A. radiation.
   B. strength of the explosion.
   C. high incidence of burn injury.
   D. all of the above.

_____ 5. The site of a nuclear detonation is generally radiation free from moments after the blast until _____ hour(s) postignition.
   A. 1
   B. 6
   C. 12
   D. 48

_____ 6. In addition to an explosive agent, the "dirty bomb" contains which one of the following?
   A. chemical agent
   B. radioactive material
   C. biological agent only
   D. both chemical and biological agents

_____ 7. A volatile chemical agent does which one of the following?
   A. gathers in low spots like a subway
   B. converts quickly to a gas from a liquid
   C. causes blistering and respiratory injury
   D. interrupts the transmission of central nervous system impulses

_____ 8. The chemical agent that produces the SLUDGE signs is a:
   A. vesicant.
   B. biotoxin.
   C. nerve agent.
   D. pulmonary agent.

_____ 9. One of the most deadly toxic agents known is a:
   A. vesicant.
   B. biotoxin.
   C. nerve agent.
   D. pulmonary agent.

_____ 10. Which one of the following agents is most likely to produce blistering?
   A. vesicant
   B. biotoxin
   C. nerve agent
   D. pulmonary agent

_____ 11. Which one of the following is the most likely and most dependable clue to the release of a chemical agent?
   A. strange smell
   B. cloud of vapor
   C. multiple patients with similar signs and symptoms
   D. large numbers of dead insects found crushed on your windshield

_____ **12.** Which one of the following statements about the time of release of a biological agent is CORRECT?
   A. The patient's breath usually has a strange odor.
   B. You can see a cloud of vapor above storage containers.
   C. Multiple patients immediately complain of similar symptoms.
   D. There may be no indication of an agent being released at all.

_____ **13.** Who most likely will recognize a biological agent release?
   A. Emergency department personnel
   B. Hazardous materials team
   C. EMT-Intermediates
   D. First responders

_____ **14.** Which one of the following is the recommended and most effective form of protection against an infectious biological agent?
   A. standard precautions
   B. self-contained breathing apparatus
   C. 10 percent hypochlorite solution
   D. Mark I kit

_____ **15.** The victim of a chemical or nuclear attack needs which one of the following before you begin care?
   A. iodine tablets
   B. proper decontamination
   C. application of a HEPA respirator
   D. administration of the Mark I kit contents

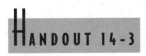ANDOUT 14-3

Student's Name _____

CHAPTER 14 SCENARIO

Review the following real-life situation. Then answer the questions that follow.

It is a warm, summer weekend and your community's annual street festival is in full swing. Officials report that this is the largest turnout in the festival's history. You are dispatched to the main grandstand area, where a large crowd has gathered to hear a highly publicized band performance. Tony and Hilda are on duty and are dispatched to the festival's first aid station for a burn patient. Upon arriving at the first aid station, you are advised there are additional patients, all presenting with similar signs and symptoms. After calling for additional assistance, you begin to evaluate and triage the patients. Common signs and symptoms include burns to exposed arms and legs, some blistering; rhinorrhea, cough, and dyspnea; and nausea and vomiting.

1. Given your initial assessment of the scene and patients, what is the probable mechanism of injury?

2. How should additional ambulances respond to the scene? How should the other spectators be managed?

3. What treatment should be provided for these patients?

EVALUATION

REINFORCEMENT

Student's Name _____

CHAPTER 14 REVIEW

Write the word or words that best complete each sentence in the space(s) provided.

1. Called _____ _____ _____ _____, the chemical, biological, and nuclear weapons used by terrorists are meant to create a maximum number of casualties.

2. The use of violence to provoke fear and influence behavior for political, social, religious, or ethnic goals is called a _____ act.

3. A special subset of explosives, _____ agents have less explosive power but greater heat and burn potential.

4. Radioactive dust and particles that threaten the lives of people far from the epicenter of a nuclear detonation are called _____.

5. A(n) _____ _____ is an instrument used to detect and measure the radiation given off by an object or area.

6. A(n) _____ is an instrument that measures the cumulative amount of radiation absorbed.

7. A conventional explosive device that distributes radioactive material over a large area is called a(n) _____ _____.

8. The term _____ refers to the ease by which a chemical changes from a liquid to a gas.

9. _____ _____ refers to the density or weight of a vapor or gas as compared to air.

10. The term _____ _____ refers to chemicals that restrict the degradation of neurotransmitters such as acetylcholine and quickly facilitate a nervous system overload.

11. The _____ _____ _____ is a two-part autoinjector set that the military uses as treatment for nerve-agent exposure.

12. A(n) _____ is an agent that damages exposed skin, frequently causing vesicles (blisters).

13. _____ agents are chemicals that primarily cause injury to the lungs.

14. A(n) _____ is a poison that is produced by living organisms but is itself not alive.

15. A(n) _____ agent is either a living organism or a toxin produced by a living organism that is deliberately distributed to cause disease and death.

©2009 Pearson Education, Inc.
Paramedic Care: Principles & Practice, Vol. 5, 3rd. Ed.

Chapter 14 Answer Key

Handout 14-2: Chapter 14 Quiz

1. D	5. A	9. B	13. A
2. C	6. B	10. A	14. A
3. B	7. B	11. C	15. B
4. D	8. C	12. D	

Handout 14-3: Chapter 14 Scenario

1. Exposure to a chemical agent, most likely a vesicant.
2. Approach from an upwind direction. Spectators and others should be evacuated to an area away from the scene and evaluated for exposure to the chemical.
3. Immediate decontamination by irrigating exposed areas with low-pressure water. Apply loose sterile dressings to burns. Consider medication for pain management.

Handout 14-4: Chapter 14 Review

1. weapons of mass destruction
2. terrorist
3. incendiary
4. fallout
5. Geiger counter
6. dosimeter
7. dirty bomb
8. volatility
9. Specific gravity
10. nerve agent
11. Mark I kit
12. vesicant
13. Pulmonary (or choking)
14. biotoxin
15. biological